THE AFFECTIVE DISORDERS

THE **Affective Disorders**

edited by *John M. Davis, M.D., Ph.D.* and *James W. Maas, M.D.*

American Psychiatric Press, Inc.   *Washington, D.C.*

Library of Congress Cataloging in Publication data
Main entry under title:
The Affective Disorders

   Includes bibliographical references and index.
   1. Affective disorders. I. Davis, John M.,
1933-   . II. Maas, James W. [DNLM: 1. Affective
disorders—Congresses. WM 171 A2559 1981]
RC537.A315 1983   616.85'27   83-3731
ISBN 0-88048-214-1

Printed in the U.S.A.

Contents

Contents

Contents

Contributors

EDITORS

John M. Davis, M.D., Ph.D.
Director of Research
Illinois State Psychiatric Institute
Chicago, Illinois

James Maas, M.D.
Professor of Psychiatry
University of Texas
Health Science Center at San Antonio

OTHER CONTRIBUTORS

Darrell R. Abernethy, M.D., Ph.D.
Assistant Professor of Psychiatry and
   Medicine
Tufts University School of Medicine
Boston, Massachusetts

Hagop Souren Akiskal, M.D.
Professor of Psychiatry
Associate Professor of Pharmacology
Director, Affective Disorders Program
University of Tennessee
College of Medicine
Staff Psychiatrist
Sleep Disorders Center
Baptist Memorial Hospital
Memphis, Tennessee

Richard I. Altesman, M.D.
Director, Outpatient Psychopharma-
   cology Service
McLean Hospital
Belmont, Massachusetts
Instructor, Harvard Medical School
Boston, Massachusetts

Nancy C. Andreasen, M.D., Ph.D.
Professor of Psychiatry
Department of Psychiatry
The University of Iowa
Iowa City, Iowa

Jose L. Ayuso-Gutierrez, M.D.
Professor of Psychiatry
Clinic Hospital
Universidad Complutense
Madrid, Spain

Ross J. Baldessarini, M.D.
Professor of Psychiatry
Harvard Medical School
Associate Director
Mailman Research Laboratories
McLean Affiliate of Massachusetts
   General Hospital
Belmont, Massachusetts

Giovanni B. Cassano, M.D.
Direttore Seconda Cattedra
Clinica Psichiatrica Delluniversita
  Degli Studi
Policlinico S. Chiara
Pisa, Italy

Gaston Castellanos, M.D.
Head of Biological Psychiatry
National Institute of Neurology
Members of the Mexico University's
Institute of Biomedical Research
Mexico City, Mexico

Paula J. Clayton, M.D.
Professor and Head
Department of Psychiatry
University of Minnesota
Minneapolis, Minnesota

Bruce M. Cohen, M.D.
Chief, Clinical Biochemistry
  Laboratory
Mailman Research Center
Belmont, Massachusetts
Assistant Professor of Psychiatry
Harvard Medical School
Boston, Massachusetts

Robert M. Cohen, M.D., Ph.D.
Deputy Chief
Clinical Neuropharmacology Branch
National Institute of Mental Health
Bethesda, Maryland

Jonathan O. Cole, M.D.
Chief, Psychopharmacology Program
McLean Hospital
Belmont, Massachusetts

John Corcella, M.D.
Associate Professor of Psychiatry
Marshall University
School of Medicine
Huntington, West Virginia

Marcia Divoll, R.N., B.S.
Clinical Research Supervisor
Division of Clinical Pharmacology
Instructor in Psychiatry
Tufts University School of Medicine
Boston, Massachusetts

Albert Dresse, M.D.
Professor of Psychopharmacology
University of Liege
Institute of Pathology
Laboratory of Pharmacology
Brussels, Belgium

David L. Dunner, M.D.
Professor
Department of Psychiatry and Behav-
  ioral Sciences
University of Washington
Chief of Psychiatry
Harborview Medical Center
Seattle, Washington

Pola Engel-Sittenfeld, Ph.D.
Psychiatric Klinik
University of Munich
Nussbaumstr. Munich
Federal German Republic

Eva Estrada, Ph.D.
National Institute of Neurology
Members of the Mexico University's
Institute of Biomedical Research
Mexico City, Mexico

Daniel J. Fredman, M.D.
Michael Reese Hospital
Chicago, Illinois

Robert O. Friedel, M.D.
Chief of Psychiatry
Medical College of Virginia
Richmond, Virginia

Jean-Michel Gaillard, M.D.
University of Geneva
Geneva, Switzerland

Alexander H. Glassman, M.D.
Chief, Clinical Psychopharmacology
New York State Psychiatric Institute
Professor of Clinical Psychiatry
College of Physicians and Surgeons
Columbia University
New York, New York

Frederick K. Goodwin, M.D.
Branch Chief
Clinical Psychobiology Branch
National Institute of Mental Health
Bethesda, Maryland

David J. Greenblatt, M.D.
Chief
Division of Clinical Pharmacology
New England Medical Center Hospital
Professor of Psychiatry and Associate
    Professor of Medicine
Tufts University School of Medicine
Boston, Massachusetts

Waldemar Greil, M.D.
Oberarzt
Psychiatric Klinik
University of Munich
Nussbaumstr, Munich
Federal German Republic

Paul Grof, M.D., Ph.D.
Hamilton Psychiatric Hospital
Hamilton, Canada

Jon E. Gudeman, M.D.
Associate Professor of Psychiatry
Harvard Medical School
Boston, Massachusetts

Leo E. Hollister, M.D.
Professor of Medicine and Psychiatry
Stanford University Medical Center
Palo Alto, California

Garland Johnson, Ph.D.
Research Scientist
The Upjohn Company
Kalamazoo, Michigan

Helmfried Klein, M.D.
Chief, Psychiatric Clinics
University of Munich
Nussbaumstr, Munich
Federal German Republic

David J. Kupfer, M.D.
Professor of Psychiatry
Western Psychiatry Institute and
    Clinic
University of Pittsburgh
School of Medicine
Department of Psychiatry
Pittsburgh, Pennsylvania

Yves Lecrubier, M.D.
Department Psychiatrie
Groupe Hopitalier
Pitie-Salpetriere
Paris, France

Robert D. Linden, M.D.
University of Chicago
Chicago, Illinois

Dott. Carlo Maggini
Assitente Clinica Psichiatrica
Universita Degli Studi
Policlinico S. Chiara
Pisa, Italy

Dierdre B. Montgomery
Research Fellow
Academic Department of Psychiatry
St. Mary's Hospital
London, England

Stuart A. Montgomery, B.S.C., M.D.
Hons Cons and Senior Lecturer in
    Psychiatry
Academic Department of Psychiatry
St. Mary's Hospital Medical School
London, England

John J. Mooney, M.D.
Instructor in Psychiatry
Harvard Medical School
Boston, Massachusetts

Dennis L. Murphy, M.D.
Chief, Clinical Neuropharmacology
    Branch
National Institute of Mental Health
Bethesda, Maryland

Alexander Nies, M.D.
Chief, Psychiatry Service
Veterans Administration Medical
    Center
Newington, Connecticut

Paul J. Orsulak, Ph.D.
Assistant Professor of Psychiatry
Harvard Medical School
Associate Director
Neuropsychopharmacology Labor-
    atory
Massachusetts Mental Health Center
Technical Director
New England Deaconess Hospital
Boston, Massachusetts

John Overall, Ph.D.
University of Texas
Medical School
Houston, Texas

David Pickar, M.D.
Chief, Section of Clinical Studies
Clinical Neuroscience Branch
National Institute of Mental Health
Bethesda, Maryland

Alain Puech, M.D.
Assistant Head
Department of Pharmacology
Faculte de Medecine
Pitie Salpetriere
Paris, France

Donald S. Robinson, M.D.
Professor and Chairman
Department of Pharmacology
Marshall University
School of Medicine
Huntington, West Virginia

Alan H. Rosenbaum, M.D.
Director of Inpatient Services
Henry Ford Hospital
Detroit, Michigan

Benjamin F. Roy, M.D.
Staff Psychiatrist
Clinical Neuropharmacology Branch
National Institute of Mental Health
Bethesda, Maryland

A. John Rush, M.D.
Associate Professor
Affective Disorders Unit and Department of Psychiatry
University of Texas
Health Science Center
Dallas, Texas

Alan F. Schatzberg, M.D.
Assistant Professor of Psychiatry
Harvard Medical School
Boston, Massachusetts
Associate Psychiatrist and Co-Director
Affective Disease Program
McLean Hospital
Belmont, Massachusetts

Joseph J. Schildkraut, M.D.
Professor of Psychiatry
Harvard Medical School
Director, Neuropsychopharmacology Laboratory
Massachusetts Mental Health Center
Director
Psychiatric Chemistry Laboratory
New England Deaconess Hospital
Boston, Massachusetts

J. Scuvee-Moreau, Ph.D.
Department of Pharmacology
University of Liege
Belgium

Richard I. Shader, M.D.
Department of Psychiatry
Tufts University Medical School
Boston, Massachusetts

Larry J. Siever, M.D.
Director
Outpatient Clinic at Bronx Veterans Administration Medical Center
Associate Professor
Mount Sinai School of Medicine
New York, New York

Pierre Simon, Ph.D.
Chief, Pharmacology and Clinical Psychopharmacology
Department of Pharmacology
Faculte de Medecine
Pitie Salpetriere
Paris, France

Natraj Sitaram, M.D.
Director, Affective Disorders Unit
Lafayette Clinic
Associate Professor of Psychiatry
Wayne State University
Detroit, Michigan

Fridolin Sulser, M.D.
Professor of Pharmacology
Vanderbilt University
School of Medicine
Tennessee Neuropsychiatric Institute
Nashville, Tennessee

Rene Tissott, M.D.
University Clinic of Psychiatry
Geneva, Switzerland

Thomas A. Wehr, M.D.
Chief, Clinical Research Unit
Clinical Psychobiology Branch
National Institute of Mental Health
Bethesda, Maryland

Myrna M. Weissman, Ph.D.
Professor of Psychiatry and Epidemi-
    ology
Director, Depression Research Unit
Yale University
School of Medicine
Department of Psychiatry
Depression Research Unit
New Haven, Connecticut

Daniel Widlöcher, M.D.
Chief, Department of Psychiatry
Salpetriere
Paris, France

Anna Wirz-Justice, Ph.D.
Visiting Scientist to Clinical Psycho-
    biology Branch
National Institute of Mental Health
Biochemist from Psychiatrische Univ.
    Klinik
Basel, Switzerland

Introduction

Depression, the most common of the psychiatric disorders, is a heterogeneous group properly called the affective disorders. Progress in psychopharmacology and growing understanding of the etiology of these disorders make the clinician particularly reliant upon researchers to lead the way in initiating new therapies. This book promises to be an outstanding reference work for clinical psychiatrists, family practitioners, gerontologists and pharmacologists. The chapters, each written by recognized authorities, present the most recent developments in and theories of pathogenesis, biochemistry and management of affective disorders.

The Upjohn Company was privileged to host an outstanding faculty from Europe, Latin America and North America for a scientific symposium on these timely and important subjects. Three days in a setting free from the everyday demands of practice, laboratory and teaching provided a unique opportunity for challenging and productive exchange of ideas. The text which follows is based upon the papers presented in Augusta, Michigan in October, 1981, and reflects the vigorous, creative dialogue that took place among world leaders in the specialties of psychiatry and psychopharmacology.

Robert P. Purpura, M.D.
Medical Manager, Psychopharmacology
The Upjohn Company

PART ONE

Symptomatology, Etiology, Epidemiology

1

A Review of the New Antidepressant Medications

John M. Davis, M.D., Daniel J. Fredman, M.D., and Robert D. Linden, M.D.

Over the past few years, a variety of new antidepressant medications have been evaluated using double-blind methodology. Some of these drugs, such as trimipramine, maprotiline, and amoxapine, have already been released for clinical use. Another drug, trazodone, is in the final phase of investigation, and its release is expected within the next year. Several other new antidepressants are in earlier phases of investigation and should be released sometime within the next few years. The practicing psychiatrist, then, needs information on the efficacy and safety of several new antidepressant agents. Although their release by the FDA reflects a general set of standards, some psychiatrists may desire further information as to the relative efficacy of the new medications, and whether these new drugs offer any particular advantages, such as fewer side effects or a faster onset of action. Approximately 100 random assignment double-blind studies were examined and compiled, and are discussed in this chapter. Clinicians can look at the tabulated results of these studies and judge for themselves the efficacy of the new medications.

The new antidepressants are also relevant to our theoretical understanding of depression. Our present theories of depression, the norepinephrine and serotonin theories, are derived largely from the effects of drugs on biogenic amines. The tricyclic antidepressants, for example, are potent inhibitors of the active reuptake of norepinephrine and serotonin [1-4] in the brain, and are, therefore, hypothesized to potentiate these amines. According to the norepinephrine (NE) or serotonin (5-HT) theories of depression, one would anticipate that the new antidepressants would also potentiate NE or 5-HT. Alternatively, if an antidepressant is efficacious and has no known effect on NE or 5-HT, it may constitute significant evidence against these theories. In addition to the clinical focus, this chapter will review both clinically available and experimental drugs to see how well the NE or 5-HT theories stand up to this aspect of hypothesis testing.

Maprotiline is a norepinephrine reuptake inhibitor. It was the first tetracyclic antidepressant released by the FDA. Several controlled, double-blind studies have shown it to be superior to placebo and as effective as the standard antidepressants, amitriptyline, imipramine, and doxepin (Table 1).[5-41] The effective daily dosage in depression usually ranges from 75 to 150 mg in single or divided doses. Young or elderly patients may require a lower total daily dosage. Considering the large number of double-blind studies comparing this drug to standard drugs and placebo, there is little

Table 1 Maprotiline vs. Standard Tricyclic

			Percent Improvement with Drugs		
Study		N	Maprotiline	Standard Tricyclic	Difference
1.	Trick	21	83	89	−6
2.	Mathur	30	80	60	+20
3.	Murphy	61	56	41	+15
4.	Liebling	19	70	89	−19
5.	Forrest	184	89	82	+7
6.	Weissman	66	77	81	−4
7.	Amin	20	40	70	−30
8.	Scandinavian Collaborative Study (8 Hospitals)	208	62	64	−2
9.	Marais	24	100	83	+17
10.	Collaborative vs. Outpatient (unpublished)	124	90	87	+3
11.	Levin	44	91	64	+27
12.	International Collaborative	417	66	74	−8
13.	Jones (unpublished)	32	75	88	−13
14.	Middleton	26	64	75	−11
15.	Kessell and Holt	73	72	73	−1
16.	Guz	57	75	62	+13
17.	Angst	23	67	64	+3
18.	Collaborative Outpatient Studies (unpublished)	99	73	77	−4
19.	Collaborative Inpatient Studies (unpublished)	71	81	60	+21
20.	Lehman	39	68	55	+13
	Overall	1,638	73	73	0

Table 2 Amoxapine vs. Placebo

			Percent Good Result		
Study		N	Amoxapine	Placebo	Difference
1.	Steinbook	14	90	100	−10
2.	Wilson	13	75	40	+35
3.	Gallant	24	83	67	+16
4.	Smith	50	69	42	+27
5.	Kiev	47	88	83	+5
6.	Fabre	38	83	35	+48
Overall		186	81	57	+24

doubt that maprotiline is an effective antidepressant. It has become available for clinical use this year.

Amoxapine is another drug that has been released for use this year. It is a dibenzoxazepine derivative that is both a NE and 5-HT reuptake inhibitor. Amoxapine has been found to be efficacious in a number of double-blind studies comparing it to standard antidepressants. In comparison to placebo and standard tricyclics, amoxapine was shown to be 24% more effective than placebo and 6% more effective than the standard tricyclics (Tables 2&3).[42–64] It is doubtful that the drug is superior to the standard antidepressants, but rather it appears equivalent in efficacy. In terms of anticholinergic side effects, a review of eight double-blind studies comparing amoxapine to standard tricyclics demonstrated 7% less incidence of dry mouth in the amoxapine group (Table 4). The incidence of dry mouth is here taken as one indication of the propensity of a medication to induce anticholinergic side effects.

Interestingly, amoxapine has a chemical structure similar to that of the antipsychotic agent loxapine. Amoxapine's pharmacological properties, however, are characteristic of an antidepressant, insofar as amoxapine has the ability to potentiate catecholamines, to antagonize reserpine and tetrabenazine-induced depression, to antagonize reserpine-induced hypothermia in mice and to potentiate the lethal effects of yohimbine.[43] Additional effects are, however, similar to those of neuroleptics in producing sedation, decrease in motor activity, transitory suppression of avoidance reaction, and inhibition of stereotyped behavior induced by amphetamines in rats.[45]

Trazodone, a triazolopyridine derivative, represents a new class of antidepressants that selectively inhibits serotonin reuptake. It also produces a down-regulation of NE receptor sites. Down-regulation can be defined as a receptor subsensitivity to NE and to the beta-adrenergic agonist isoproterenol. This noradrenergic subsensitivity is linked to a

3

Table 3 Amoxapine vs. Standard Tricyclic

			Percent Good Result		
Study		N	Amoxapine	Standard Tricyclic	Difference
1.	Steinbook	19	90	89	+1
2.	Wilson	17	75	56	+19
3.	Smith	50	69	58	+11
4.	Kiev	48	88	79	+9
5.	Fabre	41	83	70	+13
6.	Sethi	50	76	80	−4
7.	Bagadia	48	59	62	−3
8.	Sathananthan	20	80	70	+10
9.	Takahashi	102	81	68	+13
10.	Paprocki	38	86	82	+4
11.	de Souza Campos	44	90	71	+19
12.	Fruensgaard	34	91	91	0
13.	Yamhure	53	82	100	−18
14.	Aberg	58	83	97	−14
15.	de Paula	46	63	45	+18
16.	Kaumeier	48	83	50	+23
17.	Holden	21	90	64	+26
18.	Burrows	16	88	75	+13
19.	Donlon	31	71	65	+6
Overall		784	79	73	+6

reduction in the density of beta-adrenergic receptors, a subpopulation of central NE receptors, without a change in their binding affinity.[65] Though the mechanism of action producing down-regulation is unclear, down-regulation may be an indication of a functional increase in NE available at the receptor site and would, therefore, be consistent with the NE and 5-HT hypotheses.

Trazodone has been well studied and is likely to be released for general use within the near future. An extensive review of 30 random assignment double-blind studies reveals trazodone to be 32% more effective than placebo and 4% more effective than standard tricyclics (Tables 5&6).[65–90] One would conclude that it is equally effective to the standard tricyclics. The effective daily dose ranges from 50 to 800 mg, usually given at bedtime.[68,75] Unlike the standard antidepressants, trazodone has no anticholinergic side effects, though infrequently reported side effects include lethargy, nausea, and headache.

Trimipramine, which has been on the market since 1979, has not been as extensively studied as the previously mentioned antidepressants.[91–102] In five double-blind studies, it was shown to be 18% more efficacious than the standard tricyclics (Table 7). Based upon this, trimipramine appears to be superior to the standard tricyclic. However, the trend reported by Rickels in his large, carefully controlled study gives preference to the standard tricyclic amitriptyline (Table 8).[100] Overall, some ambiguity exists as to the precise efficacy of trimipramine, but it appears roughly comparable to the standard tricyclics.

Chlorimipramine has been used in Europe and England for a number of years. Chlorimipramine blocks serotonin reuptake in vitro, and is often considered to act relatively specifically on the serotinergic system. In man, however, chlorimipramine is metabolized to desmethylchlorimipramine, which blocks the reuptake of norepinephrine. Plasma-level studies indicate that there are substantial levels of desmethylchlorimipramine after administration of chlorimipramine.[103]

These and other studies of 3-methoxy-4-hydroxyphenylglycol (MHPG) indicate that in man sufficient amounts of desmethylchlorimipramine are formed so that chlorimipramine can also be considered to affect the noradrenergic system.[104] Chlorimipramine has been the subject of many double-blind studies, and there is no doubt that it is an effective antidepressant. In a review of eight random assignment double-blind studies, it was found to be almost equal in efficacy to the standard tricyclics (Table 9).[104–121]

An interesting trend in clinical studies shows that chlorimipramine appears to have an antiobsessive effect.[122–124] This is an important finding because obsessive-compulsive disorder can be very severe and resistant to treatment. Yaryura-Tobias suggests an organic basis for obsessive-compulsive illness, in which a decrease in serotonin may be present.[122] In his double-blind study comparing chlorimipramine to placebo, Escobar demonstrated the usefulness of this drug in phobic states.[125] Previous open

Table 4 Amoxapine Side Effects

			Percent Incidence Dry Mouth		
Study	N	Amoxapine	Standard Tricyclic	Difference
1. Bagadia	48	95	92	−3
2. Takahashi	114	56	66	−10
3. de Souza Campos	60	6	7	−1
4. Aberg	53	0	16	−16
5. Kaumeier	48	0	4	−4
6. Sethi	30	76	77	−1
7. Smith	60	27	33	−6
8. Sathananthan	20	0	10	−10
Overall	433	35	42	−7

Table 5   Trazodone vs. Placebo

		Percent Good Result		
	N	Trazadone	Placebo	Difference
Non-U.S. Studies				
1. Vinci	48	73	6	+67
2. Cianchetti	58	51	24	+27
3. Antonelli	53	72	14	+58
4. Eckmann	90	69	33	+36
5. Eckmann	90	76	29	+47
6. Escobar	25	62	50	+12
Subtotal Non-U.S. Studies	364	68	27	+41
U.S. Studies				
1. Goldberg	80	81	58	+23
2. Kellams	18	56	0	+56
3. Feighner	27	53	0	+53
4. Fabre	18	56	11	+45
5. Gerner	25	42	23	+19
6. Newton	173	42	30	+12
Subtotal U.S. Studies	341	54	31	+23
Overall	705	61	29	+32

studies in both the United States and abroad also produced favorable results, suggesting that this agent is effective in the treatment of phobic patients.[126–128]

Adverse reactions with chlorimipramine include the following: agitation, confusion, drowsiness, dry mouth, insomnia, tremor, tachycardia, and hypotension or hypertension.[129] A daily dose ranging from 50 to 200 mg administered in divided doses is recommended. Chlorimipramine has also been shown to be effective when administered intravenously; the chief advantage claimed is an acceleration of onset of therapeutic effect.[130,131] It has been also claimed to be effective in phobic and obsessional states.[132]

Lofepramine is a norepinephrine reuptake inhibitor that is an analogue of imipramine. It is metabolized to desmethylimipramine, which is also a major metabolite of imipramine. Studies have shown it to be similar to imipramine in antidepressant effect.[133–138] In the double-blind studies reviewed, lofepramine was found to be 5% less efficacious than the standard tricyclics, but we concluded it is equally effective (Table 10). However, lofepramine has a reduced (15%) incidence of dry mouth (Table 11) consistent with its being metabolized to desmethylimipramine (desipramine), which is the least anticholinergic of the standard tricyclics.

Mianserin is a tetracyclic compound which has some interesting properties.[139-170] At low doses it does not inhibit the uptake of NE, 5-HT, or dopamine, nor is it a monoamine oxidase inhibitor (MAOI).[167] Mianserin appears to act through a presynaptic mechanism to increase norepinephrine turnover.[168] Thus, mianserin is consistent with the norepinephrine theory, even though its mechanism of action is quite different from those of the standard antidepressants. It also seems to have minimal cardiovascular toxicity and a lower anticholinergic side effect profile as compared to the standard antidepressants.[144,169] A review of 12 double-blind studies demonstrated 13% less dry mouth side effects with mianserin (Table 12). It is now used commercially in many countries and has been investigated in numerous controlled double-blind studies compared to the standard tricyclics amitriptyline and imipramine. A review of nine double-blind studies revealed mianserin to be somewhat less effective (10%) than the

Table 6   Trazodone vs. Standard Tricyclic

		Percent Improvement		
	N	Trazodone	Standard Tricyclic	Difference
Non-U.S. Studies				
1. de Gregorio	74	57	62	−5
2. Vinci	49	73	75	−2
3. Cianchetti	59	51	36	+15
4. Cioffi	24	42	25	+17
5. Peterova	20	80	60	+20
6. Eckmann	90	69	49	+20
7. Pariante	34	71	59	+12
8. Agnoli	82	78	76	+2
9. Mazzei	39	84	75	+9
10. Al-Yassiri	25	92	54	+38
11. Escobar	28	62	93	−31
12. Pierce (single-blind)	35	62	63	−1
Subtotal Non-U.S. Studies	559	67	61	+6
U.S. Studies				
1. Goldberg	76	81	71	+10
2. Kellams	19	56	20	+36
3. Feighner	35	53	28	+25
4. Fabre	19	56	60	−4
5. Gerner	21	42	33	+9
6. Newton	184	42	55	−13
Subtotal U.S. Studies	354	54	53	+1
Overall	913	62	58	+4

Table 7 Trimipramine vs. Standard Tricyclic

| Study | N | Percent Good Result | | |
		Trimipramine	Standard Tricyclic	Difference
1. Evans	68	42	40	+2
2. Lean and Sidhu	40	65	30	+35
3. Salzmann	27	62	29	+33
4. Burke	26	69	54	+15
5. Rifkin	38	84	58	+26
Overall	199	60	42	+18

Table 8 Trimipramine and Amitriptyline in Neurotic Depressed Outpatients: Summary of Rickels Study (100)

| Sample | Results | Covariate Adjusted | | | |
| | | Group Mean | | | Trend |
		TRI	AMIT	PLA	Flavor
122 depressed	1. Hamilton Depression Scale	.48	.36	.67	A
outpatients;	2. Physicians Questionnaire	1.97	1.84	2.33	A
data at week 4[a]	3. Zung Depression Scale	2.13	2.07	2.37	A
	4. Global Estimate of Psychopathology	2.75	2.62	3.28	A
	5. Global End Point (Physicians)	5.27	5.22	4.65	T
	6. Global End Point (Patients)	3.6	3.29	2.63	A

[a] In scale 1–4, a low number indicates a good response, and in scale 5–6, a high number means a good response.

Table 9 Clomipramine vs. Standard Tricyclic

| Study | N | Percent Good Result | | |
		Clomipramine	Standard Tricyclic	Difference
1. Gore	45	87	82	+5
2. Kampman	53	71	52	+19
3. Rickels	121	53	69	−16
4. Arfwidsson	40	39	59	−20
5. Mulginigama	34	83	44	+39
6. Poldinger	57	47	48	−1
Overall	350	l	62	−1

Table 10 Lofepramine vs. Standard Tricyclic

| | | Percent Good Result | | |
| | | | Standard | |
Study	N	Lofepramine	Tricyclic	Difference
1. D'Elia	49	58	78	−20
2. McClelland	41	86	85	+1
3. Wright and Hermann	40	15	35	−20
4. Goncalves and Wegemer	30	60	33	+27
Overall	160	55	60	−5

Table 11 Lofepramine vs. Standard Tricyclic: Incidence of Dry Mouth

| | | Percent Incidence | | |
| | | | Standard | |
Study	N	Lofepramine	Tricyclic	Difference
1. D'Elia	62	26	48	−22
2. Obermair and Poldinger	40	5	10	−5
Overall	102	18	33	−15

Table 12 Mianserin vs. Standard Tricyclic: Incidence of Dry Mouth

| | | Percent Incidence | | |
| | | | Standard | |
Study	N	Mianserin	Tricyclic	Difference
1. DeBuck	36	6	39	−33
2. Murphy	101	43	37	+6
3. Murphy	106	24	47	−23
4. Saletu	37	0	35	−35
5. Conti	137	13	27	−14
6. Jaskari	154	22	37	−15
7. Pinder	65	13	32	−19
8. Pinder	62	43	24	+19
9. Hoc	36	35	84	−49
10. Khan	56	25	25	0
11. Wheatly	79	10	20	−10
12. Blaha	48	4	20	−16
Overall	917	21	34	−13

Table 13 Mianserin vs. Standard Tricyclic

			Percent Improvement		
Study	N	Mianserin	Standard Tricyclic	Difference
1. Blaha	48	57	60	−3
2. DeBuck	32	76	80	−4
3. Murphy	84	44	37	+7
4. Kretschmar	36	55	19	+36
5. Conti	137	51	66	−15
6. Pinder	65	68	71	−3
7. Pinder	62	43	71	−28
8. Perry	28	60	77	−17
9. Svestka	82	55	88	−33
Overall	574	54	64	−10

standard tricyclics (Table 13). This is a statistically significant difference, although additional studies are needed. Mianserin has been shown to be clearly superior to placebo.[146,164] In reviewing three double-blind studies, it was found to be 42% more effective than placebo (Table 14). The dosage range is 30–150 mg/day and is usually administered at bedtime.[170]

Nomifensine is a tetrahydroisoquinoline compound that is of interest in that it inhibits both norepinephrine and dopamine reuptake.[171–192] It is unique among antidepressants in the degree to which it inhibits dopamine reuptake. In three double-blind studies, nomifensine was shown to be 56% more effective than placebo (Table 15). It manifests antidepressant activity similar to that of imipramine; a review of eight double-blind studies revealed only a 1% difference in efficacy as compared to the standard tricyclics (Table 16). A review of two large double-blind studies showed nomifensine to have 13% less dry mouth side effects than standard tricyclics (Table 17).

Viloxazine is a bicyclic tetrahydroxazine that resembles tricyclic antidepressants in its pharmacological effects; that is, reversal of reserpine

Table 14 Mianserin vs. Placebo

			Percent Improvement		
Study	N	Mianserin	Placebo	Difference
1. Hamouz	80	63	20	+43
2. Perry	28	60	69	−9
3. Russell	48	79	8	+71
Overall	156	67	25	+42

Table 15 Nomifensin vs. Placebo

| Study | N | Percent Good Result | | |
		Nomifensin	Placebo	Difference
1. Eckmann	60	90	7	+83
2. Eckmann II	64	80	23	+57
3. Kroeger	31	90	67	+23
Overall	155	80	24	+62

and tetrabenazine-induced depressive symptoms in mice, potentiation of noradrenergic phenomena, and suppression of REM sleep.[193–216] It differs from the tricyclics in that it increases the convulsive threshold and produces less anticholinergic effects.[193] Viloxazine inhibits the uptake of norepinephrine and is less effective in blocking the reuptake of serotonin. Double-blind studies have shown it to be an antidepressant comparable in efficacy to the standard tricyclics. A review of nine double-blind studies showed viloxazine to be essentially equal in efficacy to the standard tricyclics (Table 18). Reviewing seven double-blind studies, there were 11% less incidence of dry mouth side effects with those patients on viloxazine. In another double-blind study, it was found to be effective in depressed geriatric patients.[198]

Alprazolam represents a new family of triazolobenzodiazepines and has anxiolytic, hypnotic, muscle relaxant, anticonvulsant, and antiaggressive properties qualitatively similar to diazepam, although it is from three to five times more potent than diazepam.[217] Schatzberg and Cole, in a recent review of the use of benzodiazepines in depressive disorders, found

Table 16 Nomifensin vs. Standard Tricyclic

| Study | N | Percent Good Result | | |
		Nomifensin	Standard Tricyclic	Difference
1. Sharma	35	44	32	+12
2. Ananth and von Steen	26	92	92	0
3. Amin	26	33	91	−58
4. Amin and Ban	19	60	67	−7
5. Angst	30	47	47	0
6. Poldinger	40	70	55	+15
7. Van Scheyen	20	45	33	+12
8. Grof	24	42	33	+9
Overall	220	54	55	−1

Table 17 Nomifensin vs. Standard Tricyclic Incidence of Dry Mouth

Study	N	Nomifensin	Standard Tricyclic	Difference
1. Ananth	30	60	87	−27
2. Poldinger	40	10	0	+10

some evidence to indicate that drugs of this class may have specific antidepressant activity.[218] Recent studies using this agent have demonstrated its usefulness in outpatients with neurotic depression. Feighner reported that alprazolam demonstrated a more rapid onset of action than imipramine, with equivalent antidepressant effect (Table 19).[220] In addition, alprazolam was better tolerated and produced fewer side effects. Another unpublished study comparing alprazolam to imipramine, amitriptyline, doxepin, and placebo found alprazolam to be superior to placebo in the treatment of depression (Table 20).[221] Combining the result using the test of Fleiss, the superiority of alprazolam over placebo was significant to 2×10^{-6}. Interestingly, these reports are in contrast to what is reported for other benzodiazepines. In addition, alprazolam was found to be significantly better than placebo on all major parameters of antidepressive efficacy. Fewer overall cardiovascular or anticholinergic side effects were seen with those patients on alprazolam, as compared to the tricyclic group.

Bupropion is a phenylaminoketone compound that has been studied in a limited number of double-blind studies.[222] These studies are well done and suggest that the drug is an effective antidepressant.[223-228] Bupropion is neither a tricyclic nor an MAOI, and has demonstrated none of the

Table 18 Viloxazine vs. Standard Tricyclic

Study	N	Percent Good Result		Difference
		Viloxazine	Standard Tricyclic	
1. Floru	50	76	60	+16
2. Santonastaso	26	54	69	−15
3. Picho	119	64	56	+8
4. Kiloh	57	30	58	−28
5. Peat	23	54	60	−6
6. Elwan	51	83	67	+16
7. McEvoy	22	90	67	+23
8. Lennox	29	88	92	−4
9. Davies	22	55	45	+10
Overall	399	64	62	+2

Table 19 Alprazolam vs. Placebo

| Study | N | Percent Good Result | | |
		Alprazolam	Placebo	Difference
1. Feighner	344	75	49	+26
2. Upjohn	164	70	62	+8
Overall	508	73	53	+20

anticholinergic, cardiovascular, or sedative side effects common to those agents.[223-225] It has been found to exert little or no inhibition of the reuptake of serotonin or norepinephrine in rat brain synaptosomes; however, it has been found to be a significant inhibitor of dopamine reuptake.[228] More recently, it has been shown that bupropion caused a significant reduction of noradrenergic beta receptor density;[229] that is, there is a down-regulation of the noradrenergic receptor sites. The daily dosage of this drug ranges from 300 to 600 mg.[222]

Iprindole is neither a norepinephrine reuptake inhibitor nor an MAOI. Furthermore, it does not inhibit the reuptake of either serotonin or dopamine. Three double-blind studies have provided evidence of its efficacy.[230-232] As with bupropion, iprindole has been postulated to down-regulate the noradrenergic receptor site in the brain.[229] This implies some action on norepinephrine, although the exact mechanism by which this occurs is not yet known.

Zimelidine is a bicyclic compound that has been shown to be a powerful inhibitor of the reuptake of serotonin.[233] Clinical efficacy has been observed in a dosage range from 50 to 150 mg per day.[234]

Fluoxetine is another bicyclic compound that has been shown to be a potent inhibitor of 5-HT reuptake.[235-238] Results from open-label clinical trials have indicated efficacy with a dose of the drug ranging from 40 to 80 mg per day.

Table 20 Alprazolam vs. Standard Tricyclic

| Study | N | Percent Good Result | | |
		Alprazolam	Standard Tricyclic	Difference
1. Feighner	382	75	72	+3
2. Upjohn	282	70	77	−7
Overall	664	73	74	−1

Fluvoxamine, unlike the bicyclics zimelidine and fluoxetine, is of the family of (2-amino-ethyl) oxame ethers of the aralkyl ketones. It is a potent reuptake inhibitor of serotonin, but has a negligible effect on norepinephrine reuptake.[239] No anticholinergic activity has been noted with this agent; and, in addition, a specific antidepressant effect was demonstrated in several open-label clinical studies.[240-242] The dosage ranges from 50 to 300 mg per day. More information from controlled studies is needed before a conclusion as to its efficacy can be drawn.

Ciclazindol is a tetracyclic compound that has potential antidepressant and anoretic properties in man.[243] It has been found to have both norepinephrine and dopamine reuptake inhibiting properties.[243,244] Structurally, it resembles the antiobesity drug, mazindol. Ciclazindol antagonizes reserpine and tetrabenazine depressant effects and potentiates the effect of sympathomimetic amines in mice.[244] Further double-blind studies are required in the evaluation of this agent.

Melitracen is an imipramine-like compound with pharmacological properties similar to imipramine. It has been claimed to be most effective in endogenous depression.[245] Double-blind studies have demonstrated its potential as an effective antidepressant.[246,247] Effective daily doses of melitracen range from 75 to 250 mg, with an average of 150 mg.[247]

Butriptyline is another of the new tricyclic compounds with pharmacological properties similar to those of the standard tricyclics. It has been shown to have some antidepressant effect in at least one double-blind study.[248] Further double-blind studies are warranted.

Tandamine is a thiopyranoindole compound that is a norepinephrine reuptake inhibitor.[249] At least one study has shown it additionally to have reuptake inhibitory properties on dopamine.[250] Tandamine is only a weak reuptake inhibitor of 5-HT.[251] The drug has been well tolerated in clinical trials, and no anticholinergic or cardiovascular side effects have been noted.[249,251] Effective dosage ranges have yet to be determined; and double-blind studies are required to establish the effectiveness of this agent.

In summary, there are numerous new antidepressant medications that are in various stages of investigation. It is hoped that the busy clinician can examine the tables in this paper and judge the efficacy of several of the new drugs. Because some of the new antidepressants are of equivalent efficacy to the tricyclic antidepressant, and have a lower incidence of anticholinergic and cardiovascular side effects, they may be valuable in many clinical situations.

References

1. Glowinski J and Axelrod J. Inhibition of uptake of tritiated noradrenaline in the intact rat brain by imipramine and structurally related compounds. *Nature* 204:1318, 1964.

2. Rosloff BN and Davis JM. Effects of iprindole on norepinephrine turnover and transport. *Psychopharmacologia* 40:53–64, 1974.

3. Fuxe K and Ungerstedt U. The effect of imipramine on central 5-hydroxy-tryptamine neurons. *J Pharm Pharmacol* 20:150–51, 1968.

4. Lindrbrink P, Jonsson G and Fuxe K. The effect of imipramine-like drugs and antihistamine drugs on the uptake mechanisms in the central noradrenaline and 5-hydroxytryptamine neurons. *Neuropharmacology* 10:521–36, 1971.

5. Amin M et al. A double-blind comparative clinical study with Ludiomil (CIBA 34,276 Ba) and amitriptyline in newly admitted depressed patients. *Current Therapeutic Research* 15:691–99, 1973.

6. Angst J et al. "A Double-Blind Comparative Study on the Effectiveness of Maprotiline (Ludiomil) and Imipramine (Tofranil) in Endogenous Depression." In *Depressive Illness. Diagnosis, Assessment, Treatment*, edited by Kielholz, P. Berne: Hans Huber, 1972. pp. 245–52.

7. Balestrieri A et al. Clinical comparative evaluation of maprotiline, a new antidepressant drug. A multi-center study. *International Pharmacopsychiatry* 6:236, 1971.

8. Crawford R et al. A clinical trial of maprotiline (Ludiomil) in the treatment of depressive patients in general practice and the psychiatric clinic. *Journal of International Medical Research* 3(Suppl. 2):89, 1975.

9. Forrest WA. A comparison between daily and nightly dose regimen of amitriptyline and maprotiline (Ludiomil) in the treatment of reactive depression in general practice. *Journal of International Medical Research* 3(Suppl. 2):120, 1975.

10. Forrest WA. "Maprotiline (Ludiomil) in Depression: A Report on a Hospital-Monitored Release Study." In *Research and Clinical Investigation in Depression*, edited by Murphy, JE. Northampton: Cambridge Medical Publications, 1976a, p. 77.

11. Guz H. "A Controlled Double-Blind Between Patient Trial Comparing CIBA 34,276 Ba with Imipramine in Depressive State." In *Depressive Illness. Diagnosis, Assessment, Treatment*, edited by Kielholz, P. Berne: Hans Huber, 1972. pp. 234–44.

12. Kay NE and Davies B. A controlled trial of maprotiline (Ludiomil) and amitriptyline in general practice. *Medical Journal of Australia* 1:704, 1974.

13. Kessell A and Holt NF. A controlled study of a tetracyclic antidepressant - maprotiline (Ludiomil). *Medical Journal of Australia* 1:773, 1975.

14. Kielholz P. *Depressive illness. Diagnosis, Assessment, Treatment*. Berne: Hans Huber, 1972.

15. Lauritsen B. Continental hospital studies with maprotiline (Ludiomil). *Journal of International Medical Research* 3(Suppl. 2):61, 1975.

16. Lauritsen B and Madsen H. A multinational double-blind trial with a new antidepressant (Ludiomil) and amitriptyline. *Acta Psychiatrica Scandinavica* 50:192, 1974.

17. Lehmann HE et al. A double-blind comparative clinical trial with maprotiline (Ludiomil) and imipramine in newly-admitted depressed patients. *Current Therapeutic Research* 19:463, 1976.

18. Levin A. Maprotiline and amitriptyline in the treatment of depressive illness. A double-blind comparison. *South African Medical Journal* 48:47, 1974.

19. Levine S. A controlled comparison of maprotiline (Ludiomil) with imipramine avoiding observer bias. *Journal of International Medical Research* 3(Suppl. 2):75, 1975.

20. Liebling LI. Once-daily dosage study with maprotiline (Ludiomil). *Journal of International Medical Research* 3(Suppl. 2):109, 1975.

21. Mathur GN. A double-blind comparative clinical trial with maprotiline (Ludiomil) and amitriptyline. *Journal of International Medical Research* 3(Suppl. 2):71, 1975.

22. Marais GFT. Clinical evaluation of the antidepressants maprotiline and amitriptyline. A double-blind controlled trial. *South African Medical Journal* 48:1530, 1974.

23. Middleton RSW. A comparison between maprotiline (Ludiomil) and imipramine in the treatment of depressive illness in the elderly. *Journal of International Medical Research* 3(Suppl. 2):79, 1975.

24. Murphy JE. A double-blind general practice trial of maprotiline (Ludiomil) against amitriptyline in the treatment of reactive depression. *Journal of International Medical Research* 3(Suppl. 2):97, 1975.

25. Murphy JE and Forrest WA. A comparison between maprotiline (Ludiomil) and amitriptyline in the treatment of depressive reaction in general practice. *Journal of International Medical Research* 3(Suppl. 2):108, 1975.

26. Reiger W et al. Maprotiline (Ludiomil) and imipramine in depressed inpatients. A controlled study. *Journal of International Medical Research* 3:413, 1975.

27. Roy JY et al. Evaluation comparative de la dibencycladine (Ludiomil) et de l'imipramine chez le deprime psychotique. *International Journal of Clinical Pharmacology* 7:54, 1973.

28. Singh AN et al. Maprotiline (Ludiomil) (CIBA 34,276 Ba) and imipramine in depressed outpatients: A double-blind clinical study. *Current Therapeutic Research* 19:451, 1976.

29. Trick KS. Double-blind comparison of maprotiline with amitriptyline in the treatment of depressive illness. *Int Pharmacopsychiatry* 10:193–98, 1975.

30. Vaisanen E et al. Maprotiline and Doxepin in the treatment of depression. A double-blind multicenter comparison. *Acta Psychiat Scand* 57:193–201, 1978.

31. Ayd F. Maprotiline: An effective tetracyclic antidepressant. *Int Drug Therapy Newsletter*, Vol. VIII, No. 5 and 6, pp. 17–24, 1973.

32. Arvin M et al. A double-blind comparative clinical trial with Ludiomil (CIBA 34,276-Ba) and Amitriptyline in newly-admitted depressed patients. *Current Therapeutic Research*, Vol. 15, No. 10, pp. 691–99, 1973.

33. Brunner H et al. Cardiovascular effects of preparation CIBA 34,276-Ba and Imipramine. *Agents and Actions*, Vol. 2, No. 2, pp. 69–82, 1971.

34. Dell AJ. A comparison of Maprotiline (Ludiomil) and Amitriptyline (1). *J Int Med Res* 5(Suppl. 4):22–24, 1977.

35. Mindham BAE. A comparison of Maprotiline (Ludiomil) and Amitriptyline (2). *J Int Med Res* 5(Suppl. 4):25–33, 1977.

36. New drug shows promise in depressive patients. *JAMA* 220(5):661–62, May 1, 1972.

37. Logue L and Sachais B. Comparison of Maprotiline with Imipramine in severe depression: A multicenter controlled trial. *Clin Res*, p. 592A, 1977.

38. Pinder RM et al. Maprotiline: A review of its pharmacological properties and therapeutic efficacy in mental depressive states. *Drugs* 13:321–52, 1977.

39. Weissman MM et al. A double-blind trial of maprotiline (Ludiomil) and amitriptyline in depressed outpatients. *Acta Psychiatrica Scandinavica* 52:225, 1975.

40. Molnar G. Maprotiline—A double-blind study of a new tetracyclic antidepressant in severe depression. *Can Psychiat Assoc J* 22:19–23, 1977.

41. VanDer Velde C. Maprotiline versus imipramine and placebo in neurotic depression. *J Clin Psychiatry* 42:138–41, 1981.

42. Aberg A and Holmberg G. Controlled trial of a new antidepressant, Amoxapine, in comparison with Amitriptyline. *Curr Ther Res* 22:304–15, 1977.

43. Bagadia VN et al. A double-blind controlled study of Amoxapine and Imipramine in cases of depression. *Curr Ther Res* 26:417–29, 1979.

44. Burrows GD, Norman TR, and Davies BM. A comparative study of Amoxapine and Amitriptyline for depressive illness. *Australian Family Physician* 9:763-66, 1980.

45. Chermat R, Simon P, and Boissier JR. Amoxapine in experimental psychopharmacology: A neuroleptic or an antidepressant. *Arzneim-Forsch Drug Res* 29:814–20, 1979.

46. Donlon PT, Biertuemphel H, and Willenbring M. Amoxapine and Amitriptyline in the outpatient treatment of endogenous depression. *J Clin Psychiatry* 42:11–15, 1981.

47. Fabre L et al. Double-blind placebo-controlled comparison of Amoxapine and Imipramine in depressed out-patients. *Curr Ther Res* 22:611–19, 1977.

48. Fruensgaard K et al. Amoxapine versus Amitriptyline in endogenous depression: A double-blind study. *Acta Psychiat Scand* 59:502–8, 1979.

49. Gallant DM et al. Amoxapine: A double-blind evaluation of antidepressant activity. *Curr Ther Res* 15:56–59, 1973.

17

50. Hekimian LJ, Friedhoff A, and Deever E. A comparison of the onset of action and therapeutic efficacy of Amoxapine and Amitriptyline. *J Clin Psychiatry* 39:633–37, 1978.

51. Holden JM, Kerry RJ, and Orme JE. Amoxapine in depressive illness. *Curr Med Res Opin* 6:338–41, 1979.

52. Kaumeier HS and Haase HJJ. A double-blind comparison between Amoxapine and Amitriptyline in depressed in-patients. *Int J Clin Pharmacol, Therapy and Toxicology* 18:177–84, 1980.

53. Kiev A and Okerson L. Comparison of the therapeutic efficacy of Amoxapine with that of Imipramine. *Clin Trials J* 16:68–72, 1979.

54. Paprocki J et al. A double-blind comparison of Amoxapine and Imipramine in depression. *A Falha Medica* 74, No. 2, 1977.

55. de Paula J et al. Amoxapine and Amitriptyline: A double-blind study in depressed patients. *A Falha Medica* 75:165–69, 1977.

56. Rickels K et al. Amoxapine and Imipramine in the treatment of depressed outpatients: A controlled study. *Am J Psychiatry* 138:20–24, 1981.

57. Sathananthan GL et al. Amoxapine and Imipramine: A double-blind study in depressed patients. *Curr Ther Res* 15:919–22, 1973.

58. Sethi BB et al. Amoxapine and Amitriptyline: A double-blind study in depressed patients. *Curr Ther Res* 25:726–37, 1979.

59. Smith RC. Amoxapine, Imipramine, and placebo in depressive illness. *Curr Ther Res* 21:502–6, 1975.

60. de Souza Campos J et al. A double-blind comparative study between Amoxapine and Imipramine in the treatment of depression. *A Falha Medica* 75:No. 2, 1977.

61. Steinbook RM et al. Amoxapine, Imipramine and placebo: A double-blind study with pretherapy urinary 3-methoxy 4-hydroxy-phenylglycol levels. *Curr Ther Res* 26, 1979.

62. Takahashi Ryo et al. Comparison of efficacy of Amoxapine and Imipramine in a multi-clinic double-blind study using the WHO Schedule for a standard assessment of patients with depressive disorders. *J Int Med Res* 7:7–18, 1979.

63. Wilson C et al. A double-blind clinical comparison of Amoxapine, Imipramine and placebo in the treatment of depression. *Curr Ther Res* 22:620–27, 1977.

64. Yamhue A and Villalobos A. Amoxapine—A double-blind comparative clinical study and Amitriptyline in depressed, hospitalized patients. *Curr Ther Res* 21:502–6, 1977.

65. Sulser F. Current antidepressants. *Psychiatric Annals*, Vol 10, No. 9:28s–33s, 1980.

66. Al-Yassiri and Bridges PK. Trazodone efficacy and safety in endogenous depression: A double-blind comparison with imipramine. *Neuropharmacology* 19:1171–93, 1980.

67. Antonelli F et al. "Trazodone in the Treatment of Neurosis." In *Modern Problems of Pharmacopsychiatry*, Vol. 9, edited by Ban T. and Silvestrini B. Basel: Karger, 1974. pp. 127–39.

68. Cassano GB, Castrogiovanni P, and Conti L. "Clinical Evaluation of Trazodone in the Treatment of Depression." In *Modern Problems of Pharmacopsychiatry*, Vol. 9, edited by Ban, T. and Silvestrini, B. Basel: Karger, 1974. p. 199.

69. Cianchetti C and Gainotti G. Studio clinico controllato dell'attivita' antidepressiva e ansiolitica di un nuovo psicofarmaco L'AF-1161. *Gazz Int Med Chir* 72:1–10, 1968.

70. Cioffi F et al. Ulteriori dati sull'azione antidepressiva di un nuovo psicofarmaco L'AF-1161. *Rass Int Clin Ter* 49:1483–87, 1969.

71. DeGregorio M and Dionisio A. A controlled clinical study of a new antidepressant (trazodone). *Panminerva Med* 13, 1971.

72. Eckmann F et al. "Clinical Trials with Thrombrance: Results of Double-Blind Studies." In *Trazodone, A New Broad-Spectrum Antidepressant*, edited by Gershon S et al. Amsterdam: Excerpta Medica, 1980. pp. 69–74.

73. Escobar JI et al. Controlled clinical trial with trazodone, a novel antidepressant. A South American Experience. *J Clin Pharmacology* 20:124–30, 1980.

74. Fabre L, McClendon D, and Gainey A. Trazodone efficacy in depression: A double-blind comparison with imipramine and placebo in day-hospital type patients. *Curr Ther Res* 25:827–34, 1979.

75. Feighner JP. Trazodone, a triazolopyridine derivative, in primary depressive disorder. *J Clin Psychiatry* 41:250–55, 1980.

76. Fleiss JL. *Statistical Methods for Rates and Proportions.* New York: John Wiley & Sons, 1973.

77. Gerner R et al. Treatment of geriatric depression with trazodone, imipramine and placebo: A double-blind study. *J Clin Psychiatry* 41:216–20, 1980.

78. Gershon S, Rickels K, and Silvestrini B, eds. *Trazodone: A new broad-spectrum antidepressant.* Proceedings of a symposium held in Vienna during the 11th Congress of the Collegium Internationale Neuro-Psychopharmacologicum, July 9–14, 1978. Amsterdam: Excerpta Medica, 1980.

79. Goldberg H and Finnerty R. Trazodone in the treatment of neurotic depression. *J Clin Psychiatry* 41:430–34, 1980.

80. Kellams J, Klapper M, and Small J. Trazodone, a new antidepressant: Efficacy and safety in endogenous depression. *J Clin Psychiatry* 40:390–95, 1979.

81. LaPierre YD, Sussman P, and Ghandiran A. Differential antidepressant properties of trazodone and amitriptyline in agitated and retarded depression. *Curr Ther Res* 28:845–56, 1980.

82. Mazzei M, Marri FM, and Fabiani F. Relazione clinica su uno studio sperimentale con un nuovo psicofarmaco: L'AF-1161 (trazodone). *Riv Neurobiol* 17:238–60, 1971.

83. Murphy JE and Ankier SI. An evaluation of trazodone in the treatment of depression. *Neuropharmacology* 19:1217–18, 1980.

84. Newton R and Gershon S. Retrospective analysis of anticholinergic side effects in patients given trazodone, imipramine, or placebo for treatment of endogenous depression: Multiclinic study. (Submitted for publication.)

85. Pariante F. Un nuovo antidepressivo 'il trazodone': Valutazione della sua attivita con studio double-blind con crossover. *Riv Neuropsichiat Scien Aff* 17:1, 1971.

86. Peterova E. "Comparison of the Clinical Antidepressant Effects of Trazodone and Imipramine: A Preliminary Report." In *Trazodone, A New Broad Spectrum Antidepressant*, edited by Gershons S et al. Amsterdam: Excerpta Medica, 1980. pp. 58–59.

87. Pierce D. A comparison of trazodone and doxepin in depression. *Neuropsychopharmacology* 19:1219–20, 1980.

88. Rickels K. "Evaluation of Trazodone in the Treatment of Depressive Syndrome." Study Report NEWT-RE-07433. Mead Johnson Research Center, Evansville, Indiana, August 18, 1978.

89. Agnoli A et al. Psychopharmacological effects of trazodone. *Journal de Pharmacologie Clinique* 2:219–25, 1973.

90. Vinci M. Contributo clinico alla terapia delle depressioni endogene con un derivato della triazolpiridina. *Osped Psichiat* 39:416–33, 1971.

91. Pecknold et al. Trimipramine and Amitriptyline: Comparison in anxiety-depression. *Curr Ther Res* 26:497–504, 1979.

92. Burns BH. Preliminary evaluation of a new antidepressant, Trimipramine, by a sequential method. *Brit J Psychiat* 111:1155–57, 1965.

93. Evans JI. General practitioner clinical trials: Two new psychotropic drugs. *Practitioner* 198:135–39, 1967.

94. Rifkin et al. Comparison of Trimipramine and Imipramine: A controlled study. *J Clin Psychiatry* 41:124–29, 1980.

95. Malitz unpublished, Department of Experimental Psychiatry, New York State Psychiatric Institute. Data on file, Ives Laboratories, Inc.

96. Lehmann H et al. "The effects of Trimipramine on Geriatric Patients." In *Trimipramine, A New Antidepressant*, edited by Lehmann H, Berthiaume, and Ban T. 1964, pp. 69–76.

97. Kristof FE, Lehmann HE, and Ban TA. Systematic studies with Trimipramine—A new antidepressant drug. *Canad Psychiat Assn J* 12:17–20, 1967.

98. Burke BV, Sainsbury M, Meyo BA. A comparative trial of amitriptyline and trimipramine in therapy of depression. *Med Journal of Australia* 1:1216–18, 1967.

99. Hunter JW et al. A controlled cross-over study of Trimipramine and Amylobarbitone. *Brit J Psychiat* 113:667–70, 1967.

100. Rickels K et al. Amitriptyline and Trimipramine in neurotic depressed patients: A collaborative study. *Am J Psychiatry* 127:208–18, 1970.

101. Lean TH and Sidhu MS. Comparative study of Imipramine (Tofranil) and Trimipramine (Surmontil) in depression associated with gynaecological conditions. *Proc Obstet Gynaecol* 3:222–28, 1978.

102. Salzman MM. A controlled trial of trimipramine, a new antidepressant drug. *Brit J Psychiat* 111:1105–6, 1965.

103. Lingjaerde O. Inhibition of platelet uptake of serotonin in plasma from patients treated with clomipramine and amitriptyline. *Eur J Clin Pharmacol* 15:335–40, 1979.

104. Mulgirigama LD et al. An assessment of uptake inhibition of 5-Hydroxytryptamine, Dopamine, and Noradrenaline in a double-blind clinical trial of Clomipramine and Maprotiline in depressed outpatients. (In press.)

105. Symes MH. Monochlorimipramine: A controlled trial of a new antidepressant. *Brit J Psychiat* 113:671–72, 1967.

106. McClure DJ, Low GL, and Gant M. Clomipramine HCl—A double-blind study of a new antidepressant drug. *Can Psychiat Assoc J* 18:403–8, 1973.

107. Rickels K et al. Clomipramine and Amitriptyline in depressed outpatients. *Psychopharmacologia* 34:361–76, 1974.

108. Arfwidsson L et al. Comparison of Chlorimipramine and Imipramine in ambulatory treatment of depression. *Acta Psychiatrica Scandinavica* 48:367–76, 1972.

109. Kampman R, Ummikko-Pelkonen A, and Kuha S. Tricyclic antidepressants in the treatment of depressions: A double-blind comparison of Chloripramine (Anafranil) and Amitriptyline. *Acta Psychiat Scand* 58:142–48, 1978.

110. Buns et al. Inhibition of 5-HT uptake into neurons and platelets in mice treated chronically with clorimipramine and femoxetine. *Psychopharmacology* 64:149–53, 1979.

111. Lidbrink P, Jonsson G, and Fuxe K. The effect of imipramine-like drugs and antihistamine drugs on uptake mechanisms in the central noradrenalin and 5-HT neurons. *Neuropharmacol* 10:521, 1971.

112. McClure DJ, Low GL, and Gant M. Clomipramine HCl—a double-blind study of a new antidepressant drug. *Can Psychiat Assoc J* 18:403–8, 1973.

113. Gore CP. Clomipramine (Anafranil), Tofranil (Imipramine) and placebo: A comparative study in relation to electroconvulsive therapy. *J Int Med Res* 1:347–51, 1973.

114. Rack PH. A comparative clinical trial of oral Clomipramine (Anafranil) against Imipramine. *J Int Med Res* 1:332–37, 1973.

115. Hynes MV. A comparative clinical trial of oral Clomipramine (Anafranil) against Amitriptyline. *J Int Med Res* 1:338–42, 1973.

116. Harding MB. A comparative clinical trial of oral Clomipramine (Anafranil) against Amitriptyline. *J Int Med Res* 1:353–56, 1973.

117. Brander M. Methods for the Evaluation of Antidepressive substances with special reference to Monochlorimipramine (or 34586). *Schweizer Archiv Fur Neurologie und Psychiatrie* 93:137, 1964.

118. Van Scheyen JD et al. Controlled study comparing Nomifensine and Clomipramine in unipolar depression, using the Probenecid technique. *Brit J Clin Pharmac* 4:1795–1845, 1977.

119. Murphy JE. A comparative trial of a combination of Clomipramine (Anafranil) and Insidon and Limbitrol. *J Int Med Res* 1:382–85, 1973.

120. Kampman R et al. Tricyclic antidepressants in the treatment of depressions: A double-blind comparison of Clomipramine (Anafranil) and Amitriptyline. *Acta Psychiat Scand* 58:142–48, 1978.

121. Poldinger W et al. Vergleichende Klinische Erfahrungen mit Chlorimipramin und Ketimipramin. *Arzneimittel-Forsch* 19:492–93, 1969.

122. Yaryura-Tobias JA, Neziroglu MA, and Bergman L. Chlorimipramine, for obsessive-compulsive neurosis: An organic approach. *Curr Ther Res* 20:541–48, 1976.

123. Renynghe de Voxvrie G. L'Anafranil dans l'obession. *Acta Neurol Belg* 68:787–92, 1968.

124. Capstick N. Chlorimipramine in obsessional states. *Psychosomatics* 12:322–35, 1971.

125. Escobar JI and Landbloom RP. Treatment of phobic neurosis with clomipramine: A controlled clinical trial. *Curr Ther Res* 20:680–85, 1976.

126. Carey MS et al. The use of clomipramine in phobic patients. *Curr Ther Res* 17:107–10, 1975.

127. Wasman D. An investigation into the use of anafranil in phobic and obsessional disorders. *Scottish Med Jour* 20:61s–66s, 1975.

128. Colgan A. A pilot study of anafranil in the treatment of phobic states. *Scottish Med Jour* 20:55s–60s, 1975.

129. Geigy Investigator's Manual Information Booklet.

130. Madalena JC. The treatment of depressive states with monochlorimipramine in slow intravenous perfusion and by the oral route. *Hospital* (Rio de J) 74:147, 1968.

131. Bieber H and Kugler J. Die behandlung von depressiven kranken mit chlorimipramin infusionen. *Arch Psychiat Nervenkr* 219:L329–38, 1969.

132. Sivers B et al. Comparative clinical evaluation of lofepramine and imipramine. *Acta Psychiat Scand* 55:21–31, 1974.

133. d'Elia G et al. Comparative clinical evaluation of Lofepramine and Imipramine. *Acta Psychiat Scand* 55:10–20, 1977.

134. McClelland HA et al. The comparative antidepressant value of Lofepramine and Amitriptyline. *Acta Psychiat Scand* 60:190–98, 1979.

135. Angst J et al. Klinische prufung von lofepramin in Vergleich zu Imipramin. *Int Pharmacopsychiat* 10:65–71, 1975.

136. Wright Von S and Hermann L. A double-blind comparative study on the effects of Lofepramine and Amitriptyline in depressive out-patients. *Drug Res* 26:1167–69, 1976.

137. Obermair W and Poldinger W. Doppelblind-vergleich der wirkungen eines neven trizyklischen antidepressivums (Lofepramine) und eines tetrazyklischen antidepressivums (Maprotilin). *Int Pharmacopsychiat* 12:65–71, 1977.

138. Goncalves N and Wegener G: Wirkungsvergleich von Lofepramin und Mianserin an depressiven Patienten und Doppelblind. *Beldingungen Int Pharmacopsychiat* 14:3120–318, 1979.

139. Murphy JE and Bridgman KM. A comparative clinical trial of Mianserin (normal) and Amitriptyline in the treatment of depression in general practice. *J Int Med Res* 6:119–206, 1978.

140. Conti L et al. "Clinical Experience with Mianserin." In *Progress with the Pharmacotherapy of Depression: Mianserin HCl.*, edited by Drykonnigen G et al. Proc. of a Symposium held in Barcelona, Sept. 4, 1978. p. 65–73. Amsterdam: Excerpta Medica, 1979.

141. Coppen A et al. Mianserin in the prophylactic treatment of bipolar affective illness. *J of Pharmacopsychiat* 12:95–99, 1977.

142. Ghose K, Coppen A, and Turner P. Autonomic actions and interactions of Mianserin Hydrochloride (Org. 6B94) and Amitriptyline in patients with depressive illness. *Psychopharmacology* 49:201–4, 1976.

143. Zis AP and Goodwin FK. Novel antidepressants and the biogenic amine hypothesis of depression—the case for Iprindole and Mianserin. *Arch Gen Psychiatry* 36:1097–1107, 1979.

144. Peet M, Tienari P, and Jaskari MO. A comparison of the cardiac effects of Mianserin and Amitriptyline in man. *Pharmakopsychiat* 10:309–12, 1977.

145. Smith AHW, Naylor GS, and Moody JP. Placebo-controlled double-blind trial of Mianserin Hydrochloride. *Br J Clin Pharmac* 5:675–705, 1978.

146. Russell GFM et al. Comparative double-blind trial of Mianserin Hydrochloride (Organon GB94) and Diazepam in patients with depressive illness. *Br J Clin Pharmac* 5:575–655, 1978.

147. Hamer AWF et al. Mianserin and Intracardiac conduction. *IRCS Medical Science* 7:220, 1979.

148. Montgomery S et al. Differential effects on suicidal ideation of Mianserin, Maprotiline and Amitriptyline. *Br J Clin Pharmac* 5:775–805, 1978.

149. Blaha L, Pinder RM, and Stolemeijer SM. Double-blind comparative trial of Mianserin versus Clomipramine. *Current Medical Research and Opinion* 6(Suppl. 7):99–106, 1980.

150. Hopman H. Mianserin, in out-patients with depressive illness, in dosage up to 130 mg daily. *Current Medical Research and Opinion* 6(Suppl. 7):107–14, 1980.

151. Kopera H. Mianserin drug interactions and anticholinergic effects. Progress in the pharmacotherapy of depression, Mianserin HCl. *Excerpta Medica* pp. 49–55, 1979.

152. Viansanen E et al. Mianserin Hydrochloride (org. gb94) in the treatment of obsessional states. *J Int Med Res* 5:289–91, 1977.

153. Wheatley D. Controlled clinical trial of a new antidepressant (ORG,GB 94) of novel chemical formulation. *Am Ther Res* 18:849–55, 1975.

154. Pinder RM et al: Double-blind, multi-center trial comparing the efficacy and side-effects of mianserin and clomipramine in depressed in-patients and outpatients. Int. Pharmacopsychiatry 15:218–27, 1980.

155. Saletu B and Guenberger J. Changes in clinical symptomatology and psychometric assessments in depressed patients during mianserin and combined amitriptyline/chloridazepoxide therapy: A double-blind comparison. *Curr Med Res Opin* 6(Suppl. 7):52–62, 1980.

156. Jaskari MO et al. The treatment of depression: Comparative study of the effect of Mianserin, Tolvin, and Amitriptyline. *Ther G G N* 118:806–18, 1979.

157. Pull et al. Double-blind multicenter trial comparing mianserin and imipramine. *Acta Psychiat Belg* 78:827–32, 1978.

158. Perry GF et al. Clinical study of mianserin, imipramine and placebo in depression: Blood level and MHPG correlation. *Brit J Clin Pharmacol* 5(Suppl. 1):355–415, 1978.

159. Saletu B et al. "Double-Blind Clinical and Psychological Test Investigations in Depressed Out-Patients with Mianserin and Limbitrol." In *Progress in the pharmacotherapy of depression: Mianserin HCl*, edited by Drykoningen et al. Amsterdam: Excerpta Medica, 1979. pp. 8–18.

160. Svestka J et al. Controlled comparison of mianserin with imipramine in endogenous depressions. *Activ Nerv Sup* 21:147–48, 1979.

161. Hoc J. Comparative double-blind clinical trial with mianserin and nortriptyline. *Acta Psychiatrica Belgica* 78:833–40, 1978.

162. Murphy et al. Mianserin in the treatment of depression in general practice. *Practitioner* 217:135–38, 1976.

163. DeBuck R. A comparison of the efficacy and side effects of mianserin and clomipramine in primary depression: A double-blind randomized trial. *Curr Med Res Opin* 6(Suppl. 7):88–98, 1980.

164. Hamouz W et al. A double-blind group comparative trial of mianserin and diazepam in depressed outpatients. *Pharmakopsychiat* 13:79–83, 1980.

165. Khan MC and Moslehuddin K. A double-blind comparative trial of mianserin and maprotiline in the treatment of depression. *Curr Med Res Opin* 6(Suppl. 7):63–71, 1980.

166. Kretschmar JH. Mianserin and amitriptyline in elderly hospitalized patients with depressive illness: A double-blind trial. *Curr Med Res Opin* 6(Suppl. 7):144–51, 1980.

167. Leonard BE. Some effects of a new tetracyclic antidepressant compound, (org GB 94), on the metabolism of monoamines in rat brain. *Psychopharmacologia* 36:221–36, 1974.

168. Leonard BE. Some effects of Mianserin on monoamine metabolism in the rat brain. *Br J Clin Pharmacol* 5:11s–12s, 1978.

169. Vogel HP et al. Mianserin versus Amitriptyline. *Int Pharmacopsych* 11:25–31, 1976.

170. Feighner JP. Pharmacology: New antidepressants. *Psychiat Ann* 10:35s–41s, 1980.

171. Amin MM, Ban TA, and Lehmann HE. Nominfensin in the treatment of depression: A report on the Canadian part of a transcultural study. *Psychop Bull* 114:35–37, 1978.

172. Amin MM, Ban TA, and Pecknold JC. Nominfensin in the treatment of depression: A standard-controlled clinical study. *Psychopharm Bull* 14:37–39, 1978.

173. Acebal E et al. A double-blind comparative trial of nomifensin and desimipramine in depression. *Europ J Clin Pharmacol* 10:109–13, 1976.

174. Ananth J and Von Der Steen N. A double-blind controlled comparative study of nomifensin in depression. *Curr Ther Res* 23:213–21, 1978.

175. Angat J et al. Ergebnisse eines offenen und eines doppelblind versuches von Nomifensin im Vergleich zu Imipramin. *Arch Psychiat Nervenki* 219:265–76, 1974.

176. Poldinger W and Gommel G. Differences in effect between nomifensin and nortriptyline. *Int Pharmacopsychiat* 13:58–68, 1978.

177. Van Scheyen JD, Van Praag HM, and Korf J. Controlled study comparing nomifensine and clomipramine in unipolar depression, using the probenecid technique. *Brit J Clin Pharm* 4:179S–84S, 1977.

178. Taeuber K. Comparison of nomifensine and placebo. *Brit J of Clin Pharmacology* 4:209S-213S, 1977. (See also the following references quoted by Taeuber:)

   a) Eckmann F. "Klinische Untersuchungen mit dem Antidepressivum Nomifensin." In *Systematization Provocation and Therapy of Depressive Psychoses*, edited by Walcher W. pp. 199–204, Second Int Symp braz. April 1973, Vienna: Hollinek, 1974.

   b) Kroeger R and Eckmann F. "Klinische Untersuchungen mit Nomifensin. Bericht uber Einen Doppelblindvergleich Zwischen Nomifensin und Placebo: Wirkungsnachweis bei Endogenen und Involutiven Depressionen." In *Alival Symposium Uber Ergebnisse der Experimentellen und Klinischen Prufung.* Berlin, 1976. Stuttgart and New York: F.K. Schattauer, 1977.

   c) Bruckner GW and Jansen W. "Nomifensin: Anwendung bei Altersdepressionen." In *Alival Symposium uber Ergebnisse der Experimentellen und Klinischen Prufung,* Berlin, 1976. Stuttgart und New York: F.K. Schattauer, 1977.

179. Forrest A, Hewett A, and Nicholson P. Controlled randomized group comparison of nomifensine and imipramine in depressive illness. *Brit J of Clin Pharmacol* 4:215S–220S, 1977.

180. Moizeszowicz J and Segundo S. Controlled trial of nomifensin and viloxazine in the treatment of depression in the elderly. *J Clin Pharmacology* 1977.

181. Sharma SD. A double-blind clinical evaluation of nomifensine. *Curr Ther Res* 27:157–63, 1980.

182. Grof P et al. Dopaminergic agonist nomifensine compared with amitriptyline: A double-blind clinical trial in acute primary depressions. *Brit J Clin Pharm* 4:221S–25S, 1977.

183. McClelland HA, Kerr TA, and Little JC. A clinical comparison of nomifensine and amitriptyline. *Brit J of Pharmacol* 4:233S–36S, 1977.

184. Habermann W. A review of controlled studies with nomifensine, performed outside the U.K. *Brit J of Clin Pharm* 4:237S–41S, 1977.

a) Andersen T. "Doppelblindunters Uchung des Praparate Nomifensin und Doxepin in Einer Reprasentativen Patientengruppe Mitklinisch Behandelten Depressionen." In *Alival Symposium uber Ergebnisse der Experimentellen und Klinischen Prufung*, Berlin, 1–2 October 1976. Stuttgart and New York: F.K. Schattauer, 1976.

b) Levin E. "Neurotische Depressionen: Ein Indikationsgebiet von Alival." In *Alival Symposium uber Ergebnisse der Experimentellen und Klinischen Prufung*, Berlin, 1–2 October 1976. Stuttgart and New York: F.K. Schattauer, 1977.

185. Ong SBY and Lee CT. A double-blind comparison of nomifensine and amitriptyline in the treatment of depression. *Acta Psychiat Scand* 63:198–207, 1981.

186. Hunt P et al. Nomifensine, a new potent inhibitor of dopamine uptake into synaptosomes from rat brain corpus striatum. *J Pharm Pharmacol* 26:370–71, 1974.

187. McCawley A. A double-blind evaluation of nomifensine and imipramine in depressed outpatients. *Am J Psychiatry* 136:841–42, 1979.

188. Franchin EA. Ensaio clinico em 30 pacientes de una nova medicaio antidepressiva: Nomifensin. *Rev Bras Clin Ter* 2:317–22, 1973.

189. Leon P and Osorio M. Efficacy and tolerance of a new psychotherapeutic antidepressant - nomifensin. *Acta Medica Peruana* 3:202–6, 1974.

190. Pecknold JD et al. A clinical trial with nomifensin, a new antidepressant drug. *Int J Clin Pharmacol* 11:304–8, 1975.

191. Schacht R and Heptner W. Effect of nomifensin, a new antidepressant on the uptake of noradrenaline and serotonin and on release of noradrenalin in rat brain synaptosomes. *Biochem Pharmacol* 23:3413–22, 1974.

192. Angst J et al. Ergebnisse eines offenen und eines doppelblind - versuches von nomifensin imvergleich zu imipramine. *Arch Psychiat Nervenkr* 219:265–76, 1974.

193. Bayliss PFC and Duncan SM. The clinical pharmacology of viloxazine hydrochloride — a new antidepressant of novel chemical structure. *Br J of Clin Pharm* 1:431–37, 1974.

194. Bayliss PFC et al. An open study of two dose levels of 'vivalan' (viloxazine hydrochloride ici 58,834) in depression general practice. *J Int Med Res* 2:253–59, 1974.

195. Bayliss PFC et al. A double-blind controlled trial of 'vivalan' (viloxazine hydrochloride) and imipramine hydrochloride in the treatment of depression in general practice. *J Int Med Res* 2:260–64, 1974.

196. Floru L and Tegeler J. Eine vergleichende Untersuchung der beiden antidepressiva viloxazin und imipramin. *Pharmakopsychiat* 12:313–20, 1979.

197. Magnus RV. A placebo controlled trial of viloxazine with and without tranquilizers in depressive illness. *J Int Med Res* 3:207–13, 1975.

198. Nugent D. A double-blind study of viloxazine (vivalan) and amitriptyline in depressed geriatric patients. *Clinical Trials Journal* 6:1:13–17, 1979.

199. Santonastaso P, Maistrello I, and Battistin L. Comparison of vivalan (viloxazine hydrochloride) with imipramine in the treatment of depression. *Acta Psychiat Scand* 60:137–43, 1979.

200. Wheatley D. Viloxazine: A new antidepressant. *Curr Ther Res* 16:8:821–28, 1974.

201. Peet M. A clinical trial of ici 58,834 - a potential antidepressant. *J Int Med Res* 1:624–26, 1973.

202. Elwan O. A comparative study of viloxazine and imipramine in the treatment of depressive states. *J Int Med Res* 8:7–17, 1980.

203. Lennox IG. Viloxazine and amitriptyline in depressive illness. *The Practitioner* p. 153–56, 1976.

204. Davies B et al. A sequential trial of viloxazine (vivalon) and imipramine in moderately depressed patients. *Med J Aust* 1:521–22, 1977.

205. McEvoy J et al. Viloxazine in the treatment of depressive neurosis: A controlled clinical study with doxepin and placebo. *Brit J Psychiat* 137:440–43, 1980.

206. Moizeszowicz J and Segundo S. Controlled trial of nomifensin and Viloxazine in the treatment of depression in the elderly. *J Clin Pharmacology*, 1977.

207. Amin MM et al. Viloxazine in the treatment of depression: Psycho-physical measures and clinical response. *Psychopharm Bull* 14:33–35, 1978.

208. Murphy JE. Vivalin. *Journal Int Med Research* 3:122–25, 1975.

209. Kiloh LG et al. Double-blind comparative trial of viloxazine and amitriptyline in patients suffering from endogenous depression. *Aust and New Zealand Journal of Psychiatry* 13:357–60, 1979.

210. Blackburn TP et al. Effects of viloxazine, its major metabolites, on biogenic amine uptake mechanisms in vitro and in vivo. *Eur J Pharmacol* 52:367–74, 1978.

211. Pichot P et al. A controlled, multicenter therapeutic trial of viloxazine. *J Int Med Res* 3:80s–86s, 1975.

212. Tsegos IK and Ekdawi MY. A double-blind controlled study of viloxazine and imipramine in depression. *Curr Med Res Opin* 2:455–60, 1974.

213. DeWilde J. Double-blind controlled trial of viloxazine and imipramine in the treatment of hospital depressed patients. *Acta Therapeutica* 3:49–56, 1977.

214. Wheatley D. Viloxazine — a new antidepressant. *Curr Ther Res* 16:821–28, 1974.

215. Nugent D. A double-blind study of viloxazine and amitriptyline in depressed geriatric patients. *Clin Trials J* 16:13–17, 1979.

216. Pinder RM et al. Viloxazine: A review of its pharmacological properties and therapeutic efficacy in depressive illness. *Drug* 13:401–21, 1977.

217. Upjohn Laboratories Data.

218. Schatzberg A and Cole J. Benzodiazepines in depressive disorders. *Arch Gen Psychiatry* 35:1359–65, 1978.

219. Fabre L. Pilot open-label study with alprazolam in outpatients with neurotic depression. *Curr Ther Res* 19:661–68, 1976.

220. Feighner J. Benzodiazepines as antidepressants. *Mod Prob Pharmacopsychiat* 18:197–213, 1982.

221. Upjohn Labs; Alprazolam Summary.

222. Fabre LF and McLendon DM. A double-blind placebo controlled study of bupropion (Wellbatrin) in the treatment of depressed inpatients. *Curr Ther Res* 23:393–402, 1978.

223. Fann WE et al. Clinical trial of bupropion HCl in treatment of depression. *Curr Ther Res* 23:222–29, 1978.

224. Soroko FE et al. Bupropion hydrochloride (+) d-t-butylamine-3-chloropro-biophenoid HCl: A novel antidepressant agent. *Comm D Pharm Pharmacol* 29:767–70, 1977.

225. Peck AW et al. A comparison of bupropion hydrochloride with dexampheta-mine and amitriptyline in health subjects. *Br J Clin Pharmacol* 7:469–78, 1979.

226. Brodie H. Clinical investigator's manual (Wellbatrin), unpublished, Bur-roughs Wellcome Company, 1976.

227. Fann WE et al. Clinical trial of bupropion HCl in treatment of depression. *Curr Ther Res* 23:222–29, 1978.

228. Soroko FE et al. Bupropion hydrochloride, a novel antidepressant agent. *J Pharmacol* (in press).

229. Pandey G and Davis JM. Treatment with antidepressants, sensitivity of betareceptors and affective illness. New York: John Wiley & Sons, 1980.

230. Johnson J and Maden JG. A new antidepressant — pramindole — a double-blind controlled trial. *Clin Trials J* 4: 787–90, 1967.

231. Sutherland MS et al. Comparison of effects of pramindole and imipramine. *Clin Trials J* : 857–60, 1967.

232. Sterlin C et al. A preliminary investigation of wy-3263 versus amitriptyline in depressions. *Curr Ther Res* 10:576–82, 1968.

233. Coppen A et al. Inhibition of 5-HT reuptake by amitriptyline and zimelidine and its relationship to their therapeutic action. *Psychopharmacology* 63:125–29, 1979.

234. Aberg A and Holmberg G. Preliminary clinical test of zimelidine, a new 5-HT uptake inhibitor. *Acta Psychiat Scand* 59:45–58, 1979.

235. Lemberger L et al. Fluoxetine, a selective serotonin uptake inhibitor. *Clin Pharmacol Ther* 23:421–29, 1978.

236. Rowe H et al. Pharmacologic effects in man of a specific serotonin-reuptake inhibitor. *Science* 199:436, 1978.

237. Fuller RW, Perry KW, and Molloy BB. Effect of an uptake inhibitor on serotonin metabolism in a brain: studies with 3-(p-trifluoromethylphenoxy)-N-methyl-3-phenylpropylamine. *Life Sci* 15:1161–71, 1974.

238. Lemberger L et al. The effect of lilly compound 94939, a potential antidepressant, on biogenic amine uptake in man. *Br J Clin Pharmacol* 3:215–18, 1976.

239. Claassen V et al. Fluvoxamine, a specific 5-HT uptake inhibitor. *Br J Pharmacol* 60:505–16, 1977.

240. Wright JH and Denber HCB. Clinical trial of fluvoxamine: a new serotonergic antidepressant. *Curr Ther Res* 23:83–89, 1978.

241. Saletu B et al. Fluvoxamine — a new serotonin reuptake inhibitor: first clinical and psychometric experiences in depressed patients. *J Neural Trans* 41:17–36, 1977.

242. Itil TM et al. Fluvoxamine, a new antidepressant. *Prog Neuro-Psychopharmacol* 1:309–22, 1977.

243. Oh WMS et al. Influence of ciclazindol on monoamine uptake and cns function in normal subjects. *Psychopharmacol* 60:177–81, 1979.

244. Ghose K et al. Antidepressant activity and pharmacological interactions of ciclazindol. *Psychopharmacol* 57:109–14, 1978.

245. Ayd FJ. Melitracen: A tricyclic antidepressant. *Int Drug Ther Newsletter* 3:37–38, 1968.

246. Thorell LH and Wretmark G. A comparative study of N7001 (Metrisil) and imipramine on a series of depressive patients. *Acta Psychiat Scand* 50:508–15, 1974.

247. Francesconi G et al. Controlled comparison of melitrocen and and amitriptyline in depressed patients. *Curr Ther Res* 20:529–40, 1976.

248. Levinson B. Butriptyline hydrochloride and imipramine hydrochloride in the treatment of non-psychotic depression — a double-blind trial. *SA Med J* 48:873–75, 1974.

249. Saletu DT and Bymaster FP. Tandamine — a new norepinephrine reuptake inhibitor. *Int Pharmacopsychiat* 12:137–52, 1977.

250. Wong DT and Bymaster FP. An inhibitor of dopamine uptake, LR5182. *Life Sciences* 23:1041–48, 1978.

251. Pugsley T and Lippmann W. Effects of tandamine and pirandamine, new potential antidepressants, on the brain uptake of NE and 5-HT and related activity. *Psychopharmacology* 47:33–41, 1976.

2

Biological Discrimination of Subtypes of Depressions

Joseph J. Schildkraut, M.D., Alan F. Schatzberg, M.D., Paul J. Orsulak, Ph.D., John J. Mooney, M.D., Alan H. Rosenbaum, M.D., and Jon E. Gudeman, M.D.

The biological heterogeneity of depressive disorders was discussed in an early review of the catecholamine hypothesis of affective disorders which described how various alterations in catecholamine metabolism might be of importance in the pathophysiology of certain types of depressions.[1] This focus on catecholamine metabolism was acknowledged to be a reductionistic oversimplification of an extremely complex biological state (which undoubtedly involved abnormalities in many other neurotransmitter or neuromodulator systems, as well as endocrine changes and other biochemical abnormalities). Nonetheless, in that review more than 15 years ago, it was suggested that different subgroups of patients with depressive disorders might be characterized by differences in the metabolism of norepinephrine and the physiology of noradrenergic neuronal systems, including alterations in noradrenergic receptor sensitivity.[1] Since that time, studies by our research group,[2–8] as well as other investigators have provided data supporting this possibility, and this literature has been reviewed recently.[9]

It is now generally acknowledged that urinary 3-methoxy-4-hydroxyphenylglycol (MHPG) is a major metabolite of norepinephrine originating in the brain.[10–12] However, urinary MHPG may also derive in part from the peripheral sympathetic nervous system, and the exact fraction of urinary MHPG deriving from norepinephrine originating in the brain remains uncertain.[13–15] Despite this uncertainty, measurements of urinary MHPG

This work was supported in part by Grant No. MH15413 from the National Institute of Mental Health.

31

levels, nonetheless appear to be of value in exploring the pathophysiology of depressions, in defining subgroups of depressive disorders, and in predicting differential responses to various antidepressant drugs.

In longitudinal studies of patients with naturally occurring or amphetamine-induced bipolar manic-depressive episodes, many investigators have found that levels of urinary MHPG were lower during periods of depression and higher during periods of mania or hypomania than during periods of remission.[16-23] However, not all depressed patients excrete comparably low levels of MHPG, and the possibility that urinary levels of MHPG as well as other catecholamine metabolites might provide a biochemical basis for differentiating among the depressive disorders has been explored by a number of investigators.[24,25]

Our research group initially reported that urinary MHPG levels were significantly lower in patients with bipolar manic-depressive depressions than in patients with unipolar nonendogenous chronic characterological depressions and the finding of reduced urinary MHPG levels in patients with bipolar manic-depressive depressions has been confirmed by a number of laboratories in addition to ours.[2,3,26-34] Of particular interest is the finding of one of these studies, which showed that when the peripheral contribution to urinary MHPG was reduced with carbidopa (a decarboxylase inhibitor that does not cross the blood/brain barrier), the differences in urinary MHPG levels in bipolar manic-depressive depressions and control subjects became more pronounced and statistically significant.[31]

In contrast to the reduction in urinary MHPG levels in patients with bipolar manic-depressive depressions when compared with values in unipolar depressions, as shown in Table 1, there was no difference in urinary vanillymandelic acid (VMA) levels.[2,6] This is important because in studies of depressed patients, reports that circulating MHPG may be converted to VMA raised questions concerning the specific value of urinary MHPG (for example in contrast to VMA) as an index of norepinephrine metabolism in the brain or as a biochemical marker.[14,15]

Table 1 Baseline Urinary MHPG and VMA Levels in Depressive Disorders

Depressive Subgroup	MHPG	VMA
Bipolar Manic-Depressive	$1,209 \pm 89^a$	$4,041 \pm 211$
Unipolar Endogenous	$1,950 \pm 177$	$3,782 \pm 246$
Unipolar Nonendogenous	$1,814 \pm 92$	$3,540 \pm 232$

Source: The data in this table are taken from Schildkraut JJ et al. Toward a biochemical classification of depressive disorders I: Differences in urinary excretion of MHPG and other catecholamine metabolites in clinically defined subtypes of depressions. *Arch. Gen. Psychiat.* 35:1427–33, 1978.
Note: Urinary MHPG and VMA levels are presented as means ± standard errors of the means, and expressed in $\mu g/24$ hours.
$^a p$ <.001 when compared to unipolar nonendogenous group.

Application of Multivariate Discriminant Function Analysis to Data on Urinary Catecholamines and Metabolites in Depressed Patients

Although MHPG was the only catecholamine metabolite that showed a pronounced difference when values in bipolar manic-depressive depressions and unipolar nonendogenous chronic characterological depressions were compared in our early studies,[2] multivariate discriminant function analysis was used to explore the possibility that the other catecholamine metabolites might provide further information that would aid in differentiating among subtypes of depressions.[3] By applying stepwise multivariate discriminant function analysis to data on urinary catecholamines and metabolites, we generated an empirically derived equation that provided an even more precise discrimination between bipolar manic-depressive and unipolar nonendogenous chronic characterological depressions than did urinary MHPG alone. In generating this equation, a metric was established so that low scores were related to patients with bipolar manic-depressive depressions, whereas high scores were related to patients with unipolar nonendogenous depressions. Preliminary validation of this equation was then obtained in a sample of patients whose data had not been used in the derivation of the equation.[3] This discrimination equation for computing the Depression-type (D-type) score was of the form:

$$\text{D-type score} = C_1(\text{MHPG}) - C_2(\text{VMA}) + C_3(\text{NE})$$
$$- C_4 \frac{(\text{NMN} + \text{MN})}{\text{VMA}} + C_0$$

While this discrimination equation was generated mathematically to provide the best least squares fit of the data (the terms were not selected by the investigators), the inclusion of VMA as well as other urinary catecholamines and metabolites (of peripheral origin) in this empirically derived equation may be correcting for that fraction of urinary MHPG that comes from peripheral sources rather than from the brain.[3] Moreover, several years ago we suggested that the fourth term—the ratio $\frac{\text{NMN} + \text{MN}}{\text{VMA}}$—might be inversely related to monoamine oxidase (MAO) activity, because normetanephrine and metanephrine could be converted to VMA by deamination.[3] Indeed, such an inverse correlation has recently been documented between this ratio $\frac{\text{NMN} + \text{MN}}{\text{VMA}}$ and platelet MAO activity, in 90 patients from whom we obtained concurrent measurements ($r = -.29$; $p < .005$). In addition to confirming that this fourth term of the D-type equation is related to platelet MAO activity, this correlation (although modest) also suggests that measurement of platelet

MAO activity may provide functionally relevant information with respect to monoamine metabolism, in that it logically relates to a ratio of levels of nondeaminated:deaminated urinary catecholamine metabolites.

As described in a paper published several years ago, to evaluate the contribution of each of the terms in this 4-term discrimination equation, we derived discrimination equations based on 1-, 2-, and 3-terms, as well as on 4-terms, using the biochemical data obtained from the initial series of patients with bipolar manic-depressive and unipolar nonendogenous depressions that had been used to derive the 4-term discrimination equation.[3] D-type scores based on these equations were then generated in the validation sample for a series of depressed patients whose biochemical data had not been used to derive the equations.

D-type scores in the patients with bipolar manic-depressive depressions and schizoaffective depressions (without histories of chronic asociality as described in references 2 and 3) were then compared to the scores in patients with unipolar nonendogenous depressions using the 1-, 2-, 3-, and 4-term discrimination equations. As shown in Figure 1, the 1-term equation based on MHPG alone tended to separate these groups with some overlap; the 2-term equation based on MHPG and VMA provided a better discrimination between the groups but some overlap remained; the 3-term equation based on MHPG, VMA and NE removed all overlap between the two groups; and the 4-term equation based on MHPG, VMA, NE and $\dfrac{NMN + MN}{VMA}$ improved on the discrimination by providing a very wide separation of the D-type scores in these two groups without any overlap. It should be reemphasized that these groups were composed only of patients from the validation sample whose biochemical data had not been used to derive these equations.[3]

We have subsequently obtained D-type scores on more than 80 additional depressed patients whose data were not used in the original derivation of this equation (that is, in selecting the terms and determining the coefficients and constant) or in its preliminary validation (as previously described). In light of the findings (described later) that patients with unipolar depressive disorders appear to be biochemically heterogeneous with respect to urinary MHPG levels, we were particularly interested in the distribution of D-type scores in the newly studied patients with "unipolar" depressions diagnosed according to our system of classification on the basis of clinical histories and presenting signs and symptoms.[2] Recent analyses of these data showed that the D-type scores (computed using the original D-type equation with the previously derived coefficients and constant) segregated these newly studied patients with unipolar depressions into two widely separated groupings: one with D-type scores < 0.5, that is, in the range of values comparable to that previously observed in bipolar manic-

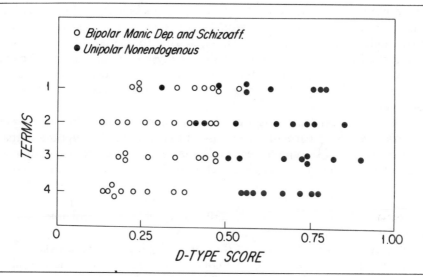

Figure 1 D-type scores computed using 1-, 2-, 3-, and 4-term discrimination equations: preliminary validation series

Source: Reproduced from Schildkraut JJ et al. Toward a biochemical classification of depressive disorders II: Application of multivariate discriminant function analysis to data on urinary catecholamines and metabolites. *Arch. Gen Psychiat.* 35:1436–39, 1978.

Note: Depression-type (D-type) scores were computed using 1-, 2-, 3-, and 4-term discrimination equations as described in the text. The resulting D-type scores were compared between patients with bipolar manic-depressive and schizoaffective depressions and patients with unipolar nonendogenous depressions.

depressive depressions;[3] and another with considerably higher D-type scores.

On the basis of earlier findings, we had hypothesized that low D-type scores in patients with so-called unipolar depressions might aid in the identification of those patients having latent bipolar disorders even prior to the first clinical episode of mania or hypomania. Consistent with this hypothesis, pilot follow-up data from our studies have shown that a number of the patients who had low D-type scores (in the range usually seen in bipolar manic-depressive depressions) with an initial diagnosis of unipolar depression when they were initially studied, went on to develop their first manic, hypomanic, or schizoaffective psychotic episode several months to several years after their biochemical studies were completed. Thus, our findings suggest that low D-type scores can predict subsequent occurrences of manic or manic-like episodes even in the absence of such a history.

Relatively few patients with typical bipolar manic-depressive depressions could be included in our recent studies, because most patients with this diagnosis now receive maintenance lithium treatment, which ethically could not be discontinued to study such patients biochemically. However, many of the patients in this newly studied series had depressive disorders that could not be assigned unambiguously to one of the diagnostic categories in our classification system, usually because of the presence of clinical features suggesting the possibility of a bipolar disorder or a schizophrenia-related disorder (with chronic asocial, eccentric, or bizarre behavior).

In this series of patients with diagnostically unclassifiable depressive disorders, we were particularly interested in exploring the hypothesis that patients with low D-type scores would show clinical features suggestive of a bipolar disorder even though the clinical diagnosis of a definite bipolar disorder could not be made in these patients. In support of this hypothesis, we found that of the 8 diagnostically unclassifiable depressed patients with lowest D-type scores, 7 met the criteria for at least a probable bipolar disorder in our classification system, and for at least a probable bipolar I or bipolar II diagnosis according to Research Diagnostic Criteria (RDC).[35] In contrast, of the 29 remaining patients with diagnostically unclassifiable depressions, only 7 showed comparable evidence for bipolarity (chi square $= 8.2; p < .01$).

Urinary MHPG Levels in Unipolar Depressive Disorders

In contrast to the relatively consistent findings showing that patients with bipolar manic-depressive depressions have low urinary MHPG levels, consistent findings have not been obtained in studies of patients with unipolar depressions in whom low, normal, or high urinary MHPG levels have been reported.[29,30,32,33,36–39] These discrepancies may be explained by diagnostic heterogeneity. Previously reported findings from our laboratory revealed a wide range of urinary MHPG levels in patients with unipolar depressive disorders,[2] and these findings have been confirmed and extended in our more recent investigations. In that previously reported series of 16 patients with unipolar endogenous depressions, the mean value of urinary MHPG was 1,950μg/24 hours.[2] And in a subsequent study of an enlarged sample (Table 2), 26 of 50 patients with unipolar depressions had urinary MHPG levels > 1,950μg/24 hours, while only 3 of 20 patients with bipolar manic-depressive or schizoaffective depressions had MHPG levels > 1,950μg/24 hours (chi square = 6.6; $p < .025$).[6]

A scatter plot of MHPG levels in this series of 70 depressed patients revealed a natural break in MHPG levels around 2,500μg/24 hours, suggesting the existence of a subgroup of unipolar depressions with MHPG levels > 2,500μg/24 hours. For example, in this series, 17 of 50 patients with unipolar depressions had urinary MHPG levels > 2,500μg/24 hours, whereas only 1 of the 20 patients with bipolar manic-depressive or

Table 2 Baseline Urinary MHPG Levels in Subtypes of Depressive Disorders

Group	N	Age (years)	MHPG (µg/day)
Bipolar Manic-Depressive and Schizoaffective	20	37 ± 3	1,373 ± 110[a,b]
Unipolar	50	42 ± 2	2,147 ± 104
Controls	26	44 ± 3	1,921 ± 117

Source: The data in this table are taken from Schatzberg AF et al. Toward a biochemical classification of depressive disorders V: Heterogeneity of unipolar depressions. *Am. J. Psychiat.*, in press.
Note: Urinary MHPG levels and ages are presented as means ± standard errors of the means.
[a] $p < .001$ when compared to unipolar group.
[b] $p < .01$ when compared to control group.

schizoaffective depressions had MHPG levels > 2,500µg/24 hours (chi square = 4.9; $p < .05$).

Thus, the data from this series of patients with unipolar depressive disorders further substantiate the biochemical heterogeneity of unipolar depressions, demonstrating that some patients have low MHPG levels (comparable to values seen in the bipolar manic-depressive or schizoaffective depressions), while others have high MHPG levels (sometimes higher than control values), and still others have MHPG levels in an intermediate range. However, as reflected in Table 2, urinary MHPG levels in most depressed patients fall within the broad range of values observed in normal control subjects.[6,40] Therefore, while urinary MHPG levels may help to differentiate among subtypes of depressive disorders once a clinical diagnosis of depression has been made, urinary MHPG levels cannot be used to make a diagnosis of depression per se.

Additional support for this heterogeneity comes from data on the distribution of urinary MHPG levels in a series of 102 patients with unipolar major depressive disorders that revealed a clustering of patients with urinary MHPG levels above 2,500µg/24 hours, in addition to clusters occurring at lower MHPG levels.[41] Moreover, the distribution of pretreatment urinary MHPG levels in an independent series of more than 200 patients with unipolar major depressive disorders, included in a collaborative multicenter study of urinary MHPG levels as predictors of responses to oxaprotiline (BA49802), amitriptyline, or placebo (coordinated by Mark Roffman, Ph.D. of Ciba-Geigy in conjunction with our laboratory), revealed a similar pattern with a clustering of depressed patients having urinary MHPG levels > 2,500µg/24 hours. In contrast, a comparable discrete clustering (peaking) of values > 2,500µg/24 hours with relatively few values between 2,300 and 2,500µg/24 hours, was not observed when urinary MHPG levels were examined in a comparison series of more than 100 control subjects.

The existence of a biologically meaningful subgroup of unipolar depressions with elevated urinary MHPG levels is also supported by our findings in a study of patients with very severe unipolar depressions, which revealed a subgroup of patients with very high urinary MHPG levels (> 2,500μg/24 hours) who also had very high levels of urinary free cortisol (UFC > 200μg/24 hours).[8] To rule out the possibility that the high UFC and urinary MHPG levels observed in this series of severely depressed patients might be secondary to anxiety, we studied urinary MHPG and UFC levels in patients with moderate to severe anxiety states, and did not observe comparably elevated MHPG levels or markedly elevated UFC levels (> 200μg/24 hours) in these patients with anxiety disorders. However, the very high UFC levels observed in our series of severely depressed patients might be related to the severity of the depression, because preliminary data from a study of UFC levels in patients with less severe depressions revealed few patients with markedly elevated UFC levels.[42]

A possible explanation of our finding of a subgroup of severely depressed patients with high urinary MHPG levels and markedly elevated UFC levels is that, in these patients, high urinary MHPG and UFC levels may occur as a secondary response to an increase in cholinergic activity. This possibility is consistent with the hypothesis that central cholinergic factors may play a role in the etiology of depressive disorders,[43-45] and is particularly intriguing in view of the findings of other investigators that (1) physostigmine, an anticholinesterase, and other pharmacological agents that increase brain cholinergic activity exacerbate depressive symptoms in depressed patients and induce depressive symptoms in normal controls;[43,46,47] (2) physostigmine produces an increase in plasma cortisol levels in normal controls;[47] (3) physostigmine can overcome suppression of the hypothalamic-pituitary-adrenocortical axis by dexamethasone in normal subjects, thereby mimicking the abnormal escape from dexamethasone suppression seen in some patients who show cortisol hypersecretion;[48] and (4) physostigmine produces an increase in cerebrospinal fluid levels of MHPG in normal subjects.[49] Thus, the markedly elevated UFC levels that we have observed in some patients with severe unipolar depressive disorders could result from an increase in cholinergic activity, and the elevated urinary MHPG levels in these patients could represent a secondary noradrenergic response to such cholinergic hyperactivity. This formulation suggests that the anticholinergic effects of certain antidepressant drugs may contribute to their antidepressant effects in patients with this subtype of depressive disorder.

Thus, the findings of our recent studies further substantiate the biochemical heterogeneity of the unipolar depressive disorders, and suggest that there may be at least three subtypes of unipolar depressions that can be discriminated on the basis of differences in urinary MHPG levels. Subtype I, with low pretreatment urinary MHPG levels, may have low norepinephrine output as the result of a decrease in norepinephrine synthesis or a decrease in its release from noradrenergic neurons. In contrast, Subtype II, with intermediate urinary MHPG levels, may have normal norepinephrine output but abnormalities in other biochemical systems. And Subtype III, with high urinary MHPG levels, may have high norepinephrine output in response to alterations in noradrenergic receptors and/or to an increase in cholinergic activity, as previously described. Further studies will be required and currently are in progress to confirm these findings and to explore the possible pathophysiological abnormalities that may be associated with these subtypes of unipolar depressive disorders.

Urinary MHPG Levels as Predictors of Differential Responses to Antidepressant Drugs

Studies from a number of laboratories have indicated that pretreatment levels of urinary MHPG may aid in predicting responses to certain tricyclic and tetracyclic antidepressant drugs. Specifically, depressed patients with low pretreatment urinary MHPG levels have been found to respond more favorably to treatment with imipramine,[5,25,50–54] desipramine,[25] nortriptyline,[55] or maprotiline,[4,54] than do patients with high MHPG levels. In contrast, some studies[50,52,56,57] have found that depressed patients with high pretreatment levels of urinary MHPG respond more favorably to treatment with amitriptyline than do patients with lower MHPG levels, but this has not been observed in all studies.[58–61] Further research clearly will be required to account for these differences in findings. Nevertheless, it should be stressed that the findings of these studies do point to differences between amitriptyline and imipramine, in that low pretreatment urinary MHPG levels have been shown to predict more favorable responses to imipramine in many studies, whereas this has not been found in any of the studies of amitriptyline.

Our recently published prospective studies have confirmed that patients with relatively low urinary MHPG levels ($\leq 1,950\mu g/24$ hours) respond more favorably to treatment with imipramine (Table 3) or maprotiline (Table 4) than do patients with higher MHPG levels.[4,5] Because our findings suggested that there may be at least three subtypes of unipolar depressive disorders that could be discriminated on the basis of differences in pretreatment urinary MHPG levels,[6] data from these two studies of pretreatment urinary MHPG levels as predictors of responses to imipramine and maprotiline were combined to provide us with a large enough series of patients to compare treatment responses in these three subtypes. While further studies (currently in progress) of a larger series of patients

Table 3 Baseline Urinary MHPG Levels and Response to Imipramine After Four Weeks

	% HDRS[a] Reduction from Baseline ≥ 60%	
	Yes	No
MHPG ≤ 1,950 μg/24 hours	9	4
MHPG > 1,950 μg/24 hours	3	8
	Fisher Exact—$P = .05$	

Source: The data in this table are taken from Schatzberg AF et al. Toward a biochemical classification of depressive disorders IV: Pretreatment urinary MHPG levels as predictors of antidepressant response to imipramine. *Communications in Psychopharmacology* 4:441–45, 1980.
[a] HDRS refers to scores on the Hamilton Depression Rating Scale.

are required for confirmation, our findings suggest that depressed patients with elevated MHPG levels (> 2,500μg/24 hours) may be more responsive to treatment with imipramine or maprotiline than are patients with intermediate MHPG levels (1,951–2,500μg/24 hours), though neither group is as responsive to these drugs as are patients with low pretreatment urinary MHPG levels (≤1,950μg/24 hours). Moreover, as described in a recently published paper, we observed that patients with low pretreatment urinary MHPG levels responded rapidly to relatively low doses of maprotiline, whereas those patients with higher MHPG levels required significantly higher doses and longer periods of drug administration.[4]

Table 4 Baseline Urinary MHPG Levels and Response to Maprotiline After Four Weeks

	% HDRS[a] Reduction from Baseline ≥ 60%	
	Yes	No
MHPG ≤ 1,950 μg/24 hours	8	4
MHPG > 1,950 μg/24 hours	3	13
	Chi Square = 4.74; $P < .05$	

Source: The data in this table are taken from Schatzberg AF et al. Toward a biochemical classification of depressive disorders III: Pretreatment urinary MHPG levels as predictors of response to treatment with maprotiline. *Psychopharmacology* 75:34–38, 1981.
[a] HDRS refers to scores on the Hamilton Depression Rating Scale.

The complex effects on noradrenergic, dopaminergic, and other neurotransmitter systems, including alterations in various indices of presynaptic and postsynaptic receptor functions that are observed after chronic administration of various antidepressant drugs,[62–71] suggest that specific empirical trials will be required to assess the value of urinary MHPG levels — or any other biochemical measure — as clinically useful predictors of responses to a specific antidepressant drug. For example, it has recently been reported that patients with normal or high urinary MHPG levels who show suppression of cortisol in response to dexamethasone respond favorably to treatment with mianserin, whereas patients with low urinary MHPG levels whose cortisol secretion is not suppressed by dexamethasone do not respond to mianserin.[72]

Studies of Monoaminergic Receptors and Related Measures in Depressed Patients

Patients with affective disorders may show alterations in the sensitivity of one or another type of monoaminergic receptor.[1,73,74] Many antidepressant drugs have been found to alter the sensitivity of various neurotransmitter or neuromodulator receptors in brain after chronic treatment,[62–71,75–78] and the changes in receptor function coincide with the course of clinical improvement during antidepressant therapy. Pharmacological challenges producing peripheral effects (such as changes in blood pressure) and neuroendocrine responses (such as release of cortisol or growth hormone) that are under central control mechanisms, have been undertaken to clarify both the central noradrenergic receptor function[63,79] and the relationships between central cholinergic, noradrenergic, and other neurotransmitter or neuromodulator systems.[45,80,81] These results suggest that alterations in receptor sensitivity may play a role in both the pathophysiology of the depressive disorders and the mechanisms of action of various antidepressant drugs.

Adrenergic receptors on human blood cells have been suggested as a readily available source of material for the study of adrenergic receptors in psychiatric patients.[82] β-adrenergic receptors have been identified on leukocytes, and one group of investigators found the specific binding of the β-adrenergic antagonist,[3]H-dihydroalprenolol to lymphocytes, was decreased in depressed and manic patients when compared to control subjects and euthymic patients.[85] Moreover, β-adrenergic receptor mediated stimulation of cAMP production by isoproteronol was reduced in leukocytes[83,84] and lymphocytes[85] from depressed patients. While it has been cautioned that the decreased β-adrenergic receptor function in lymphocytes from depressed patients may reflect homeostatic regulation of peripheral β-adrenergic receptors in response to increases in plasma

41

catecholamines,[85] β-adrenergic stimulants (for example, salbutamol) have been reported to be rapidly effective in the treatment of depressed patients.[87]

Human platelets possess α_2-adrenergic receptors, which suppress the activity of platelet adenylate cyclase.[88–91] Neither basal nor α-adrenergic receptor mediated suppression of prostaglandin stimulated cAMP production has been found to be altered in platelets in depressed patients.[92–94] However, depressed patients have been reported to have greater platelet α_2-adrenergic receptor numbers than control subjects in several recent studies, but not in all.[95–99] This discrepancy could possibly reflect differences in platelet α_2-adrenergic receptors across subgroups of depressed patients.

[3]H-imipramine binds to high affinity sites in the brain, and platelets and cellular uptake regulation sites for serotonin have been labeled with ^{3}H-imipramine.[100–106] A highly significant decrease in the number of ^{3}H-imipramine binding sites with no significant change in the apparent affinity constant was observed in platelets from depressed patients when compared with those from control subjects.[102,107,108] Decreased platelet serotonin uptake has been observed in patients with depressive disorders,[109–111] and it has been proposed that decreased platelet ^{3}H-imipramine binding observed in depressed patients may reflect a deficiency in the platelet serotonin transport mechanism in these patients.[108]

Ongoing laboratory research during the past several years has enabled us to develop and refine a blood fractionation and platelet homogenization procedure that provides high yields of platelet membrane vesicles, as well as free intact platelet mitochondria from relatively small clinically obtainable blood samples.[112–114] Using this procedure, we have isolated partially purified platelet membrane vesicles containing both α_2-adrenergic receptors and membrane-bound adenylate cyclase, which is coupled to prostaglandin receptors and receptors for α_2-adrenergic agonists.[114] We have examined and compared the binding of adrenergic agonists, partial agonists, and antagonists using this membrane preparation.[114] Also, we have studied the regulation by monovalent cations and guanine nucleotides of (1) α_2-adrenergic agonists (both high and low affinity) and antagonist binding to platelet membranes, and (2) platelet membrane adenylate cyclase activity.[114] This preparative procedure also enables us to isolate leukocytes and measure β-adrenergic receptor binding for agonist and antagonist ligands as well as β-adrenergic stimulated adenylate cyclase activity in the leukocytes from these same blood specimens. We are currently beginning to apply these procedures to studies of adrenergic receptor functions in patients with various subtypes of depressive disorders examined before and after treatment with antidepressant drugs. In particular, we shall be testing the hypothesis that there will be differences in the properties of platelet α_2-adrenergic receptors and/or leukocyte β-adrenergic receptors when groups of depressed patients with low and high urinary MHPG levels (or low and high D-type scores) are compared.

Practical Clinical Applications of this Research and the Development of the Psychiatric Chemistry Laboratory

For several years our research laboratory provided collaborating physicians with determinations of urinary MHPG levels as well as other relevant biochemical measurements for use in their clinical practices. However, the number of requests soon became overwhelming and in 1977, in cooperation with the Department of Pathology at the New England Deaconess Hospital, our group established the Psychiatric Chemistry Laboratory as a model academic clinical laboratory facility for the integration and translation of biochemical research into clinical psychiatric practice.[115] In addition to providing specialized clinical laboratory tests for use in psychiatry, an explicit aim of the Psychiatric Chemistry Laboratory has been to provide consultation and educational services to assist physicians in using and interpreting these tests.

In summary, we have now reached a point where the clinical laboratory can be used in psychiatry, as it is in other fields of medicine, both to assist in making more specific diagnoses and to aid in prescribing more effective forms of treatment. For example, one may draw an analogy between the pneumonias and the depressions, in that both are disorders diagnosed on the basis of clinical data. In the case of pneumonias, the physician makes a diagnosis on the basis of history and physical examination (including the chest X-ray). Having made the diagnosis, sputum cultures can then be obtained from the clinical laboratory to aid in determining the specific type of pneumonia that the patient may have, and the specific antibiotic or other forms of treatment that may be most effective. Similarly, in the case of depressions, the physician diagnoses depression on the basis of clinical history coupled with physical and mental status examinations. Having made a diagnosis of depression, a physician can then use clinical laboratory tests to obtain further information to assist in determining the type of depression the patient may have, and the forms of treatment most likely to be effective in the care of that patient. While none of the biochemical tests we have today will insure that the physician can select a clinically effective treatment on the first trial, the use of these clinical laboratory tests can increase the probability of doing so. Considering the time it takes for antidepressant drugs to exert their clinical effects, even a small increase in the percentage of patients who receive an effective drug on the first clinical trial of treatment would represent a major advance in the treatment of patients with depressive disorders.

References

1. Schildkraut JJ. The catecholamine hypothesis of affective disorders: A review of supporting evidence. *Am. J. Psychiat.* 122:509–22, 1965.

2. Schildkraut JJ et al. Toward a biochemical classification of depressive disorders I: Differences in urinary MHPG and other catecholamine metabolites in clinically defined subtypes of depressions. *Arch. Gen. Psychiat.* 35:1427–33, 1978.

3. Schildkraut JJ et al. Toward a biochemical classification of depressive disorders II: Application of multivariate discriminant function analysis to data on urinary catecholamines and metabolites. *Arch. Gen. Psychiat.* 35:1436–39, 1978.

4. Schatzberg AF et al. Toward a biochemical classification of depressive disorders III: Pretreatment urinary MHPG levels as predictors of response to treatment with maprotiline. *Psychopharmacology* 75:34–38, 1981.

5. Schatzberg AF et al. Toward a biochemical classification of depressive disorders IV: Pretreatment urinary MHPG levels as predictors of antidepressant response to imipramine. *Communications in Psychopharmacology* 4:441–5, 1980–81.

6. Schatzberg AF et al. Toward a biochemical classification of depressive disorders V: Heterogeneity of unipolar depressions. *Am. J. Psychiat.* 139:471–5, 1982.

7. Gudeman JE et al. Toward a biochemical classification of depressive disorders VI: Platelet MAO activity and clinical symptoms in depressed patients. *Am. J. Psychiat.* 139:630–33, 1982.

8. Rosenbaum AH et al. Toward a biochemical classification of depressive disorders VII: Urinary free cortisol and urinary MHPG in depressions. *Am. J. Psychiat.* In press.

9. Schildkraut JJ et al. "The Role of Norepinephrine in Depressive Disorders. " In *Depression and Antidepressants,* edited by E. Friedman. New York : Raven Press, in press.

10. Maas JW and Landis DH. *In vivo* studies of metabolism of norepinephrine in central nervous system. *J. Pharmacol. Exper. Ther.* 163:147–162, 1968.

11. Schanberg SM et al. 3-Methoxy-4-hydroxyphenylglycol sulfate in brain and cerebrospinal fluid. *Biochem. Pharmacol.* 17:2006–08, 1968

12. Schanberg SM et al. Metabolism of normetanephrine-H^3 in rat brain-identification of conjugated 3-methoxy-4-hydroxyphenylglycol as major metabolite. *Biochem. Pharmacol.* 7:247–54, 1968.

13. Maas JW et al. 3-Methoxy-4-hydroxyphenylethyleneglycol production by human brain *in vivo*. *Science* 205:1025–27, 1979.

14. Blombery PA et al. Conversion of MHPG to vanillylmandelic acid. *Arch. Gen. Psychiat.* 37:1095–98, 1980.

15. Mardh G, Sjoquist B, and Anggard E. Norepinephrine metabolism in man using deuterium labelling: The conversion of 4-hydroxy-3-methoxyphenyl-

glycol to 4-hydroxy-3-methoxy-mandelic acid. *J. Neurochem.* 36:1181–85, 1981.

16. Greenspan K et al. Catecholamine metabolism in affective disorders III. MHPG and other catecholamine metabolites in patients treated with lithium carbonate. *J. Psychiat Res.* 7:171-83, 1970.

17. Schildkraut JJ et al. Amphetamine withdrawal: Depression and MHPG excretion. *Lancet* 2:485–86, 1971.

18. Schildkraut JJ et al. Catecholamine metabolism in affective disorders: A longitudinal study of a patient treated with amitriptyline and ECT. *Psychosomatic Med.* 34:470, 1972; plus erratum *Psychosomatic Med.* 35:274, 1973.

19. Watson R, Hartmann E, and Schildkraut JJ. Amphetamine withdrawal: Affective state, sleep patterns and MHPG excretion. *Amer. J. Psychiat.* 129:263–69, 1972.

20. Bond PA, Jenner FA, and Sampson GA. Daily variations of the urine content of 3-methoxy-4-hydroxyphenylglycol in two manic-depressive patients. *Psychological Med.* 2:81–85, 1972.

21. Bond PA et al. Urinary excretion of the sulfate and glucuronide of 3-methoxy-4-hydroxyphenyl-ethyleneglycol in a manic-depressive patient. *Psychological Med.* 5:279–85, 1975.

22. DeLeon-Jones FD et al. Urinary catecholamine metabolites during behavioral changes in a patient with manic-depressive cycles. *Science* 179:300–302, 1973.

23. Post RM et al. Alterations in motor activity, sleep and biochemistry in a cycling manic-depressive patient. *Arch. Gen. Psychiat.* 34:470–77, 1977.

24. Maas JW, Fawcett JA, and Dekirmenjian H. 3-Methoxy-4-hydroxyphenyl-glycol (MHPG) excretion in depressive states. *Arch. Gen. Psychiat.* 19:129–34, 1968.

25. Maas JW, Fawcett JA, and Dekirmenjian H. Catecholamine metabolism, depressive illness and drug response. *Arch. Gen. Psychiat.* 26:252–62, 1972.

26. Schildkraut JJ et al. MHPG excretion and clinical classification in depressive disorders. *Lancet* 1:1251–52, 1973.

27. Schildkraut JJ et al. MHPG excretion in depressive disorders: Relation to clinical subtypes and desynchronized sleep. *Science* 181:762–64, 1973.

28. Maas JW, Dekirmenjian H, and DeLeon-Jones F. "The Identification of Depressed Patients Who Have a Disorder of Norepinephrine Metabolism and/or Disposition." In *Frontiers in Catecholamine Research—Third International Catecholamine Symposium,* edited by Usdin E and Snyder S. New York: Pergamon, 1973. pp. 1091–96.

29. DeLeon-Jones F et al. Diagnostic subgroups of affective disorders and their urinary excretion of catecholamine metabolites. *Am. J. Psychiat.* 132:1141–48, 1975.

30. Goodwin FK and Post RM. "Studies of Amine Metabolites in Affective Illness and in Schizophrenia: A Comparative Analysis." In *Biology of Major Psychoses,* edited by Freedman DX. New York:Raven Press, 1975. pp. 299–332.

31. Garfinkel PE et al. CNS monoamine metabolism in bipolar affective disorders. *Arch. Gen. Psychiat.* 34:735–39, 1977.

32. Goodwin FK and Potter WZ. "Norepinephrine Metabolite Studies in Affective Illness." In *Catecholamines: Basic and Clinical Frontiers*, edited by Usdin E, Kopin I and Barchas J, volume 2. New York: Pergamon Press, 1975. pp. 1863–65.

33. Beckmann H and Goodwin FK. Urinary MHPG in subgroups of depressed patients and normal controls. *Neuropsychobiology* 6:91–100, 1980.

34. Edwards DJ et al. MHPG excretion in depression. *Psychiatry Research* 2:295–305, 1980.

35. Spitzer RL, Endicott J, and Robins E. Research diagnostic criteria. Rationale and reliability. *Arch. Gen. Psychiat.* 35:773–78, 1978.

36. Maas JW. Clinical and biochemical heterogeneity of depressive disorders. *Annals of Internal Medicine* 88:556–663, 1978.

37. Taube SL et al. Urinary 3-methoxy-4-hydroxyphenylglycol and psychiatric diagnosis. *Am. J. Psychiat.* 135:78–82, 1978.

38. Casper RC et al. Neuroendocrine and amine studies in affective illness. *Psychoneuroendocrinology* 2:105–13, 1977.

39. Garfinkel PE, Warsh JJ, and Stancer HC. Depression: New evidence in support of biological differentiation. *Am. J. Psychiat.* 136:535–39, 1979.

40. Hollister LE et al. Excretion of MHPG in normal subjects. Implications for biological classification of affective disorders. *Arch. Gen. Psychiat.* 35:1410–415, 1978.

41. Schildkraut JJ et al. "Biochemical Discrimination of Subgroups of Depressive Disorders Based on Differences in Catecholamine Metabolism." In *Biological Markers in Psychiatry and Neurology*, edited by Hanin I and Usdin E. New York: Pergamon Press, 1982. pp 22–33.

42. Rosenbaum AH et al. "Urinary Free Cortisol and MHPG Levels in Anxious Patients and Normal Controls." Paper read at Society of Biological Psychiatry Annual Meeting, May 1981, New Orleans.

43. Janowsky DS et al. A cholinergic-adrenergic hypothesis of mania and depression. *Lancet* 2:632–35, 1972.

44. Sitaram N and Gillin JG. Development and use of pharmacological probes of the CNS in man: Evidence of cholinergic abnormality in primary affective illness. *Biological Psychiatry* 15:925–55, 1980.

45. Risch SC, Kalin NH, and Janowsky DS. Cholinergic challenges in affective illness: Behavioral and neuroendocrine correlates. *J. Clin. Psychopharmacol.* 1:186–92, 1981.

46. Garver DL and Davis JM. Biogenic amine hypothesis of affective disorders. *Life Sci.* 24:383–94, 1979.

47. Risch SC et al. Mood and behavioral effects of physostigmine on humans are accompanied by elevations in plasma β-endorphin and cortisol. *Science* 209:1545–46, 1980.

48. Carroll BJ et al. Neurotransmitter studies of neuroendocrine pathology in depression. *Acta Psychiatric Scand.* 61:(Supplement 80), 183–99, 1980.

49. Davis KL et al. Neurotransmitter metabolites in cerebrospinal fluid of man following physostigmine. *Life Sci.* 21:933–36, 1977.

50. Beckmann H and Goodwin FK. Antidepressant response to tricyclics and urinary MHPG in unipolar patients. *Arch. Gen. Psychiat.* 32:17–21, 1975.

51. Steinbook RM et al. Amoxapine, imipramine and placebo: A double-blind study with pretherapy urinary 3-methoxy-4-hydroxyphenylglycol levels. *Current Therap. Res.* 26:490–96, 1979.

52. Cobbin DM et al. Urinary MHPG levels and tricyclic antidepressant drug selection. *Arch. Gen. Psychiat.* 36:1111–15, 1979.

53. Maas J et al. "Neurotransmitter Metabolites and the Therapeutic Response to Antidepressant Drugs." Paper presented at the 12th Congress of the College Internationale Neuro-psychopharmacologicum, 22–26 June 1980, Goteborg, Sweden.

54. Rosenbaum AH et al. MHPG as a predictor of antidepressant response to imipramine and maprotiline. *Am. J. Psychiat.* 137:1090–92, 1980.

55. Hollister LE, Davis KL, and Berger PA. Subtypes of depression based on excretion of MHPG and response to nortriptyline. *Arch. Gen. Psychiat.* 37:1107–10, 1980.

56. Schildkraut JJ. Norepinephrine metabolites as biochemical criteria for classifying depressive disorders and predicting responses to treatment: Preliminary findings. *Am J. Psychiat.* 130:696–99, 1973.

57. Modai I et al. Response to amitriptyline and urinary MHPG in bipolar depressive patients. *Neuropsychobiology* 5:181–84, 1979.

58. Saachetti E et al. 3-Methoxy-4-hydroxyphenylglycol and primary depression: Clinical and pharmacological considerations. *Biol. Psychiat.* 14:473–84, 1979.

59. Coppen A et al. Urinary 4-hydroxy-3-methoxyphenylglycol is not a predictor for clinical response to amitriptyline in depressive illness. *Psychopharmacology* 64:95–97, 1979.

60. Spiker DG et al. Urinary MHPG and clinical response to amitriptyline in depressed patients. *Am. J. Psychiat.* 137:1183–87, 1980.

61. Roffman M. Ciba-Geigy collaborative study, unpublished data—personal communication.

62. Sulser F, Vetulani J, and Mobley PK. Mode of action of antidepressant drugs. *Biochem. Pharmacol.* 27:257–61, 1978.

63. Charney DS, Menkes DB, and Heninger GR. Receptor sensitivity and the mechanism of action of antidepressant treatment. *Arch. Gen. Psychiat.* 38:1160–80, 1981.

64. Waldmeier PC. Noradrenergic transmission in depression: Under or overfunction? *Pharmakopsychiat.* 14:3–9, 1981.

65. Heninger GR. "The Monoamine Receptor Sensitivity Hypothesis of Antidepressant Drug Action." Abstracts of the American College of Neuropsychopharmacology Annual Meeting, December 1981. p. 39.

66. Frazer A, Lucki I, and Heydorn W. "Antidepressant Drugs: Effects on Monoamine Receptors and Monoamine Responsiveness." Abstracts of the American College of Neuropsychopharmacology Annual Meeting, December 1981. p. 39.

67. deMontigny C and Blier P. "Pre- and Postsynaptic Effects of Antidepressant Treatments on Monoaminergic Systems." Abstracts of the American College of Neuropsychopharmacology Annual Meeting, December 1981. p. 40.

68. Svensson TH and Scubee-Moreau J. "Sensitivity *In Vivo* of Central α_2- and Opiate Receptors After Chronic Treatment with Various Antidepressants." Abstracts of the American College of Neuropsychopharmacology Annual Meeting, December 1981. p. 40.

69. Davis M. "Agonist Induced Changes in Behavior as a Measure of Functional Changes in Receptor Sensitivity Following Chronic Administration of Antidepressant Drugs." Abstracts of the American College of Neuropsychopharmacology Annual Meeting, December 1981. p. 41.

70. Pandey GN et al. "Antidepressant Treatment and Central Adrenergic and Histamine Receptors." Abstracts of the American College of Neuropsychopharmacology Annual Meeting, December 1981. p. 41.

71. Charney DS and Heninger GR. "Receptor Sensitivity and the Etiology and Treatment of Depressive Illness." Abstracts of the American College of Neuropsychopharmacology, December 1981. p. 42.

72. Cairncross KD, Cobbin DM, and Pohlen GJ. Letter to Editor. *Brit. Med. J.* 283:991, 1981.

73. Bunney WE et al. A neuronal receptor sensitivity mechanism in affective illness (a review of evidence). *Communications in Psychopharmacology* 1:393–405, 1977.

74. Cohen RM et al. Presynaptic noradrenergic regulation during depressions and antidepressant drug treatment. *Psychiatry Research* 3:93–105, 1980.

75. Segawa T, Mizuta T, and Nomura Z. Modifications of central 5-hydroxytryptamine binding sites in synaptic membranes from rat brain after long term administration of tricyclic antidepressants. *Eur. J. Pharmacol.* 58:75–83, 1979.

76. Maggi A, U'Pritchard DC, and Enna SJ. Differential effects of antidepressant treatment on brain monoaminergic receptors. *Eur. J. Pharmacol.* 61:91–98, 1980.

77. Peroutka SJ and Snyder SH. Longterm antidepressant treatment decreases spiroperidol-labeled serotonin receptor binding. *Science* 210:88–90, 1980.

78. Enna SJ and Kendall DA. Interactions of antidepressants with brain neurotransmitter receptors. *J. Clin. Psychopharmacol.* 1:(Supplement), 125–175, 1981.

79. Siever L, Insel T, and Uhde T. Noradrenergic challenges in the affective disorders. *J. Clin. Psychopharmacology* 1:193–206, 1981.

80. Risch SC, Kalin NH, and Murphy DL. Neurochemical mechanisms in the affective disorders and neurochemical correlates. *J. Clin. Psychopharmacol.* 1:180–85, 1981.

81. Risch SC, Kalin NH, and Murphy DL. Pharmacological challenge strategies: Implications for neurochemical mechanisms in affective disorders and treatment approaches. *J. Clin. Psychopharmacology* 1:238–43, 1981.

82. Bunney WE and Murphy DL. "Strategies for the Systematic Study of Neurotransmitter Receptor Function in Man." In *Pre- and Postsynaptic Receptors*, edited by Usdin E and Bunney WE. New York: Marcel Dekker, 1975. pp. 283–313.

83. Scott RE. Effects of prostaglandins, epinephrine and NaF on human leukocyte, platelet and liver adenyl cyclase. *Blood* 35:514–16, 1970.

84. Williams LT, Snyderman R, and Lefkowitz RJ. Identification of β-adrenergic receptors in human lymphocytes by (-) ^{3}H-alprenolol binding. *J. Clin. Invest.* 57:149–55, 1976.

85. Extein I et al. Changes in lymphocyte beta-adrenergic receptors in depression and mania. *Psychiat. Res.* 1:191–97, 1979.

86. Pandey GN et al. Beta-adrenergic receptor function in affective illness. *Am. J. Psychiat.* 136:675–78, 1979.

87. Lecrubier Y et al. A beta adrenergic stimulant (salbutamol) versus clomipramine in depression: A controlled study. *Brit. J. Psychiat.* 136:354–58, 1980.

88. Hoffman BB et al. Alpha-adrenergic receptor subtypes: Quantitative assessment by ligand binding. *Life Sci.* 24:1739–46, 1979.

89. Wood CL et al. Subclassification of alpha-adrenergic receptors by direct binding studies. *Biochem. Pharmacol.* 28:1277–82, 1979.

90. Lefkowitz RF. Identification and regulation of alpha- and beta-adrenergic receptors. *Fed. Proc.* 37:123–29, 1978.

91. Fain JN and Garcia-Sainz JA. Role of phosphatidylinositol turnover in alpha$_1$ and of adenylate cyclase in alpha$_2$ effects of catecholamines. *Life Sci.* 26:1183–94, 1980.

92. Scott M, Reading HW, and Ludon JB. Studies on human blood platelets in affective disorders. *Psychopharmacol.* 60:131–35, 1979.

93. Wang Y-C et al. Platelet adenylate cyclase responses in depression: Implications for a receptor defect. *Psychopharmacologia* (Berl.) 36:291–300, 1974.

94. Murphy DL, Donnelly C, and Moskowitz J. Inhibiton by lithium of prostaglandin E$_1$ and norepinephrine effects on cyclic adenosine monophosphate production in human platelets. *Clin. Pharmacol. Ther.* 14:810–14, 1973.

95. Garcia-Sevilla JA et al. Platelet α_2-adrenergic receptors in major depressive disorders. *Arch. Gen. Psychiat.* 38:1327–33, 1981.

96. Garcia-Sevilla JA et al. Platelet alpha$_2$ adrenoreceptors in major depressive disorders (MDD). *The Pharmacologist* 23:216 (abstr. 536), 1981.

97. Garcia-Sevilla JA et al. Tricyclic antidepressant drug treatment decreases α_2-adrenoreceptors on human platelet membranes. *Eur. J. Pharmacol.* 69:121–23, 1981.

98. Kafka MS et al. Alpha-adrenergic receptor function in schizophrenia, affective disorders, and some neurological diseases. *Communications in Psychopharmacology* 4:477–86, 1980.

99. U'Pritchard DC et al. "α_2-Adrenergic Receptors: Comparative Biochemistry of Neural and Nonneural Receptors, and *In Vitro* Analysis of Psychiatric Patients." In *Biological Markers in Psychiatry and Neurology.* New York: Pergamon Press, 1982. pp 205–17.

100. Langer SZ et al. High-affinity ^{3}H-imipramine binding in rat hypothalamus: Association with uptake of serotonin but not of norepinephrine. *Science* 210:1133–35, 1980.

101. Rehavi M et al. Demonstration of specific high affinity binding sites for ^{3}H-imipramine in human brain. *Life Sci.* 26:2273–79, 1980.

102. Langer SZ et al. High-affinity binding of ^{3}H-imipramine in brain and platelets and its relevance to the biochemistry of affective disorders. *Life Sci.* 29:211–20, 1981.

103. Briley MS, Raisman R, and Langer SA. Human platelets possess high-affinity binding sites for ^{3}H-imipramine. *Eur. J. Pharmacol.* 58:347–48, 1979.

104. Talvenheimo J, Nelson PJ, and Rudnick G. Mechanisms of imipramine inhibition of platelet 5-hydroxytryptamine transport. *J. Biol. Chem.* 254:4631–35, 1979.

105. Paul SM et al. Demonstration of specific "high affinity" binding sites for ^{3}H-imipramine in human platelets. *Life Sci.* 26:953–59, 1980.

106. Paul SM et al. Does high affinity ^{3}H-imipramine binding label serotonin reuptake sites in brain and platelet? *Life Sci.* 28:2753–60, 1981.

107. Briley MS et al. Tritiated imipramine binding sites are decreased in platelets of untreated depressed patients. *Science* 209:303–05, 1980.

108. Paul SM et al. Depressed patients have decreased binding of tritiated imipramine to platelet serotonin "transporter." *Arch. Gen. Psychiat.* 38:1315–17, 1981.

109. Coppen A and Ghose K. Peripheral α-adrenoreceptor and central dopamine receptor activity in depressive patients. *Psychopharmacology* 59:171–77, 1978.

110. Tuomisto J, Tukiainen E, and Ahlfors UG. Decreased uptake of 5-hydroxytryptamine in blood platelets from patients with endogenous depression. *Psychopharmacol.* 65:141–47, 1979.

111. Meltzer HY et al. Serotonin uptake in blood platelets of psychiatric patients. *Arch. Gen. Psychiat.* 38:1322–26, 1981.

112. Mooney JM et al. An improved method for the recovery of mitochondrial monoamine oxidase from human platelets using colchicine and nitrogen decompression. *Biochemical Medicine* 26:156–66, 1981.

113. Mooney JJ et al. Platelet monoamine oxidase activity in psychiatric disorders: the application of a technique for the isolation of free platelet mitochondria from relatively small blood samples. *J. Psychiat. Res.* 16:163–71, 1981.

114. Mooney JJ et al. Sodium inhibits both adenylate cyclase and high affinity trituim-labeled p-aminoclonidine binding to α_2 -adrenergic receptors in purified human platelet membranes. *Molecular Pharmacology*. 21:600–8, 1982.

115. Schildkraut JJ et al. "Clinical Laboratory Tests in Depressions and Schizophrenias." (Offered by the Psychiatric Chemistry Laboratory, in cooperation with the New England Deaconess Hospital, Department of Pathology.) Boston: New England Deaconess Hospital, 1978.

3

Clinical and Etiologic Implications of Biologic Derangements in Major Depressions

A. John Rush, M.D.

A host of biological derangements have been identified in at least some patients with affective disorders. This chapter will focus primarily on the dexamethasone suppression test (DST)[1] and the sleep EEG[2] to illustrate the potential clinical applications for specific biological tests. In principle, other biological measures could serve these same functions. Second, comments about the possible etiologic implications of these sorts of tests are provided.

Any given test procedure might serve one or more of the following functions: assist diagnosis, measure response to treatment, indicate prognosis, direct treatment selection, provide clues to the underlying pathophysiology, identify "at risk" persons prior to the expression of a clinical episode or the illness itself, and reflect the anatomical basis for the disorder (Table 1). For example, catecholamine metabolite concentrations in urine, cerebrospinal fluid and/or blood have been reported to differentiate some depressives from normals, to relate to descriptive subtypes, and/or to predict treatment response to specific antidepressants in depressed patients. One test may serve only one of these functions, or it may serve several functions. Thus, a test that relates to treatment selection may not relate to current descriptive subclassifications, or vice versa.

The author wishes to express his appreciation to Ms. Marie Marks for her secretarial support, to Kenneth Z. Altshuler, M.D., for his administrative support and to Howard P. Roffwarg, M.D., Michael A. Schlesser, M.D., Donna E. Giles, Ph.D., Frederick Bonte, M.D., Ernest Stokely, Ph.D., and C. Richard Parker, Ph.D., for their professional collaboration in various projects reported herein.

Table 1 Potential Functions of Laboratory Testing

---

1. Adjunct to diagnosis
2. Measure response to treatment
3. Reflect ultimate or immediate prognosis
4. Direct treatment selection
5. Reflect underlying pathophysiology
6. Identify "at risk" persons prior to clinical illness
7. Reflect anatomical basis for the disorder

Adjunct to Diagnosis

The DST has been reported to be of great diagnostic value in differentiating melancholic or endogenous from nonendogenous depression.[1,3] On the other hand, a few reports suggest that dexamethasone nonsuppression does *not* relate highly to this descriptive subtype and even that 15.1% of normal controls will exhibit nonsuppression.[4]

Most DST studies have relied heavily or exclusively on inpatient samples.[1,5-9] One might logically argue that laboratory test procedures for classic, psychomotor-retarded, insomniac, melancholic depressions are hardly needed as diagnostic adjuncts. On the other hand, many affectively disordered patients are difficult to diagnose. In addition, such testing in treatment-resistant patients may be helpful in pointing the way toward selecting the next treatment step.

In order to determine whether the DST might be of clinical value in a group more difficult to diagnose, we recently studied a mostly outpatient cohort ($n = 70$).[3] Based on only the 1600 post-dexamethasone cortisol value, DST nonsuppression was found in 41% of endogenous unipolar nonpsychotic major depressions diagnosed according to Research Diagnostic Criteria (RDC).[10] On the other hand, only 5% of nonendogenous nonpsychotic unipolar major depressions showed DST nonsuppression. These results are consistent with other reports[5,7] that the DST relates heavily to the presence of endogenous depression. In addition, the DST appears useful in outpatient depressions, where descriptive diagnosis is often most complex and time consuming.

The phenomenon of nonsuppression relates highly to the symptomatic episode itself.[1,5] Figures 1–3 illustrate this point in different cases. To date, we have found that of the more than 70 inpatients who initially showed DST nonsuppression on admission, over 90% converted their DST to normal suppression with clinical improvement (17-item Hamilton Depression Rating Scale [HDRS][11] of 12 or less). Those who failed to convert fared poorly in follow-up. That is, readmissions or suicide attempts were likely. This finding corroborates reports by others[12-14] that a failure to normalize the DST implies a poor prognosis in the immediate future.

Some studies have found that DST nonsuppression is much more likely in primary than secondary depressions.[15] We regard this conclusion as premature. The incidence of DST nonsuppression will depend upon the definition of primary and secondary depressions as well as on the relative proportions of endogenous and nonendogenous depressions in each of these subgroups. Our own study in a mostly outpatient sample revealed that 42% of secondary depressions ($n = 12$) exhibited nonsuppression, whereas only 30% of the primary depressions ($n = 58$) showed nonsuppression. However, if the endogenous depressions are eliminated from each of these groups, then 0% of primary ($n = 25$) and 29% of the secondary depressions ($n = 7$) showed nonsuppression.[3]

Our third point is that DST nonsuppression appears more likely in major depressions with a positive history of depression in first-degree relatives, that is, Winokur's Familial Pure Depressive Disease,[16] when compared to Depressive Spectrum Disease in inpatients [8,9,17] or to Sporadic Depressive Disease in outpatients.[3] Whether this finding reflects a genetic

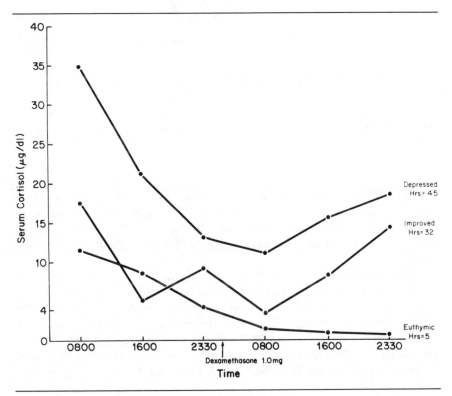

Figure 1 HPA-axis activity in a female with bipolar depression during treatment with phenelzine

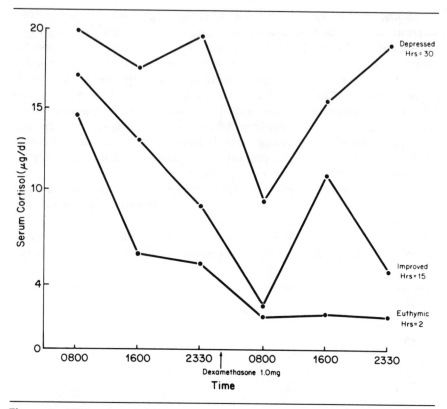

Figure 2 HPA-axis activity in a male with primary unipolar depression during treatment with desipramine

predisposition to DST nonsuppression during depression, or whether it is accounted for by a higher proportion of endogenous compared to nonendogenous depressions within the Familial Pure Depression Disease group than in the other subtypes defined by family history remains to be seen.

The need for normal control studies with the DST persists. One recent report[1] indicated that only 3 of 70 such normals (4%) showed nonsuppression with the 1.0 mg DST. However, this study employed only the 0800 and 1600 post-dexamethasone cortisol determinations. Table 2 shows the results from our own study of 23 drug-free, normal adults, 23–50 years of age.[18] Only 1 of 23 subjects showed nonsuppression (4.3%) and then only at the 2330 post-dexamethasone cortisol, following 1.0 mg of dexamethasone.

Figure 4 shows the relative theoretical specificity obtained from this normal sample assuming a hypothetical normal population (n = 23) without nonsuppression at various post-dexamethasone cortisol cutoff points. Using a radioimmunoassay, we found that a threshold or cutoff value of 4.0 μg/dl offers 96% specificity, that is, 4% false positives will occur. None of the normals showed nonsuppression at 5.0 μg/dl or above.

Furthermore, a 0.75 mg DST in normals revealed a higher incidence of false positives at all threshold values. For example, at a 5.0 μg/dl threshold and 0.75 mg of dexamethasone, 21% of normals showed nonsuppression. Even at 6.0 μg/dl, 17% showed nonsuppression (Figure 4). We conclude from these data that 1.0 mg of dexamethasone is the lowest dose that can be used for diagnostic purposes. Less than 1.0 mg is much more likely to yield false–positive results.

On the other hand, the same study revealed that various infections, allergies, and perhaps selected medications appeared to increase the probability of nonsuppression with 1.0 mg of dexamethasone in normals. Further studies of drug-free and drug-taking normals are needed.

The sleep EEG also appears to have diagnostic implications.[19] In our outpatient study, endogenous depressions exhibited significantly greater reductions in REM latency, total sleep time, Stage 2 time, and non-REM

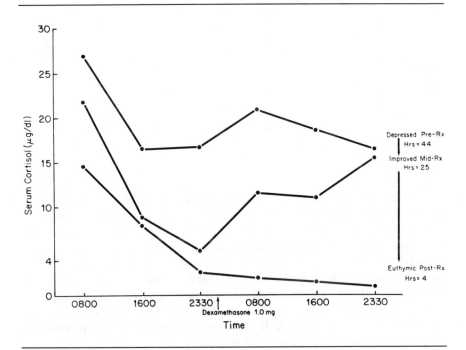

Figure 3 HPA-axis activity in a male with primary unipolar depression pre-, mid, and post-18ECT treatments

Table 2 Pre- and Post-1.0 MG DST Serum Cortisols ($n = 23$)

Subject	Pre-DST			Post-DST		
	0800	1600	2330	0800	1600	2330
1	16.3	4.8	9.9	.6	.5	.9
2	10.8	9.2	2.0	1.1	.6	.2
3	11.7	4.4	6.6	1.8	3.5	2.5
4	16.6	9.0	2.5	1.7	1.5	1.6
5	21.3	13.0	2.3	1.3	1.1	2.7
6	20.4	10.2	4.9	1.9	1.5	1.5
7	14.2	16.0	5.7	1.8	1.8	1.5
8	8.8	4.1	2.3	.4	.4	.5
9	17.7	12.2	2.8	1.4	1.1	.9
10	18.6	7.6	6.8	1.9	1.5	4.3[a]
11	15.8	5.4	2.3	.7	.8	2.6
12	11.7	14.3	9.9	1.0	1.2	1.8
13	12.7	9.1	5.0	1.5	.6	1.9
14	14.3	10.6	2.1	1.5	1.2	1.9
15	11.4	5.1	4.9	.8	.5	—[b]
16	10.9	6.5	4.2	1.2	1.7	—[b]
17	13.2	6.5	4.6	1.5	1.3	1.0
18	10.6	6.4	2.1	1.2	.8	1.0
19	19.9	7.9	8.5	.9	1.5	1.5
20	12.3	7.2	5.2	1.8	2.5	1.6
21	20.9	15.7	6.8	1.5	1.3	1.3
22	14.3	6.3	4.0	1.8	1.5	1.5
23	19.1	8.6	4.4	3.2	2.7	2.7
ARITH MEAN	14.9	8.7	4.8	1.4	1.4	1.7
S.D.	3.8	3.5	2.4	.6	.7	.9
GEO. MEAN	—	—	4.2	1.3	1.2	1.5
S.D. RANGE	—	—	2.5–5.6	.8–2.0	.7–2.0	.8–2.8

[a] Denotes "nonsuppressor" as defined by any post-dexamethasone serum cortisol of greater than 4.0 μg-dl.
[b] Value not available.

time when compared to nonendogenous depressions (Table 3). In addition, clinicians were more likely to prescribe antidepressants to endogenous than to nonendogenous depressions. As Table 4 suggests, REM latency may provide a more sensitive but somewhat less specific indicator of endogenous depression. Figure 5 shows how DST and REM latency relate to each other, as well as to the descriptive (endogenous vs. nonendogenous) subtypes in unipolar nonpsychotic major depressions.[3] As can be seen, DST nonsuppression is nearly always associated with low REM latencies. On the other hand, a number of patients, mostly with endogenous features by RDC, show only the reduction in REM latency.

These findings are in accord with another report [20] that suggests that a laboratory test sequence, namely DST followed by sleep EEG, can provide a test battery with which to substantiate the clinical diagnosis of endogenous depression. If nonsuppression is found, endogenous depression can be diagnosed. If DST suppression is noted, then a sleep EEG is called for. Although further studies are needed, such a conclusion appears to hold in a primarily outpatient population.[3]

In the above studies, descriptive diagnostic entities have been used as the independent variable against which various biological markers have been evaluated. However, there is no theoretical basis for assuming that meaningful biological derangements *must* correspond to known descriptive entities. In fact, general medicine is replete with cases in which the laboratory test itself dictates the subclassification of an established syndrome. For instance, anemias can result from thalasemia minor, iron deficiency, or vitamin B_{12} deficiency. While clinical history may suggest which of these entities is most likely, laboratory tests provide precise confirming or disconfirming evidence for the etiological basis of the specific anemia. Thus, the failure of a biological derangement to correspond to a given descriptive entity does not necessarily invalidate the measure.

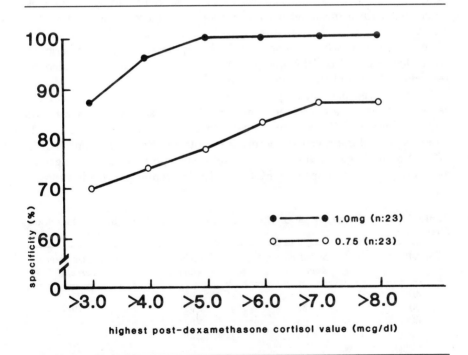

Figure 4 Specificity of the 1.0mg and 0.75mg dexamethasone suppression tests

Table 3 Endogenous vs Nonendogenous Depression by DST and Sleep Parameters

Variable	Endogenous (N = 32)	Nonendogenous (N = 38)	F	P
Hamilton Depression Rating Scale	26.7 (5.1)	21.4 (5.6)	17.0	.0001
Carroll Rating Scale	33.8 (6.3)	27.5 (7.2)	13.9	.0004
Beck Depression Inventory	30.7 (9.5)	27.5 (8.3)	2.1	NS
DST[a]	41%	5%	12.9[a]	.0003
REM Latency	56.7 (22.5)	73.0 (21.6)	9.6	.003
Total Sleep Time	347.6 (69.0)	399.3 (67.9)	9.9	.002
Non-REM Time	272.2 (51.2)	318.1 (61.5)	11.3	.001
Stage 2	159.1 (47.0)	202.8 (60.8)	11.0	.002
Treatment[a,b]	81%	50%	10.1[a]	.02

[a] Chi Square Test used.
[b] Percent prescribed antidepressant.

Treatment Response Monitoring

Both the DST and sleep EEG appear to reflect pathophysiological changes associated with a meaningful clinical response. Figure 6 shows the DST results in a small series of patients with unipolar melancholic (*DSM-III*) major depressions who evidenced DST nonsuppression prior to treatment with electroconvulsive therapy (ECT).[21] One of eight patients failed to respond to ECT and this patient continued to show DST nonsuppression. The other seven patients responded clinically and normalized their DST response during the course of treatment. Table 5 shows that significant improvements in DST occurred largely during the first half of treatment, whereas clinical improvement occurred in both the first and second halves of treatment. These findings corroborate other reports of DST changes in association with response to ECT[22] or to antidepressant medications.[23]

Table 4 REM Latencies and DST Findings as Markers for Endogenous Depressions

REM Latency	Sensitivity (Percent)	Specificity (Percent)	Confidence Interval (Percent)
40	19	95	75
50	34	92	79
60	63	87	80
62	66	79	72
65	72	58	61
DST	41	95	87

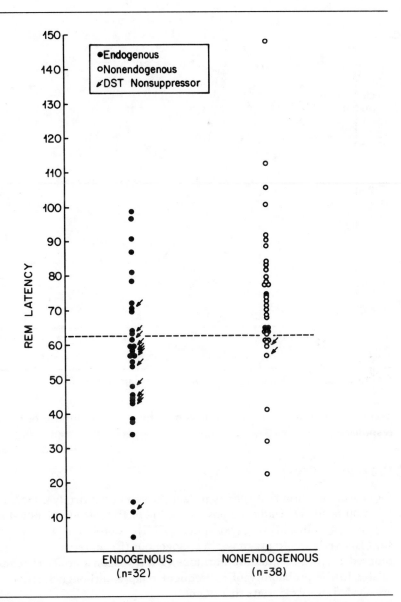

Figure 5 Relationship of REM latency to endogenous/nonendogenous depression

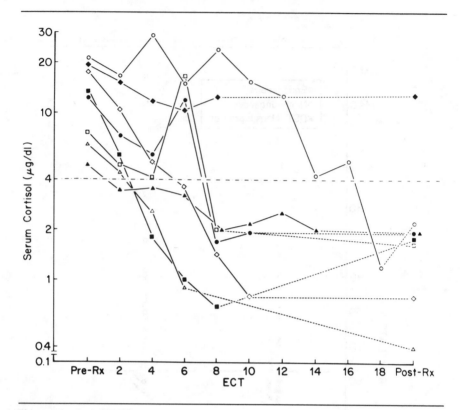

Figure 6 Serial DST among melancholic unipolars during ECT (N = 8)

They suggest that the DST response may be a useful monitor of treatment response.

Prognostic Clues

Biological measures that specify prognosis are not yet firmly established. In addition to the DST and the possible value of the sleep EEG, noted above, the thyrotropin-releasing hormone (TRH) stimulation test response[24] suggests a relation to prognosis in endogenous (E) depressions. A continued blunted thyroid-stimulating hormone (TSH) response to TRH reportedly relates to the probability of subsequent relapse, although further studies are needed to substantiate this claim.

Ideally, one would like to develop tests that could identify persons at risk for an illness before the first symptoms appear. Such tests offer the possibility of primary prevention. Findings that red blood cell membrane properties distinguish bipolar patients from normal controls, independent of illness, are suggestive that such derangements may function as markers of genetic vulnerability.[25] A recent study by our group[26] also suggests that certain structural-functional properties of red blood cell membranes—as evidenced by spectrofluorophotometric techniques—distinguish bipolar depressives from controls independent of the presence, absence, or type of symptomatic episode. Not only would such tests allow for primary prevention, but the genetic basis for the disorder would be more clearly understood.

Etiologic Implications

The majority of current investigations have focused on identifying particular biological changes associated with specific psychiatric syndromes. However, the question of whether these derangements are of etiologic import remains largely unanswered. What does dexamethasone nonsuppression or a reduced REM latency, for example, tell us about the cause(s) for endogenous depressions? Are these changes merely epiphenomenal consequences of more central pathogenetic disturbances?

If broadly similar clinical syndromes such as endogenous (or melancholic) and nonendogenous major depressions differ from each other with regard to measurable physiological or neuroendocrinological parameters, is it logical to assume that these disorders are, in fact, etiologically distinct? What experiments or naturalistic investigations can help us determine the pathogenetic relevance of the abnormalities?

Internal medicine provides several analogues of this situation. Anemias may present in clinically similar fashions: low energy, apathy, easy fatigability, pallor, and moderate exercise intolerance. The final common pathway is one of reduced production of red blood cells, or in some instances, the production of red cells that are poor carriers of oxygen. Various factors such as sex (females are more likely to have iron

Table 5 Changes During Treatment in Hrs-D and DST Responses in Unipolar Depressions that Responded to ECT[a] ($N = 7$)

	Pre-Treatment to Mid-Treatment P	Mid-Treatment to Post-Treatment P	Pre-Treatment to Post-Treatment P
HRS	<.05	<.01	<.01
0800	<.05	NS	<.01
1600	<.05	NS	<.01
2330	<.05	NS	<.01
DST	<.01	<.05	<.01

[a] Paired T-Tests

deficiency), age (B_{12} deficiency is more likely with increased age), and race (sickle cell anemia is more likely in blacks) are associated with various types of anemia. Yet, laboratory tests that evaluate pathophysiologic phenomena that lead to or precede the final common pathway bring us closer to understanding the etiology of these anemias. In other words, certain biochemical derangements relate more highly to etiologic differences than do others.

With only a small number of laboratory tests available 30 years ago, the differentiation of one anemia from another was not nearly so precise. When only serum iron levels were measurable, B_{12} deficiency and other forms of anemia were considered anemias without detectable, specific biological abnormalities. In addition, many of the various causes for iron deficiency anemias were unrecognized. The implication for depressions from the anemia analogue is that *nonendogenous* depressions may also be associated with biological abnormalities that we simply are unable to detect given our current methods.

To consider a different analogue, angina is a highly stress-related syndrome that can result in significant social and occupational impairment. There is little to biologically differentiate those with angina from normals until specific stressors, such as exercise or other demands for increased cardiac output, are introduced. When this increased demand occurs, transient electrophysiological and biochemical changes are detectable.

On the other hand, congestive heart failure usually follows a more autonomous course with symptomatic exacerbations and remissions. While early or mild cases respond to modifications in daily living, more severe cases can be fatal without acute medical treatment. Many of the biological changes found in both congestive heart failure and angina are consequences rather than causes of the disorders, yet these biological changes differentiate these two conditions. Central venous pressure, circulation time, arterial pO_2 and pCO_2, and EKG changes are examples. Clinical signs and symptoms, history of illness, and physical examination easily differentiate these two syndromes. Furthermore, treatment response patterns also distinguish the two syndromes. Although bed rest and oxygen reduce symptoms in both conditions, rotating tourniquets and using diuretics are more effective in congestive heart failure. Digitalis can be useful in both conditions, although more so in congestive heart failure. Nitroglycerin is most useful for angina. Thus, these two clinical syndromes differ with regard to history of illness, signs and symptoms, response to treatment, and laboratory tests. They may or may not, however, be etiologically distinct. That is, coronary arteriosclerosis may cause either condition. In addition, other diverse etiologies have been found for both congestive heart failure and angina pectoris.

By analogy, commonly used clinical criteria for distinguishing endogenous from nonendogenous depression may be insufficient. Specifically, the clinical endogenous-nonendogenous dichotomy may *not* imply distinct—meaning mutually exclusive—etiologies. Even the basis for believing that these two syndromes are distinct (differing histories, clinical presentations, laboratory findings, response to treatment) may be insufficient evidence for distinct etiologies. For example, dexamethasone suppressing and nonsuppressing melancholic depressions may be equivalent with regard to etiology or to treatment response. If the laboratory test differences that distinguish the two clinical syndromes are consequences of the syndromes, then one cannot use these laboratory findings to argue for distinct pathogenesis. On the other hand, if the biological abnormalities identified by laboratory testing reflect antecedents (i.e., pathogenetic) rather than consequential changes, then such data do argue for pathogenetic differences and, therefore, two syndromes.

How might we empirically evaluate the question of whether endogenous and nonendogenous depressions are etiologically distinct? One strategy would be to study remitted endogenous and nonendogenous depressions. If patients with histories of congestive heart failure or angina pectoris are evaluated when in remission with exercise stress, both may show similar EKG abnormalities if the shared etiology is coronary artery narrowing. Alternatively, new techniques analogous to visualizing the coronary arteries might provide etiologic clues if applied to remitted patients. In these instances, two clinically related but distinguishable syndromes might display the same laboratory abnormalities during *both* illness and remission. Such abnormalities should not be disregarded *a priori* because of their failure to relate uniquely to one syndrome, nor because they are not ubiquitous to all patients with a particular syndrome.

We have begun to evaluate depressed patients when ill and later when they are in clinical remission. Figures 7–9 show two groups of mostly endogenous unipolar nonpsychotic major depressions. These two groups were studied when acutely ill (pre[treatment]) and 6–7 months later (post[treatment]) after partial or complete symptomatic remission had been obtained with antidepressant medications alone or combined with psychotherapy. All patients had responded well to the treatment. After medications were stopped for 2–6 weeks, many remained in complete clinical remission (HDRS score of 7 or less). However, some became symptomatic again after antidepressants were discontinued.

At post, at least 2 drug-free weeks preceded the sleep EEG reevaluation. REM latencies (Figure 7), REM densities (Figure 8), and Stage 4 times (Figure 9) show interesting relationships to the clinical state. Two of the five patients who were symptomatic showed a near normalization of their REM latencies at post, while the other three continued to exhibit marked reductions in their REM latencies. Of the five who showed clinical

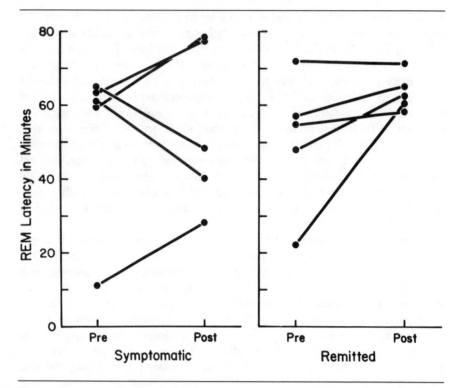

Figure 7

remission at post, four had REM latencies more than 60 minutes. Interestingly, however, only one subject exceeded 70 minutes REM latency. Thus, although clinical remission had been obtained, REM latencies were not normal.

REM density for the full night was calculated for each subject at pre and post. Clinical remission was associated with reductions in REM densities in four of five patients. On the other hand, continuing symptomatology was associated with increased REM density in three of five symptomatic subjects (Figure 8). Figure 9 shows that Stage 4 times continued to be low in those with persistent symptomatology (only one subject had a "normal" amount of Stage 4), while no change or an increase in Stage 4 time was noted in those who entered complete clinical remission. On the other hand, three of these five remitted subjects continued with low amounts of Stage 4 time.

Although these preliminary data do not allow firm conclusions, they suggest that (a) in some subjects who improve clinically, certain sleep parameters continue to be abnormal; (b) continuing symptomatology is associated with continuing abnormalities in selected sleep parameters; and (c) the presence or absence of the clinical episode (based on the signs and symptoms of depression) is not as closely related to characteristic sleep EEG changes as is, for example, the response to dexamethasone challenge. Too few nonendogenous subjects ($n = 1$) are in this sample to contrast endogenous with nonendogenous depressions.

Figure 10 illustrates another approach to the same problem. In a recently completed preliminary study using inhaled 131-Xenon and computer assisted tomographic scanning,[18,27] we studied the overall cerebral blood flow rates in bipolar and unipolar patients, first when symptomatic and later when remitted. The unipolar, endogenous group included severely ill inpatients who were diagnosed as melancholic by *DSM-III* and

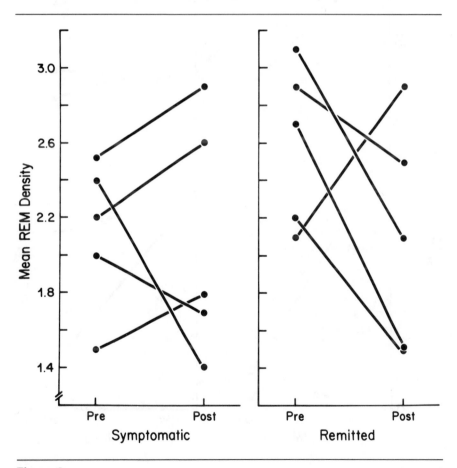

Figure 8

endogenous by RDC. All but one of these patients also exhibited DST nonsuppression.[1]

The overall blood flow as viewed from the mid-cross-sectional slice was reduced in these unipolar patients when ill, compared to both normal controls and to themselves when later remitted. (Some were studied on medication when in remission.) On the other hand, the bipolar depressed group showed near normal flow rates both when ill and later remitted. Whether these differences are due to severity, DST-nonsuppression, or

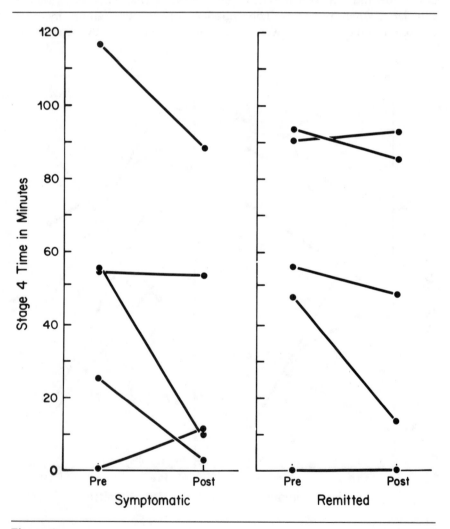

Figure 9

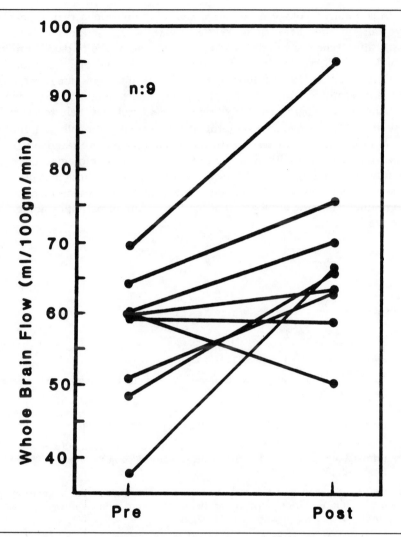

Figure 10 Unipolar endogenous melancholic depressions pre- and post-treatment

true functional anatomical-physiological differences cannot be answered without more extensive studies. Those bipolar depressives with mixed or manic symptomatology showed higher flow rates compared to age-matched controls. Further refinements in software development should shortly allow us to evaluate regional flow rates in these subjects. In addition, corrections for age, pCO_2, and other factors are needed to refine this technique before firmer conclusions can be drawn.

In summary, biological measures are being developed that appear to serve various clinical functions. While validation of descriptive diagnostic classification schemes has received the greatest emphasis to date, findings of biological discriminations of various clinical syndromes cannot by definition lead us to conclude that different etiologies are operative. Studies of remitted subjects can provide an important source of evidence regarding the etiologic basis for these disorders and may help to identify those at risk for subsequent symptomatic relapse. Additionally, studies of several biological parameters in the same subjects when ill and when in remission, may eventually allow us to tease apart those biological changes that follow as consequences of the clinical disorder from those that precede the symptomatic episode. Ultimately, biological measures may be of great help in understanding etiology, or at least the chain of pathophysiology of affective disorders.

References

1. Carroll BF et al. A specific laboratory test for the diagnosis of melancholia. *Archives of General Psychiatry* 38:15–22, 1981.

2. Kupfer DJ et al. Sleep EEG changes as predictors in depression. *American Journal of Psychiatry* 133:622–26, 1976.

3. Rush AJ et al. Sleep EEG and dexamethasone suppression test findings in unipolar major depression. *Biological Psychiatry* 17:327–41, 1982.

4. Amsterdam JP et al. The dexamethasone suppression test in outpatients with primary affective disorder and healthy control subjects. *American Journal of Psychiatry*, 139:287–91, 1982.

5. Carroll BJ, Curtis GC, and Mendels J. Neuroendocrine regulation in depression II. Discrimination of depressed from non-depressed patients. *Archives of General Psychiatry* 33:1051–57, 1976.

6. Brown WA, Johnston R, and Mayfield D. The 24-hour dexamethasone suppression test in a clinical setting: Relationship to diagnosis, symptoms and response to treatment. *American Journal of Psychiatry* 136:543–46, 1979.

7. Brown WA and Shuey I. Response to dexamethasone and subtype of depression. *Archives of General Psychiatry* 37:747–51, 1980.

8. Schlesser MA, Winokur G, and Sherman BM. Genetic subtypes of unipolar primary depressive illness distinguished by hypothalamic-pituitary-adrenal axis activity. *Lancet* 1:739–41, 1979.

9. Schlesser MA, Winokur G, and Sherman BM. Hypothalamic-pituitary-adrenal axis activity in depressive illness. Its relationship to classification. *Archives of General Psychiatry* 37:737–43, 1980.

10. Spitzer RL, Endicott J, and Robins E. Research diagnostic criteria: Rationale and reliability. *Archives of General Psychiatry* 35:773–82, 1978.

11. Hamilton M. A rating scale for depression. *Journal of Neurological Neurosurgical Psychiatry* 12:56–62, 1960.

12. Greden JF et al. Normalization of the dexamethasone suppression test. A laboratory index of recovery from endogenous depression. *Biological Psychiatry* 15:449-458, 1980.

13. Coryell W and Schlesser MA. Suicide and the dexamethasone suppression test in unipolar depression. *American Journal of Psychiatry* 138:1120–21, 1981.

14. Carroll BJ, Greden JF, and Feinberg M. "Suicide, Neuroendocrine Dysfunction and CSF 5HIAA Concentrations in Depression." In. *Recent Advances in Neuropsychopharmacology: Advances in the Bio-Science*, edited by Angrist and Betal, vol. 31. Elmsford, NY. Pergamon Press, 1981.

15. Clayton PJ. "A further look at secondary depression." In *Depression: Old Contrasts and New Approaches*, edited by Clayton, P.J. and Barrett, J. New York: Raven Press, 1982.

16. Winokur G et al. Is a familial definition of depression both feasible and valid? *Journal of Nervous and Mental Disease* 166:764–68, 1978.

17. Coryell W, Gaggney G, and Burkhardt PE. The dexamethasone and familial subtypes of depression—a naturalistic replication. *Biological Psychiatry* 17:33–40, 1982.

18. Rush AJ et al. The effect of dosage on dexamethasone suppression test in normal controls. *Psychiatry Research*, 7:277–85, 1982.

19. Kupfer DJ. REM latency: A psychobiologic marker for primary depressive disease. *Biological Psychiatry* 11:159–74, 1976.

20. Feinberg M et al. EEG studies of sleep in the diagnosis of depression. *Biological Psychiatry* 17:305–16, 1982.

21. Schlesser MA and Rush AJ. "Serial Changes in Hypothalamic-Pituitary-Adrenal Axis Activity Among Depressed Patients Receiving ECT." Paper presented to the Society for Biological Psychiatry, 1981, New Orleans, Louisiana.

22. Albala AA et al. Changes in serial dexamethasone suppression tests among unipolar depressives reviewing electroconvulsive treatment. *Biological Psychiatry* 16:551–60, 1981.

23. Greden JF et al. Dexamethasone suppression test and selection of antidepressant medications. *Journal of Affective Disorders* 3:389–96, 1981.

24. Kirkegaard N et al. Pregnostic value of thyrotrepin releasing hormone stimulation test in endogenous depression. *Acta Psychiatria Scandinavia* 52:170–77, 1975.

25. Ostrow DG et al. A heritable disorder of lithium transport in erythrocytes of a subpopulation of manic-depressive patients. *American Journal of Psychiatry* 135:9–18, 1978.

26. Pettegrew JW et al. Membrane biophysical studies of lymphocytes and erythrocytes in manic-depressive illness. *Journal of Affective Disorders* 4:237–47, 1982.

27. Rush AJ et al. "Biologic Basis for Psychiatric Disorders." In *The Clinical Neurosciences*, edited by Rosenberg, RN. London: Churchill-Livingston, in press.

4

Survey of Depressed Patients Who Have Failed to Respond to Treatment

Alan F. Schatzberg, M.D., Jonathan O. Cole, M.D., Bruce M. Cohen, M.D., Richard I. Altesman, M.D., and Celia M. Sniffin

The introduction of effective antidepressant therapies has had a major impact on the practice of medicine and on the lives of countless depressed patients. However, not all depressed patients respond to treatment.[1-3] Although the psychiatric literature has often pointed to refractory patients being nonendogenously, or atypically depressed, or as having a personality disorder,[4-7] some endogenously depressed patients also appear unaffected by these therapies and they too may actually become chronically ill. This paper reviews our clinical experience with patients referred to the McLean Hospital Affective Disease Program because of a previous failure to respond to treatment. Our experience points to two sets of factors—one that relates primarily to the treater (inappropriate treatment and appropriate but inadequate treatment, either in drug dosage or length of trial) and one that relates principally to the patient's condition (patient's type of illness does not readily respond to somatic therapy, intolerance to drug side effects, or unexplained failure to respond to seemingly adequate therapy). A treatment approach is outlined for evaluating, managing and treating so-called refractory patients.

Methodology

For this study, we reviewed the records of 110 depressed patients referred to us over a 42-month period (1974–78) because they failed to respond to treatment. All 110 had received somatic treatment for a current or past

The authors wish to acknowledge Ms. Linda Messier for preparation of the manuscript.

depressive episode, although 19 of the 110 patients had not received somatic treatment during their current depressive episodes.

The mean age of our patients was 40. Sixty-two percent were female. Thirty-two percent were single; 47% married; the remaining 21% separated, divorced or widowed. Sixty-four percent had received formal psychotherapy for at least 6 months. Although 69% had been hospitalized at some point for their illness, only 15% were inpatients when seen by us. The mean number of hospitalizations for the group was 1.7. The majority had been referred to us by psychiatrists.

In our effort to ferret out the factors involved in patients' failure to respond, data were gathered on: symptoms, organic medical and neurological diseases, duration of both current illness and episode, and previous treatments (type, dosages, length of trial, and side effects). Also, patients were classified as having an endogenous or nonendogenous syndrome by applying the system of Schildkraut et al., which our group has used for a number of years.[8,9] In this system, a diagnosis of an endogenous syndrome is made if the patient exhibits at least several of the following symptoms: anergia, anhedonia, psychomotor retardation, early morning awakening, diurnal variation, and other vegetative symptoms. *Definite* and *possible* endogenous syndromes are differentiated on the basis of the number of signs and symptoms and/or the presence (definite) or absence (possible) of autonomy—a lack of responsivity to environmental stimuli.

Criteria were also applied for a nonendogenous/chronic characterologic syndrome. These included at least several of the following: weepiness, histrionics, self-pity, anxiety, anger, reactivity (change with environmental stimuli), hypochondriasis, and emotional lability. Definite and possible nonendogenous syndromes are also discriminated on the basis of the number of signs and symptoms. The term chronic characterologic is somewhat misleading because neither chronicity nor a character disorder is required for diagnosis. Some patients may concurrently fulfill criteria for both endogenous and nonendogenous syndromes.

Data were also collected on the first antidepressant trial that the patients were prescribed after being seen by our group. These were categorized according to the nature and degree of response.

Syndrome Diagnosis

Of the 110 patients, 93 (85%) met criteria for an endogenous syndrome. Of these 93, 68 (62%) and 25 (23%) met criteria for definite or probable endogenous syndromes, respectively. Criteria for nonendogenous/chronic characterologic syndrome were met by 39 of 110 patients (36%). Of these, 17 (16%) and 22 (20%) met criteria for definite or possible syndromes, respectively. As indicated in the Methodology section, a number of

Table 1 Patient Sample: Type of Syndrome, Final Syndrome Diagnosis

	N	%
Definite Endogenous Alone	53	48
Chronic Characterologic Alone	24	22
Both	15	14
Neither	18	16
Total	110	100

Note: N = 110.

patients met criteria for both syndromes. Although generally mild in nature, 26 (24%) had a history of hypomania or mania.

For our subsequent analyses, only patients who met definite criteria for endogenous syndromes were classified as endogenous (Table 1). On the other hand, we amalgamated definite and possible chronic characterologic groups into one nonendogenous group. Patients who met criteria for both definite endogenous and for definite or probable nonendogenous/chronic characterologic were classified as having both syndromes. Those who did not meet any of these criteria were classified as exhibiting neither syndrome. Numbers and percentages of patients who fell into these categories are indicated in Table 1. Sixty-two percent of our patients met criteria for a definite endogenous depressive syndrome.

Characteristics

Understandably, the symptom profiles of our patients grossly paralleled their final clinical diagnoses. We reviewed the incidence of a number of specific symptoms or characteristics—including several relating to secondary and nonendogenous syndromes—that have been described in some studies on "resistance." We also included several endogenous items generally considered to predict good outcome. Wherever possible, incidences of similar symptoms in three major general surveys of depressed patients are presented for comparison.[10–12] As seen in Table 2, our sample did not appear to stand out in any particular or unusual way, although the incidence of suicide attempts was higher than in the comparison surveys. The incidence of alcohol abuse was within the range noted in studies on depressive illnesses.[13,14] Those affective symptoms which others believed to be uncommon in treatment-resistant patients—diurnal variation, decreased appetite/weight loss, and early morning awakening—were present in 46–67% of patients. This is in line with the high incidence of endogenous patients in our sample as well as in other surveys. As in other studies on resistance, anxiety was a prominent feature, although it was no more common than in some of the other comparison studies.

Table 2 Patient Sample: Percentage with Specific Symptoms and Characteristics

Characteristic	Present Study	Baker et al.[10]	Kiloh et al.[11]	McConaghy et al.[12]
Alcohol Abuse	12			
Drug Abuse	8			
Headaches	13			
Suicide Attempts	20	15	7	12
Schizoid Features	13			
Panic Attacks	19	36[a]		
Hypersomnia	22			
Hyperphagia	18			18
Diurnal Variation	47	46	41	59
Anxiety	83[b]		84[b]	61[b]
Weight Loss	46	61	51	37
Early Morning Awakening	46	65	37	59
Autonomy	67			
Agitation	46	67	41	37
Secondary Depression	15			13

Note: N = 110.
[a] Anxiety Attacks
[b] Subjective Anxiety

Chronicity

Our patients were relatively chronic on two counts (Table 3). Sixty-four percent had their initial onset of affective illness at least 6 years before we saw them; 46%, over 10 years before.

Psychiatric lore suggests that depressions are self-limited and relatitively short; however, many of our patients had been depressed for several years without experiencing a 3-month symptom-free period. Although 33% had been depressed in the current episode for less than 6 months, 54% had been depressed for more than 1 year; 16% had been continuously depressed for more than 10 years.

Table 3 Duration of Current Episode and Illness

		<6 Mos.	6-12 Mos.	1-5 Yrs.	6-10 Yrs.	10+ Yrs.	Total
Current Episode	N:	36	14	31	11	18	110
	%:	33	13	28	10	16	100
Illness	N:	5	7	27	20	51	110
	%:	5	6	25	18	46	100

Note: N = 110.

Prior Treatment

We coded previous trials by drug or treatment class (tricyclic, electroconvulsive therapy [ECT], etc.), dosage and length of trial when known, and response, coding simple failure to improve separately from the development of side effects that resulted in discontinuation of treatment.

In our study, we considered only tricyclic antidepressants (TCAs), monoamine oxidase inhibitors (MAOIs), and ECT as antidepressant treatments. Lithium, phenothiazines, benzodiazepines, hypnotics, stimulants, and combination drugs were not considered antidepressant treatments. Combination drugs were not grouped with the other antidepressants because we could not easily assess adequacy of dosage (see below) or the effects of any drug-drug interactions. Furthermore, although some of these treatment regimens, such as lithium, are effective in some patients, generally they have not been considered first-order antidepressants and our patients had obviously failed to show antidepressant responses to them.

Of 110 patients, 76 (69%) had in fact received at least one antidepressant drug trial during their current episode. Among the other 34 (31%), 15 (14%) had received some other drug therapy and 19 (17%) had not received any drug for the present episode but had received medication during previous episodes. Twenty-six of 110 patients (24%) received only antidepressants; 15 (14%) received only other treatments; and 50 (45%) received both antidepressant and nonantidepressant treatments.

Those patients not receiving antidepressant therapies before referral to our program were younger, more paranoid, more hypochondriacal, less depressed, and depressed for shorter periods than those treated with standard antidepressants. They also had fewer endogenous symptoms, particularly dull thinking, worthlessness, diurnal variation, and decreased ambition and enjoyment.

Our patients had been exposed to a range of other therapies such that the 170 discrete antidepressant trials represented only 51% of the total of 33 treatments. Of the other 161 treatments, 14% involved lithium carbonate, often in response to a history of hypomanic/manic symptoms. Anxiolytic trials represented 24% of all nonantidepressant treatments; antipsychotics, 41% of all nonantidepressant trials. Although the use of benzodiazepines and phenothiazines is understandable in view of the high incidence of anxiety and agitation in our sample, our patients did not demonstrate antidepressant responses to them (Table 4).

Adequacy of Treatment

For this study, we arbitrarily defined adequacy of treatment with tricyclic antidepressants or MAOIs as approximately two-thirds of the manufactur-

Table 4 Prior Nonantidepressant Therapy: Current Episode

	Lithium	Anxio-lytics	Antipsy-chotics	Combi-nation drugs	Stimu-lants	Other	Total
No. of Treatments	22	39	66	10	5	19	161
% of Total Treatments	14	24	41	6	3	12	100

Note: Patient $N = 65$; treatment $N = 161$.

er's recommended maximum daily dose, given for at least 3 weeks. The dosages were: 200 mg/day for imipramine, doxepin, and amitriptyline; 150 mg/day for desipramine; 40 mg for tranylcypramine; and 60 mg for phenelzine. (At the time of study, the recommended maximum daily dosage for desipramine was 200 mg/day.) We did not distinguish between maximum recommended dosages for inpatients versus outpatients. An adequate course of electroconvulsive therapy was defined as seven treatments.

The definitions of adequacy in this study were empirically derived to provide us with a barometer to study patterns of prescription. Recent research has indicated that serum tricyclic levels and measurement of platelet MAO inhibition may provide us with more precise methods for determining adequacy.[3,15] However, because considerable debate still continues regarding the clinical application of plasma levels for some antidepressants and because we were interested in surveying trends in current psychiatric treatment, we formulated the definitions described previously.

Applying our criteria, we found that only 39% of the 170 antidepressant trials received by our patients during their current episode met our criteria for adequacy. Furthermore, of the 76 patients who had received one or more trials on a standard antidepressant, only 15 received two or more adequate trials. These 15 patients did not differ remarkably from our total sample in endogenous/nonendogenous classification, though a few more were either classifiable as both chronic characterologic and endogenous (20% vs. 14% in overall group) or as neither (40% vs. 16% in overall group). Of the 6 "neither" patients, 4 were classifiable as "possible" but not definite endogenous depressives. Of the 15 patients, 9 had received adequate trials of ECT and 12 had received adequate trials of tricyclics. Thus, not all endogenous or depressive patients are responsive to ECT or tricyclic therapy, although some of our nonresponders might be responsive to more vigorous treatment such as higher dosages or conceivably higher blood levels.

Intolerance

The other major, and often less appreciated, reason for patients failing to respond clinically to antidepressant drugs is intolerance or marked side effects, a common factor in patient/physician decisions not to increase antidepressant dosages or to discontinue treatment. Empirically, we defined intolerance as an untoward experience on a drug that resulted in discontinuation of the trial, whether initiated by patient or physician. Often intolerance is due to autonomic side effects such as dry mouth or constipation; to agitation, including unpleasant grogginess or other presumably central anticholinergic drug effects that often occur early in treatment; or to a psychological reaction to medication.

In our sample, intolerence was noted in 30% of all antidepressant treatments (Table 5). Only 6% of the adequate dosage trials were associated with intolerance, in contrast to 47% of the inadequate trials. No significant differences among disorders in the incidence of intolerance existed. Thus, although intolerance played an important role in undertreatment for all types of patients, it accounted for only 47% of the inadequate trials. We had hypothesized that chronic characterological nonendogenous patients would report high degrees of treatment intolerance but this conjecture was not confirmed.

Among the 76 patients who received antidepressants, we identified 14 who had experienced intolerance on at least two antidepressant trials at dosages that we considered inadequate. Only 1 patient in this group had also received two adequate trials with no response. Nine of the 14 intolerant patients fulfilled criteria for definite endogenous; 2 for chronic

Table 5 Prior Antidepressant Therapy: Current Episode

	Intolerant		No Response		Response not Coded	
	R × N	%	R × N	%	R × N	%
Adequate Dose (R × N = 67; 39%)	4	2	63	37	0	0
Inadequate Dose (R × N = 101; 60%)	47	28	54	32	0	0
Dose Not Coded (R × N = 2; 1%)					2	1
Total	51	30	117	69	2	1

Note: Patient N = 76; treatment N = 170.

characterologic; 2 for both; and 1 for neither. Thus, this group paradoxically appeared more clearly endogenous than the group that had received adequate trials.

Outcome

We were able to follow a subsample of patients; the others were referred back to their therapists and were unavailable for follow-up. Data on those patients who were treated with a tricyclic antidepressant or an MAOI for at least a 4-month follow-up are presented in Table 6. Of the 57 patients treated with a tricyclic, 26 (46%) showed a sustained improvement (i.e., moderate to marked improvement lasting at least 3 months). Sixteen (28%) were intolerant to the tricyclic and 15 (26%) showed little or no improvement on tricyclic antidepressants. Thus, not all depressives are sensitive to tricyclic therapy, and intolerance was as significant a problem in our hands as it had been in those of previous treaters. However, 9 of 15 patients (60%) did respond to treatment with MAOI's.

Endogenously Depressed Patients

Our definite endogenous depressives were less sensitive to tricyclic antidepressant therapy but more sensitive to treatment with MAOIs than the literature suggests. Only 13 of 33 definite endogenous depressives responded to tricyclic antidepressant therapy. The remaining 20 definite endogenous nonresponders were almost evenly divided into intolerance or lack of improvement (Table 6). In contrast however, of 9 definite endogenous depressives treated with MAOIs, 7 responded, 1 was intolerant, and the other failed to respond.

Previous Intolerance or Nonresponse

We were able to follow 24 of the 28 patients who showed nonresponse or intolerance to two antidepressant trials. We treated 13 of the 15 patients who had failed on at least two "adequate" trials on antidepressants before coming to us. Nine of the 13 showed at least moderate improvement. Six of the 9 were markedly improved: two on MAOIs, 2 on standard tricyclics at higher dosages, 1 on lithium plus a tricyclic, and 1 on a then investigational antidepressant (maprotiline). Three were moderately improved: 2 (1 of whom had also demonstrated intolerance to two trials) on MAOI's and 1, a paranoid depressive, on a tricyclic plus an antipsychotic. Four were unchanged or only transiently helped by medication.

We were able to follow 12 of the 14 patients who had been intolerant to two antidepressants. Six were markedly improved: 1 on desipramine, the

Table 6 Outcome of Patients Treated with TCA[a] or MAOI[b]

	TCA (N= 57)			
	Endogenous (Definite)	Chronioc Characterologic (Possible or Definite)	Both	Neither
Total Treated	33	11	5	8
Improved	13	6	2	5
Intolerant	9	5	2	0
Unimproved	11	0	1	3
	MAOI (N = 15)			
Total Treated	9	3	0	3
Improved	7	1	0	1
Intolerant	1	0	0	1
Unimproved	1	2	0	1

[a] TCA = Tricyclic Antidepressant.
[b] MAOI = Monoamine Oxidase Inhibitor.

tricyclic antidepressant that has been shown to produce the fewest or least severe anticholinergic side effects; 1 on nortriptyline; 1 on maprotiline; and 3 on MAOIs. Two were moderately improved: 1 on an MAOI (as previously noted) and 1 on fluotracen, an investigational tricyclic. Four were failures on a range of treatments, although 1 responded to ECT but continued to cycle. Two have not been followed.

Thus, we feel we have been able to markedly benefit 50% of the 24 more difficult, resistant patients and to moderately help another 17%, while failing in a third. However, there still remain subgroups of patients who are less responsive to standard treatment or who cannot tolerate a variety of drugs. Further research is required to understand the psychobiology of these patients and to develop other treatment strategies.

Discussion

Our data support the observations of others that depression may become a chronic illness.[1,16] Indeed, 26% of our sample had been continuously depressed for more than 6 years. More striking is the finding that chronicity is not limited to neurotic, atypical, nonendogenous, or characterologic depressions, but that patients with endogenous or endogenomorphic depressions may also become chronically ill. Thus, in a chronically depressed patient, one must avoid ruling out on the basis of chronicity an endogenous depressive disorder that may be responsive to standard somatic therapy.

The failure to diagnose an endogenous depression may, in part, explain why 31% of our sample had not been given trials on standard antidepressants, but had often been treated with benzodiazepines and antipsychotics. This finding also supports those of Kotin et al., who found that 18% of depressed patients who were referred to their specialized NIMH program had been prescribed non-antidepressant medication (mostly phenothiazines and benzodiazepines) and that 37% had been given no medication.[17] Although phenothiazines and benzodiazepines share some role in the treatment of anxious depressives, little evidence exists that they are effective in treating endogenously depressed patients, particularly those with significant psychomotor retardation.[18] In fact, some depressed patients may even show an increase in symptoms on these drugs. Further, Weissman and Klerman have demonstrated an association between chronicity of depression and benzodiazepine usage.[16]

Yet, the choosing of an appropriate somatic therapy represents only the first step and first potential pitfall in the treatment process. Sixty-one percent of our patients who had been given standard antidepressants received inadequate trials. These findings support the earlier observations of Kotin et al., as well as two recent surveys of medical practitioners, which have all pointed to treatment with inadequate dosages of tricyclics as representing a major problem in the therapy of depressed patients.[17,19,20]

We advocate that the clinician develop a framework for diagnosing depressed patients and for choosing and prescribing specific antidepressants, one that includes selection of specific drugs and dosages, and minimum time periods. Such guidelines are readily available in the psychiatric literature.[8,21-23]

We acknowledge that drug side effects are a common problem in treatment. Half of the previous inadequate trials in our study were associated with untoward side effects. However, a number of steps may aid in keeping patients on their medications despite these side effects. A positive doctor-patient relationship may abate the patient's anxiety about any medication.[21] In regard to tricyclic antidepressants, nortriptyline appears to be relatively low in cardiotoxic and hypotensive effects and thus potentially useful in geriatric patients, and desipramine appears to have the mildest anticholinergic effects.[24-26] In cases of severe, peripheral anticholinergic effects, the addition of bethanechol, a peripheral cholinergic agent, may be a useful antidote, and the addition of a benzodiazepine may decrease agitation occurring early in treatment with amitriptyline.[27,28]

Although the tricyclic antidepressants have classically been prescribed as the first order treatment of all endogenous depressions, our data indicate that some endogenous depressed patients cannot tolerate or do not respond to these drugs but instead respond to monoamine oxidase inhibitors. Our experience is at variance with Tyrer's conclusions that endogenous depressives are not responsive to MAOI treatment.[29] It is, however, compatible with the more recent work of Paykel et al., who recently found that an endogenous/nonendogenous continuum did not separate responders from nonresponders.[30] Earlier conclusions may have been partially based on studies in which the dosage of MAOI was set too low. Recent research indicates that patients may require treatment with relatively higher dosages to attain the degree of platelet MAO inhibition that correlates with clinical response.[15]

We concur with the recent arguments of Rifkin et al., that the MAOIs deserve a new look and further study.[31] Conceivably, the index platelet MAO activity may help us determine which patients are potentially more responsive to MAOIs than to tricyclics. In this regard, our group recently described significant positive correlations in depressed patients between platelet MAO activity and certain symptoms of anxiety,[31] symptoms which Tyrer and others have argued predict response to and are ameliorated by treatment with MAOIs.[29] Thus, the presence of anxiety in chronically depressed patients may point to preferential use of MAOIs in some patients.

Measurement of urinary 3-methoxy-4-hydroxyphenylglycol (MHPG) appears useful in predicting response to specific antidepressants. For example, our group and others have described that patients with low urinary MHPG levels are more responsive to treatment with imipramine or maprotiline than are patients with high MHPG levels.[32-35] We have gone on to report that when one "trichotomizes" patients into low, intermediate, and high MHPG groups, patients with intermediate MHPG levels respond less favorably to imipramine or maprotiline than do patients with low or high MHPG levels.[36] The intermediate MHPG group had a relatively high dropout rate, suggesting that intermediate MHPG levels may predict intolerance to certain antidepressant medications. Further studies of clinical characteristics and biological measures are needed to confirm and elaborate on our findings. Ultimately, such research may lead to more precise *a priori* treatment selection and when coupled with the development of new antidepressants with distinct biochemical properties, we may be able to reduce dramatically the numbers of patients who fail to respond to treatment.

References

1. Robins E and Guze SB. "Classification of Affective Disorders: The Primary-Secondary, the Endogenous, and the Neurotic- Psychotic Concepts." In *Recent Advances in the Psychobiology of Depressive Illnesses*, edited by Williams TA, Katz

MM, Shield JA. Washington, D.C.: Department of Health, Education and Welfare. Publication No. (HSM) 70-9053, 1972.

2. Ananth J and Ruskin R. Treatment of intractable depression. *Int Pharmacopsychiatry* 9:218–29, 1974.

3. Glassman A et al. Clinical implications of imipramine plasma levels for depressive illnesses. *Arch Gen Psychiatry* 34:197–207, 1977.

4. Sethna ER. A study of refractory cases of depressive illnesses and their response to combined antidepressant treatment. *Br J Psychiatry* 124:265–72, 1974.

5. Helmchen H. Symptomatology of therapy-resistant depressions. *Pharmakopsychiat* 7:145–55, 1974.

6. Lopez-Ibor Alino JJ. Therapeutic resistant depressions: Symptoms, resistance and therapy. *Pharmakopsychiat* 7:178–87, 1974.

7. Lehmann HE. Therapy-resistant depressions: A clinical classification. *Pharmakopsychiat* 7:156–63, 1974.

8. Schildkraut JJ and Klein DF. "The Classification and Treatment of Depressive Disorders." In *Manual of Psychiatric Therapeutic Practical Psychopharmacology in Psychiatry*, edited by Shader RI. Boston: Little, Brown and Co., 1975.

9. Schildkraut JJ. *Neuropsychopharmacology and Affective Disorders.* Boston: Little, Brown and Co., 1975.

10. Baker M et al. Depressive disease: Classification and clinical characteristics. *Comp Psychiatry* 12:354–65, 1971.

11. Kiloh LG and Garside RF. The independence of neurotic depression and endogenous depression. *Br J Psychiatry* 109:451–63, 1963.

12. McConaghy N et al. The independence of neurotic and endogenous depression. *Br J Psychiatry* 113:479–84, 1967.

13. Cassidy WL et al. Clinical observations in manic depressive disease: A quantitative study of one hundred manic-depressive patients and fifty medically sick controls. *J A M A* 164:1535–46, 1957.

14. Mayfield DG and Coleman LL. Alcohol use and affective disorder. *Dis Nerv Syst* 29:467–74, 1968.

15. Ravaris CL et al. A multiple-dose, controlled study of phenelzine in depression-anxiety states. *Arch Gen Psychiatry* 33:347–50, 1976.

16. Weissman MM and Klerman GL. The chronic depressive in the community: Unrecognized and poorly treated. *Comp Psychiatry* 18:523–32, 1977.

17. Kotin J, Post RM, and Goodwin FK. Drug treatment of depressed patients referred for hospitalization. *Am J Psychiatry* 1139–41, 1973.

18. Schatzberg AF and Cole JO. Benzodiazepines in depressive disorders. *Arch Gen Psychiatry* 35:1359–65, 1978.

19. Ketai R. Family practitioners' knowledge about treatment of depressive illness. *J A M A* 235:2600–3, 1976.

20. Fauman MA. Tricyclic antidepressant prescription by general hospital physicians. *Am J Psychiatry* 137:490–91, 1980.

21. Goodwin FK. "Drug Treatment of Affective Disorders: General principles." In *Psychopharmacology in the Practice of Medicine*, edited by Jarvik ME. New York: Appleton-Century-Crofts, 1977.

22. Goodwin FK and Ebert MT. "Specific Antimanic and Antidepressant Drugs." In *Psychopharmacology in the Practice of Medicine*, edited by Jarvik ME. New York: Appleton-Century-Crofts, 1977.

23. Cole JO. "Further Notes on Drug Therapy." In *Depression: Biology, Psychodynamics, and Treatment*, edited by Cole JO, Schatzberg AF, and Frazier SH. New York: Plenum Press, 1978.

24. Smith RC et al. Cardiovascular effects of therapeutic doses of tricyclic antidepressants: Importance of blood level monitoring. *J Clin Psychiatry* 41:12(Sec 2):57–63, 1980.

25. Snyder SH and Yamamura HI. Antidepressants and the muscarinic acetylcholine receptor. *Arch Gen Psychiatry* 34:236–39, 1977.

26. Blackwell B et al. The anticholinergic activity of two tricyclic antidepressants. *Am J Psychiatry* 135:722–24, 1978.

27. Everett HC. The use of bethanechol chloride with tricyclic antidepressants. *Am J Psychiatry* 132:1202–06, 1976.

28. Feighner JP et al. A placebo-controlled multicenter trial of Limbritol versus its components (amitriptyline and chlordiazepoxide) in the symptomatic treatment of depressive illness. *Psychopharmacology* 61:217–25, 1979.

29. Tyrer P. Towards rational therapy with monoamine oxidase inhibitors. *Br J Psychiatry* 128:354–60, 1976.

30. Paykel ES et al. Depressive classification and prediction of response to phenelzine. *Br J Psychiatry* 134:572–81, 1979.

31. Gudeman JE et al. Toward a biochemical classification of depressive disorders VI. Platelet MAO activity and clinical symptoms in depressed patients. *Am J Psychiatry* 139:630–3, 1982.

32. Maas JW, Fawcett JA, and Dekirmenjian H. Catecholamine metabolism, depressive illness, and drug response. *Arch Gen Psychiatry* 26:252–62, 1972.

33. Rosenbaum AH et al. MHPG as a predictor of antidepressant response to imipramine and maprotiline. *Am J Psychiatry* 137:1090–92, 1980.

34. Schatzberg AF et al. Toward a biochemical classification of depressive disorders III. Pretreatment urinary MHPG levels as predictors of response to treatment with maprotiline. *Psychopharmacology* 75:34–38, 1981.

35. Schatzberg AF et al. Toward a biochemical classification of depressive disorders IV. Pretreatment urinary MHPG levels as predictors of response to imipramine. *Communic in Psychopharm* 4:441–5, 1981.

36. Schatzberg AF et al. Toward a biochemical classification of depressive disorders V. Heterogeneity of unipolar depressions. *Am J Psychiatry* 139:471–5, 1982.

5

Plasma Catecholamines and Dihydroxyphenylglycol (DOPEG) in Depressed Patients During Phenelzine and Amitriptyline Treatment

Donald S. Robinson, M.D., Garland Johnson, Ph.D., John Corcella, M.D., and Alexander Nies, M.D.

This chapter reviews selected findings from a clinical trial of amitriptyline and phenelzine in depressed outpatients. The experimental design of this study is a 6-week double-blind controlled trial comparing the treatment effects of the monoamine oxidase inhibitor (MAOI) phenelzine (60 mg/day) versus the tricyclic antidepressant (TCA) amitriptyline (150 mg/day). Interim results of this ongoing trial have been published elsewhere.[1] Clinical ratings were obtained at baseline and every 2 weeks during treatment using the self-rating Hopkins Symptom Checklist (SCL-90) and a Structured Depression Interview (SDI) administered by a trained interviewer.[2-4] Laboratory measures at each bi-weekly visit included plasma catecholamine and dihydroxyphenylglycol (DOPEG) levels, platelet MAO inhibition, and phenelzine or TCA plasma concentration.

Entry criteria for primary depression were met by 178 patients who, after random assignment, began antidepressant drug treatment; 74 patients completed the phenelzine treatment and 71 the amitriptyline treatment period, and were then evaluated for therapeutic response at 6 weeks (Table 1). The treatment groups were similar with respect to number of dropouts, sex, age, and initial symptom severity (Tables 1 and 2).

Overall efficacy of the two drugs was similar, and MAOI and TCA response rates were comparable. Improvement on many of the major symptom scales of the SDI was not significantly different for the two drugs

This work was supported in part by U.S. Public Health Service grants MH 32176 and MH 36179. The valuable assistance of D. Albright, D. Nicoll, D. Kennedy, C.A. Baker, and R.T. Smith is gratefully acknowledged.

Table 1 Baseline Characteristics of Drug Treatment Groups in Phenelzine-Amitriptyline Clinical Trial

	Phenelzine	Amitriptyline
Patients starting R_x	89	89
Patients completing R_x	74 (84%)	71 (80%)
Females: Males	52 : 22	53 : 18
Age[a]	36.8 ± 1.4	40.1 ± 1.5
SCL-90[a]	151 ± 7	142 ± 7
Hamilton (17-item)[a]	24.5 ± .7	24.2 ± .6
Diagnostic index[a]	6.1 ± .5	6.2 ± .5

[a] Mean ± SE

(Table 3). Also, the mean decreases in SCL-90 Total (Figure 1) and Depression (Figure 2) scales were comparable. However, a finding of significance between the MAOI and TCA was the greater improvement with phenelzine treatment on many anxiety measures. With phenelzine treatment the mean improvement at week 6 on the SCL-90 Anxiety scale was significantly greater than with amitriptyline (Figure 2).

The SDI contains 34 symptom items that can be rated and used to quantify clinical improvement; there are 10 additional demographic or historical items not useful in assessing symptom severity which are included in calculating the diagnostic index (DI), a numerical index of symptom mix or depression type.[4] Significant drug differences were

Table 2 Baseline Symptom Scores of Treatment Groups in Phenelzine-Amitriptyline Outpatient Trial

SDI Symptom Item[a]	Phenelzine (n = 74)	Amitriptyline (n = 71)
Total Depression	35.9 ± 1.4	36.2 ± 1.2
Depressed Mood	9.5 ± .4	9.4 ± .4
Retardation	8.3 ± .4	8.2 ± .4
General Somatic	7.6 ± .3	7.6 ± .3
Guilt	6.0 ± .4	6.2 ± .4
Suicidal Ideation	2.0 ± .2	1.9 ± .2
Work & Interest	2.4 ± .2	2.5 ± .2
Total Anxiety	22.1 ± 1.1	20.6 ± 1.0
Psychic	13.7 ± .7	12.2 ± .6
Situational	5.1 ± .4	5.2 ± .4
Irritability	3.3 ± .2	3.2 ± .2
Somatic Anxiety	10.1 ± .4	9.4 ± .4

[a] Structured Depression Interview (SDI) Symptom Scale scores (Mean ± SE).

apparent for 8 of these 34 SDI symptom items, 4 showing superiority of phenelzine over amitriptyline (greater improvement in psychic anxiety, reactivity of mood, symptom fluctuation, and hypomania), and 4 showing superiority of amitriptyline over phenelzine (initial insomnia, middle insomnia, terminal insomnia, and weight loss). These differential antidepressant drug effects are shown in Table 4. This number of symptom items (8 of 34) showing significant drug differences is greater than would be expected owing to chance alone, and represents true differential therapeutic properties of the two drug classes.

We have been especially interested in the measurement of plasma catecholamine and dihydroxyphenethyleneglycol (DOPEG) levels in a recent subset of patients from the clinical trial, and these interim findings will be presented in more detail. A recently developed radioenzymatic assay method was utilized for these studies which employs tritiated S-adenosyl L-methionine-[³H-methyl], catechol-O-methyltransferase, and

Table 3 Improvement with Phenelzine or Amitriptyline after 6 Wks Treatment[a]

Improvement Score[b]	Phenelzine 74 pts	Amitriptyline 71 pts
Total Depression	22.6 ± 1.6	20.6 ± 1.6
Total Anxiety	11.5 ± 1.0	9.2 ± 0.8
Somatic Anxiety	5.0 ± 0.5	4.2 ± 0.4
Hypochondriasis	8.0 ± 0.8	7.2 ± 0.7
Hamilton (17-item)	11.0 ± 0.8	12.2 ± 0.9

[a] Depressed outpatients treated with phenelzine 60 mg or amitriptyline 150 mg daily.
[b] Change in Structured Depression Interview (SDI) symptom scale scores (Mean ± SE).

rapid thin layer chromatography.[5] The sensitivity of the method is 160 pg/ml, and approximately 50μl of plasma are required for assay.

Recent evidence indicates that DOPEG may be a useful biochemical marker of central nervous system adrenergic neuronal activity.[6] DOPEG is known to be formed in brain tissue from tritiated norepinephrine and tritiated dopamine; therefore it is possible that plasma DOPEG levels directly reflect central noradrenergic turnover and release.[7] Although plasma 3-methyl-4-hydroxyphenylglycol (MHPG) levels in depressed patients have been previously reported,[8,9] to our knowledge this is the first study of plasma DOPEG levels in depressed patients.

Plasma-free DOPEG was measured pretreatment, and after 2, 4, and 6 weeks of drug treatment in 48 patients, 24 on each drug. Both amitriptyline and phenelzine treatment were associated with significant declines ($p <$ .05) in mean plasma DOPEG concentrations (Table 5). The decline in

DOPEG with phenelzine was more pronounced and significantly greater than with amitriptyline at both 4 weeks and 6 weeks of treatment. Several previous reports have documented a decrease in urinary MHPG excretion with TCAs, MAOIs, and amphetamine administration.[9-12] Beckmann and Murphy have reported on 12 patients who exhibited a marked decrease in urinary MHPG excretion during phenelzine treatment. A more recent report describes depressed urinary MHPG in several patients treated with the MAOI tranylcypromine and in a single patient who received phenelzine. In this report, rats given clorgyline or pargyline also showed a profound decrease in urinary MHPG and DHPG, with the greatest effect as expected, produced by the selective inhibitor of MAO_A, clorgyline.[11]

Although there was a relatively small number of patients in this study of this norepinephrine metabolite, we did examine for a relationship between baseline (pretreatment) plasma DOPEG and depressive sympto-

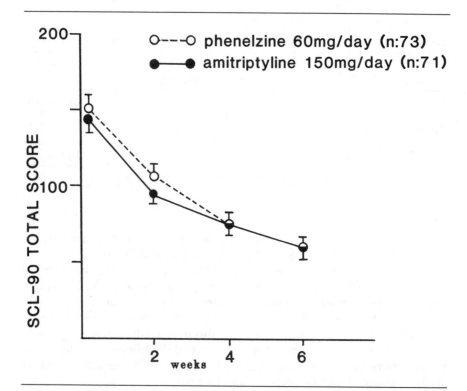

Figure 1 Changes in Symptom Check List (SCL-90) scores for depressed outpatients treated in a double-blind clinical trial with either phenelzine (Phen) 60mg (n = 73) or amitriptyline (Ami) 150mg (n = 71) daily for 6 weeks

Note: Means (± SE) of the total SCL-90 scores are shown for pretreatment and after 2, 4, and 6 weeks of drug treatment.

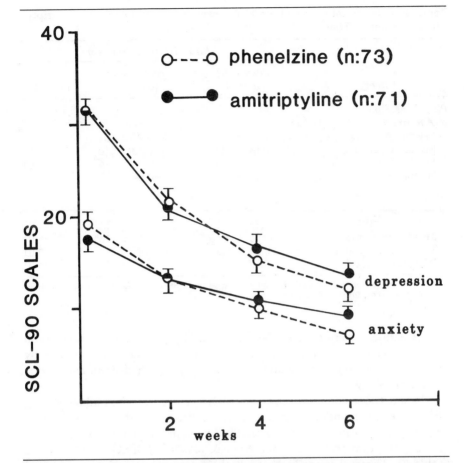

Figure 2 Changes in Symptom Check List (SCL-90) scores for depressed outpatients treated in a double-blind clinical trial with either phenelzine (Phen) 60mg (n = 73) or amitriptyline (AMI) 150mg (n = 71) daily for 6 weeks

Note: Mean (± SE) of the Depression and Anxiety scale scores are shown for pretreatment and after 2, 4, and 6 weeks of drug treatment. Improvement in the Anxiety scores after 4 and 6 weeks of phenelzine treatment is significantly greater than with amitriptyline ($p < .05$).

matology. No significant associations of DOPEG levels with type or severity of depressive symptoms were found; nor did baseline levels of plasma DOPEG predict therapeutic drug response to either phenelzine or amitriptyline.

The effects of these two drugs on plasma norepinephrine (NE) and epinephrine (E) concentrations were also assessed in a relatively small number of the same patients (Table 6). Phenelzine produced a progessive and significant decrease in plasma NE concentrations during the 6-week

Table 4 Differential Effects of Antidepressant Drugs in Phenelzine-Amitriptyline Comparative Trial

	Mean Improvement Score		
SDI Item [a]	Phenelzine (n = 74)	Amitriptyline (n = 71)	P
Phenelzine Superior to Amitriptyline			
Psychic Anxiety	7.7 ± .7	5.7 ± .6	.02
Reactivity of Mood	0.64 ± .11	0.13 ± .10	<.01
Symptom Fluctuation	0.64 ± .13	−0.08 ± .14	.01
Hypomania	0.16 ± .07	−0.04 ± .07	<.05
Amitriptyline Superior to Phenelzine			
Initial Insomnia	0.35 ± .14	0.82 ± .13	.02
Middle Insomnia	0.05 ± .14	0.69 ± .12	<.01
Terminal Insomnia	0.01 ± .14	0.55 ± .13	<.01
Weight Change	0.07 ± .12	0.52 ± .13	<.01

[a] Structured Depression Interview (SDI) symptom scale. Mean (± SE) of pretreatment minus the 6-week (improvement) score for 8 of 34 SDI items are shown.

drug treatment period. On the other hand, amitriptyline showed no consistent effect on plasma NE. Epinephrine levels declined slightly by about 30% with both drugs, and this change approached significance ($p = .10$) (Table 6).

When these changes in plasma DOPEG and catecholamines during phenelzine treatment were analyzed with regard to individual symptoms, we found significant negative correlations of improvement (as measured by several symptom scales) and the 6-week plasma DOPEG and NE levels (Table 7). These changes included both improvement in interview-rated SDI symptoms and in physician-rated global improvement. There was no

Table 5 Plasma DOPEG Levels in Depressed Patients: Effects of Phenelzine and Amitriptyline Treatment

	DOPEG (pg/ml) [a]	
	Phenelzine (n = 24)	Amitriptyline (n = 24)
Baseline	1140 ± 80	1020 ± 70
2 weeks	600 ± 100	630 ± 40
4 weeks	240 ± 20[b]	670 ± 40
6 weeks	295 ± 60[b]	620 ± 25

[a] Mean ± SE.

[b] Decrease in DOPEG is significantly greater with phenelzine than amitriptyline treatment (p <.001).

Table 6 Plasma Catecholamines in Depressed Outpatients: Effects of Phenelzine and Amitriptyline Treatment[a]

	NE (pg/ml)		E (pg/ml)	
	Phen (n = 15)	Ami (n = 11)	Phen (n = 15)	Ami (n = 11)
Baseline	560 ± 70	550 ± 60	68 ± 12	55 ± 9
2 weeks	520 ± 80	490 ± 80	61 ± 8	40 ± 9
4 weeks	390 ± 60	480 ± 70	52 ± 7	40 ± 7
6 weeks	250 ± 40[b]	700 ± 90	47 ± 7	40 ± 6

[a] Mean ± SE.
[b] Decrease in NE is significantly greater with phenelzine (Phen) than amitriptyline (Ami) treatment ($p < .01$)

relationship of plasma tricyclic antidepressant drug levels (individual or total TCA concentrations) during amitriptyline treatment and either norepinephrine or epinephrine levels. Similarly, plasma phenelzine concentrations did not correlate with plasma catecholamine or metabolite levels during MAOI treatment, but the decline in plasma DOPEG at 4 and 6 weeks did correlate significantly with the percent of platelet MAO inhibition ($p < .05$).

Discussion

This clinical trial reveals comparable efficacy overall for amitriptyline and phenelzine in the treatment of outpatients with primary depressions. Although the patient sample is heterogeneous for symptoms and typology, including patients with major depressive disorders (with and without the

Table 7 Correlations of Plasma DOPEG and NE with Clinical Improvement (%) at 6 weeks during Phenelzine Treatment

	Kendall's tau	
SDI Item[a]	DOPEG (n = 23)	NE (n = 14)
Depression	−.31*	−.42*
Total Anxiety	−.10	−.55***
Somatic Anxiety	.08	−.04
Psychomotor Change	−.29*	−.37*
Retardation	−.38**	−.28
Global Improvement[b]	−.33*	−.26

Note: Association of 6-week plasma DOPEG or NE concentration and improvement score with phenelzine treatment is significant by Kendall's tau at: *$p < .05$, **$p < .01$, ***$p < .005$.
[a] SDI = Structured Depression Interview.
[b] Physician-rated global improvement.

criteria for melancholy), the majority of patients had nonendogenous depressions of the type prevalent in the outpatient and primary care settings. It is particularly interesting that the only significant difference in treatment effect between the two drugs is the greater anti-anxiety properties of phenelzine.

These measures of plasma catecholamines and metabolites reported in this chapter are interesting for two reasons. The relationship of peripheral adrenergic activity to stress, anxiety, etc., is well known. Also, antidepressant drugs significantly affect central adrenergic neuronal activity and monoamine turnover.

The utility and significance of assessing catecholamine metabolism in urine of patients with affective disorders has been widely studied and debated.[10,13,14] Kopin and coworkers have recently shown that MHPG is extensively and rapidly converted to vanillylmandelic acid (VMA) in the periphery.[15] These authors suggest that only about 20% of urinary MHPG is derived from brain NE metabolism. Hollister et al. have recently reviewed the biological factors influencing urinary MHPG excretion and the stability of this trait within an individual during a 24-hour period.[16] These authors point out the need for additional studies to establish the utility of measuring MHPG excretion either for categorizing types of depressed patients or for predicting response to antidepressant drugs.

More recent studies of plasma catecholamine metabolites are of interest because plasma levels might obviate some of the problems of interpretation of urinary MHPG excretion. Also, Swann et al. have shown in normal volunteers that debrisoquin effectively inhibits both homovanillic acid production from dopamine and MHPG production from NE mainly in the periphery, thereby increasing the proportion of plasma MHPG derived from brain NE metabolism from 10%–30% to an estimated 75%.[17] This technique appears promising, but requires considerable study.

This chapter reports the first study of plasma DOPEG level monitoring in depressed patients before and during drug treatment. Both amitriptyline and phenelzine significantly depress plasma DOPEG concentrations, as might be predicted from their primary pharmacological actions. This finding is consistent with previous reports of antidepressant drugs lowering urinary MHPG excretion.[10–12] Our data can be interpreted in several ways. One explanation could be that the marked decline in plasma NE levels during phenelzine therapy, as well as the associated profound decrease in plasma DOPEG levels, is a reflection of the well-known peripheral sympatholytic effects of the MAOI class of drugs. This effect is presumably mediated by a primary MAOI effect on central vasomotor and cardiovascular regulatory pathways. Another reason may be that the decline in plasma NE and DOPEG is predominently a sympathetic neuronal rather than an adrenal medullary effect, because the decreases in plasma NE and DOPEG are substantially greater than the decrease in plasma E levels during drug treatment. Last, it is possible that the correlations we noted between clinical improvement with phenelzine treatment and the magnitude of the decline in plasma NE and DOPEG may primarily reflect a dosage phenomenon, constituting in essence an "epi" phenomenon. This might be true because patients within the phenelzine treatment group receiving the highest dosages (expressed as mg/kg body weight) also improved more than those receiving lower dosages. Thus, the associations of plasma catecholamine changes may primarily reflect a direct pharmacological effect of the MAOI on adrenergic systems and not physiological changes associated with improvement in anxiety or depressive symptomatology.

Because of the evidence that plasma DOPEG levels do reflect brain noradrenergic metabolism, these studies of depressed patients deserve to be continued in order to establish the importance of the catecholamine changes reported in this preliminary investigation.

Summary

In an ongoing clinical trial of the comparative efficacy of the MAOI phenelzine and the TCA amitriptyline, overall, the therapeutic effects of the two drugs appear to be similar in treating outpatients with primary depressions. The major drug difference is the greater anti-anxiety effects of phenelzine. A general trend for superiority of phenelzine over amitriptyline was seen on nearly all anxiety scales of the SCL-90 and the Structured Depression Interview.

Plasma catecholamine and DOPEG levels were measured in a recent subset of patients in the clinical trial. Both phenelzine and amitriptyline reduced plasma DOPEG concentrations, the decrease in DOPEG being significantly greater with phenelzine. The mean plasma NE concentration also declined significantly during phenelzine treatment but showed no consistent changes during amitriptyline treatment. With phenelzine treatment, the 6-week DOPEG concentrations correlated negatively and significantly with clinical improvement on several symptom scales and with global response. The association of the 6-week NE plasma concentrations and clinical improvement on several of the depression and anxiety symptom scales was rather striking. These preliminary results provide some evidence that changes in both plasma DOPEG and NE concentrations may reflect the quality of the therapeutic response to MAOI therapy. The theory that they may prove to be useful clinical markers is an interesting speculation requiring further study.

References

1. Ravaris CL et al. Phenelzine and amitriptyline in the treatment of depression. A comparison of present and past studies. *Arch. Gen. Psychiatry* 37:1075–80, 1980.

2. DeRogatis LR. *SCL-90-R Manual.* Baltimore: Johns Hopkins University, 1977.

3. Robinson DS et al. The monoamine oxidase inhibitor, phenelzine in the treatment of depressive-anxiety states. *Arch. Gen. Psychiatry* 29:407–13, 1973.

4. Nies A et al. "The Efficacy of the MAO Inhibitor, Phenelzine: Dose Effects and Prediction of Response." In *Neuropsychopharmacology.* Amsterdam: Excerpta Medica, 1975. pp. 765–70.

5. Baker CA and Johnson GA. Radioenzymatic assay of dihydroxyphenylglycol (DOPEG) and dihydroxyphenylethanol (DOPET) in plasma and cerebrospinal fluid. *Life Sciences* 29:165–72, 1981.

6. Warsh JJ et al. Brain noradrenergic neuronal activity affects 3,4-dihydroxyphenylethyleneglycol (DHPG) levels. *Life Sciences* 29:1303–7, 1981.

7. Warsh JJ et al. Rat brain and plasma norepinephrine glycol metabolites determined by gas chromatography-mass fragmentography. *J. Neurochemistry* 36:893–901, 1981.

8. Jimerson DC et al. Plasma MHPG in rapid cyclers and healthy twins. *Arch. Gen. Psychiatry* 38:1287–90, 1981.

9. Sweeney DR and Maas JW. Plasma MHPG in depressed patients. *Psychopharmacology Bull.* 16:31–32, 1980.

10. Beckmann H and Goodwin FK. Antidepressant response to tricyclics and urinary MHPG in unipolar patients. *Arch. Gen. Psychiatry* 32:17–21, 1975.

11. Edwards DJ. "Identification and Analysis of Alcoholic Metabolites Produced Via Monoamine Oxidases from Various Phenylethylamines." In *Monoamine oxidase: Structure, Function, and Altered Functions.* New York: Academic Press, Inc., 1980. pp. 403–12.

12. Beckmann H and Murphy DL. Phenelzine in depressed patients. Effects on urinary MHPG excretion in relation to clinical response. *Neuropsychobiology* 3:49–55, 1977.

13. Maas JW. Biogenic amines and depression: Biochemical and pharmacological separation of two types of depression. *Arch. Gen. Psychiatry* 32:1357–61, 1975.

14. Schildkraut JJ et al. "Recent Studies on the Role of Catecholamines in the Pathophysiology and Classification of Depressive Disorders." In *Neuroregulators and Psychiatric Disorders.* New York: Oxford Press, 1977. pp. 122–28.

15. Blomberg PA et al. Conversion of MHPG to vanillylmandelic acid. Implications for the importance of urinary MHPG. *Arch. Gen. Psychiatry* 37:1095–98, 1980.

16. Hollister LE et al. Excretion of MHPG in normal subjects. Implications for biological clarification of affective disorders. *Arch. Gen. Psychiatry* 35:1410–15, 1978.

17. Swann AC et al. Catecholamine metabolites in human plasma as indices of brain function: Effects of debrisoquin. *Life Sciences* 27:1857–62, 1980.

Transport of Tryptophan and Tyrosine Across the Blood Brain Barrier in Manic Depressive and Schizophrenic Patients

R. Tissot, M.D., Gaston Castellanos, M.D., J. M. Gaillard, M.D., and E. Estrada, Ph.D.

Summary

The uptake of tryptophan and tyrosine by the brain has been studied in six manic-depressive and eight schizophrenic patients. In an attempt to saturate the blood-brain transport mechanism, the uptake has been evaluated by measuring the arteriovenous differences (arterial plasma-internal jugular plasma) of these two amino acids before and after perfusion with L-dopa and L-5-HTP. Considering a positive difference as an uptake, and a negative one as an outflow, results show (1) in melancholia, an uptake of tryptophan and an outflow of tyrosine; (2) in mania, an uptake of tyrosine and an outflow of tryptophan; and (3) in schizophrenia, an outflow of tryptophan accompanied by either an uptake or an outflow of tyrosine. In addition, the kinetics of tryptophan binding to plasma proteins and the ratio of tryptophan–tyrosine uptake are different in manic-depressive illness and in schizophrenia. These results support the view that a disturbance in the blood-brain transport mechanism of tryptophan and tyrosine could be involved in the physiopathology of manic-depressive illness and schizophrenia.

The great number of monoaminergic hypotheses meant to explain the physiopathology of the two main genetic psychoses in man—manic-depressive psychosis and schizophrenia—reinforce our uncertainties. Four concurrent or complementary hypotheses for manic-depressive psychosis are serotoninergic,[1] catecholaminergic,[2,3] increased serotonin–catecholamines relationship,[4] and ionic hypothesis.[5,6] For schizophrenia, the dopaminergic and the increased dopamine–serotonin relationships are two apparently sound, complementary hypotheses.[4,7,8]

One member of our team proposed the following synthesis: the disturbances of the previously mentioned metabolisms could be correlated to modifications in circulating tryptophan and tyrosine uptake by the brain.[4] The proposal assumes that serotonin (5-HTP) and L-dopa are transported by the same system as tryptophan and tyrosine and that the production of 5-HT and DA from L-5-HTP and L-dopa (which have penetrated into the brain) is not limited by the stage of hydroxylation.[9] A perfusion of L-5-HTP or L-dopa, either by direct competence at the level of the transport mechanisms or by the retroactive regulation of the latter through the brain's production of 5-HT and DA, may produce important modifications in endogenous tryptophan and tyrosine uptake.[4] The work described here, carried out jointly by the psychiatric service of the Instituto Nacional de Neurologia, in Mexico, and the University Clinic of Psychiatry, in Geneva, is a first attempt to verify this model. The study investigated variations in the arteriovenous difference (arterial blood-internal jugular blood) of endogenous tryptophan and tyrosine during a constant perfusion (1.015 mg/kg/min) of L-5-HTP of L-dopa.

Method

Subjects

The present trial included 6 patients suffering from bipolar manic-depressive psychosis diagnosed by at least two qualified psychiatrists, on the evidence of various typical outbreaks. Three of them were examined during the depressive phase and the other three during the manic phase. We also studied 8 patients who had been suffering from schizophrenia for several years (either hebephrenia or paranoid schizophrenia). They, too, were diagnosed by at least two qualified psychiatrists. These patients' ages ranged from 25 to 58 years. During the week prior to the test the subjects' only medication was Valium 5 mg/kg.

Technique

The arterial blood was taken by catheterization of the femoral artery. In Geneva, the catheter to the gulf of the jugular vein was placed by direct puncture under superficial anesthesia with Pentothal. The experiment was initiated only when the subject was completely awake. Blood taken from the elbow's fold before using anesthesia and before initiating the arterial and jugular blood takings, showed a slight, though insignificant, increase in free tryptophan measurements.

In Mexico, the catheter to the gulf of the jugular vein was installed under radiological control via the femoral vein using local anesthesia. The experiment was developed as follows. In all cases, the 30-minute, constant perfusion of L-5 HTP or L-dopa (.015 mg/kg/min) (samples taken from 0–30) was ensured by a precision millimetric bomb. The synchronization of the arterial and venous blood samplings for the punctual takings were arranged through synchronic motor bombs connected along the same circuit; for the integrated blood samples, syringes were placed on a single millimetric precision bomb. The blood was immediately centrifuged; part of the plasma was filtered through millipore in order to determine free tryptophan. Then the filtered and the nonfiltered plasma were frozen to obtain the total tryptophan, the free tryptophan, and the tyrosine (by spectrofluorometry).[10-12]

Results

The global balances—the algebraic sum of the influx (plasma output) and the outflow (plasma intake) of tryptophan and tyrosine along the duration of the experiment—are shown in Table 1.

These balances are expressed in micrograms per plasma milliliters. If the arteriojugular difference is positive, the balance indicates the number of tryptophan or tyrosine micrograms that were captured (influx) during 38 minutes, per each plasma milliliter that irrigated the brain. Inversely, if the arteriojugular difference is negative, the balance indicates the number of tryptophan or tyrosine micrograms that have returned (outflow) during 38 minutes, per each plasma milliliter that irrigated the brain (Figure 1).

In individual patients the reciprocal evolution of the influx and outflow of tyrosine as a function of the influx and outflow of tryptophan, produces the correlations shown in Table 2.

In manic-depressive psychosis there is a significant negative correlation between the movements of tryptophan and tyrosine, a fact that is apparent in the total balances despite the small number of cases (Figure 1). Every tryptophan movement is accompanied by a more marked and inverse tyrosine movement: negative r and negative spikes less than 1. Yet in the case of depression, the negative spikes of the correlation coefficients are much more pronounced than in the case of mania. In other words, the small tryptophan movements are accompanied by important inverse tyrosine movements. In schizophrenia, this correlation is not significant, either positively or negatively, and the corresponding spikes are frequently close to 0.

Finally, in manic-depressive psychosis when the curve of evolution of the arteriojugular differences is positive, it is more marked in the case of free tryptophan than in the case of linked tryptophan. That is, the passing of tryptophan from the compartment of linked tryptophan to the compartment of free tryptophan is slower than the passing from the compartment of free tryptophan to out of the plasma. Inversely, in the case of negative arteriojugular difference, the increase in free tryptophan in venous blood is more pronounced than the increase in linked tryptophan. The total balance after 38 minutes results in a mean decrease of $4.7\mu g$/ml (44.7%) in the free tryptophan compartment in cases of depression, and a positive arteriojugular difference of $10.5\mu g$/ml; a medium increase of $15.3\mu g$/ml in the free tryptophan compartment (71.2%) in manias, and a negative arteriojugular difference of $21\mu g$/ml. In schizophrenia, the mean

Table 1 Balance of the Arteriojugular Differences in Patients after 38 Minutes

Manic Depressive Psychoses	Tryptophan µg/ml		Tyrosine µg/ml		Perfusion
	Positive	Negative	Positive	Negative	
Depression					
Seg	+ 1.3			− 29.7	L-5-HTP
Man	+10.2			−137.5	L-5-HTP
Gat	+10.8			−187.5	L-5-HTP
Mania					
Ja		− 2.8	+ 22.9		L-5-HTP
Ba		−27.2	+ 45.5		L-5-HTP
In		−34.6	− 52.4		L-dopa
Schizophrenia					
Pi		− 4.6	+ 14.6		L-5-HTP
Tri		−11.5	+ 8.6		L-5-HTP
Rin		−12.4		− 6.4	L-5-HTP
Lop		−12.8	+ 0.7		L-dopa
Cha		−23.2	+151.6		L-5-HTP
De		−23.7		− 66.3	L-5-HTP
Cr		−37.1		− 3.0	L-dopa
Ze		−74.5		− 5.2	L-dopa

increase in free tryptophan is $6.8\mu g$/ml (26.2%) for a negative arteriojugular difference of $25.5\mu g$/ml.

Discussion and Conclusions

The important variations in the arteriojugular difference caused respectively by the perfusion of L-5-HTP and L-dopa are not entirely different. Thus, we may assume [13-15] that tryptophan and tyrosine have a common membrane transportation system, and that L-5-HTP and L-dopa are both

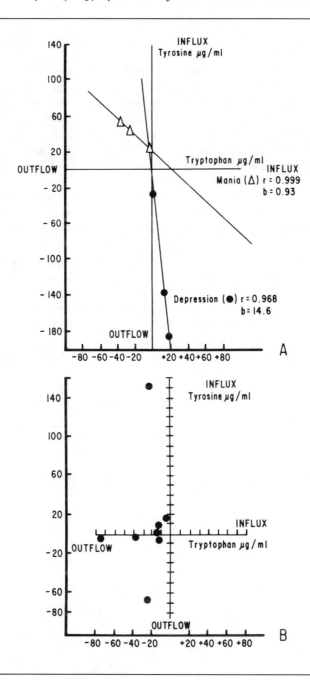

Figure 1 Arteriovenous differences balance (38 min). A, manic-depressive psychosis (n = 6). B, schizophrenia (n = 8)

competitive for tryptophan as well as for tyrosine. We believe these results eliminate the need for performing a similar number of L-dopa and L-5-HTP experiments in each syndrome.

A plasmatic arteriovenous difference of tryptophan or tyrosine between arterial blood and the internal jugular blood does not absolutely prove the existence of blood-brain movements of these amino acids. Although it is unlikely, the effect could be produced by a movement between plasma and the formed elements of the blood. As a matter of fact, in some of the subjects, we gathered blood from the femoral vein at the same time that we sampled blood from the femoral artery. Whereas the difference between arterial plasma and jugular plasma is positive, it frequently is negative between arterial plasma and the plasma from the femoral vein, or vice versa. If these differences mean plasma-blood formed element movements, they would necessarily take place in an opposite direction to the cerebral and peripheral vascular beds. Assuming we accept that the observed arteriojugular plasmatic differences show, at least partly, the blood-brain movements of the corresponding amino acids, we conclude that depression is characterized by a weak influx of tryptophan linked to a pronounced outflow of tyrosine. Mania is characterized by an influx of tyrosine linked to a tryptophan outflow, and schizophrenia by an outflow of tryptophan linked to either an influx or an outflow of tyrosine.

Our initial hypothesis (Table 3) seems thus to be partially confirmed

Table 2 Evolution for Each Case of the Movements of Tyrosine in Relation to Tryptophan

Manic Depressive Psychoses	Correlation Coefficients	Peaks
Depression		
Seg	−.739	−35.09
Man	−.960	−13.85
Gat	−.929	−19.51
Mania		
Ja	−.923	− 2.13
Ba	−.943	− 2.36
In	−.992	− 1.61
Schizophrenia		
Pi	+.668	+ 2.60
Tri	−.951	− .71
Rin	−.369	− .27
Lop	−.371	− .08
Cha	−.986	− 5.44
De	+.897	+ 2.85
Cr	+.649	+ .292
Ze	+.952	+ .11

Table 3 Hypothesis of the Brain's Uptake of Circulating Tryptophan and Tyrosine

	Uptake of Tryptophan	Uptake of Tyrosine
Depression	increased	decreased
Mania	normal or decreased	increased
Schizophrenia	decreased	increased

in the cases of manic-depressive psychosis, although we had expected a greater influx of tryptophan in cases of depression. In schizophrenia, the decrease in the tryptophan capture agrees with our hypothesis. Except in extreme cases of schizophrenia, the variations in the capture of tryptophan are clearly greater than those of tyrosine, though their correlations are very weak. On the contrary, in manic-depressive psychosis, small tryptophan variations correlated significantly to wide inverse tyrosine variations. This illness apparently shows greater inertia in the linked tryptophan/free tryptophan plasmatic balance. The latter facts could be linked to an anomaly of the free tryptophan/linked tryptophan kinetics or to a particular affinity of the tryptophan to the membrane carriers. Possibly, a tryptophan influx is linked to an almost equivalent outflow, in which case a small increase in the capture of tryptophan would result from significant increase in the influx and outflow movements that would almost be nullified. Because the amino acid transport is competitive,[13-15] it leads us to recognize the repercussion of the small variations in the 5-HT precursor capture over those of tyrosine.

Thus it seems worthwhile, on one hand, to study the kinetics of the free tryptophan/linked tryptophan plasmatic balance and, on the other, the relative importance of the simultaneous tryptophan influx and outflow in manic-depressive psychosis.

References

1. Coppen A. "Role of Serotonin in Affective Disorders." In *Serotonin and Behavior*, edited by Barchas and Usdin. New York: Academic Press, 1973. pp. 523–28.

2. Schildkraut JJ; Davis JM; and Klerman GI. "Biochemistry of Depressions." In *Psychopharmacology. A review of progress*, edited by Efron, et al. Washington, US Government Printing Office. 1968. pp. 625–48.

3. Shopsin B et al. Catecholamines and affective disorders revised: A critical assessment. *J. Nerv. Ment. Dis.* 158:369–83, 1974.

4. Tissot R. The common pathophysiology of monoaminergic psychoses: A new hypothesis. *Neuropsychobiology* 1:243–60, 1975.

5. Coppen A and Shaw DM. Mineral metabolism in melancholia. *Br. Med. J.* 2:1439–44, 1963.

6. Dick DAT et al. Sodium and potassium transport in depressive illness. *J. Physiol.* (Lond.) 227:30–32, 1972.

7. Snyder SH. Amphetamine psychosis: A "model" schizophrenia mediated by catecholamines. *Am. J. Psychiat.* 130:61–67, 1973.

8. Smythies JR. Recent progress in schizophrenia research. *Lancet* 1:136–39, 1976.

9. Lajtha A. "Transport as Control Mechanism of Cerebral Metabolite Levels." In *Brain Barrier Systems. Prog. Brain Res.*, edited by Lajtha and Ford. 29:201–18, 1968.

10. Eccleston EG. A method for the estimation of free and total acid-soluble plasma tryptophan using an ultra-filtration technique. *Clinica chim. Acta* 48:269–72, 1973.

11. Williams CH, King DJ, and Cairns J. Microestimation of tryptophan in plasma by a fluorometric procedure. *Biochem. Med.* 6:504–7, 1972.

12. Wong PWK, O'Flynn ME, and Inouye T. Micromethods for measuring phenylalanine and tyrosine in serum. *Clin. Chem.* 10:1098–1104, 1964.

13. Battistin L, Grynbaum A, and Lajtha A. The uptake of various amino acids by the mouse brain *in vivo. Brain Res.* 29:85–99, 1971.

14. Guroff G and Udenfriend S. Studies on aromatic amino acid uptake by rat brain *in vivo. J. Biol. Chem.* 237:803–6, 1962.

15. McKean CM, Boggs DE, and Peterson NA. The influence of high phenylalanine and tyrosine on the concentrations of essential amino acids in brain. *J. Neurochem.* 15:235–41, 1968.

7

Application of the Sleep EEG in Affective Disorders

David J. Kupfer, M.D.

Our current knowledge about the various types of affective disorders (unipolar-bipolar, major-minor, primary-secondary, endogenous-nonendogenous), strongly suggests that they do not simply reflect mood changes, but that they entail a dysfunction in many systems. Emphasis on psychobiology stresses an understanding of the genetic transmittal of affective disorders and stimulates a search for biological markers in affective illness. However, regardless of whether depression is "caused" by psychological or biological dysfunctioning, the diagnosis and treatment of the disease can be improved by increased knowledge on the psychobiology of mood and the biochemical systems that govern it.[1]

Many of the key symptoms in depression reflect alterations in biological systems: sleep, appetite, weight, psychomotor function, and sexual interest and activity. Because these biological systems have both peripheral and central nervous system connections, it has been hypothesized that these biological changes in depression are the cause of the illness, not simply the symptoms. Ignoring the longstanding controversy of the psychological versus the psychobiological causes of depression, measurement of changes permits objective measurements of the severity of illness; an opportunity to discover correlations between biological changes and depth of depression; and an opportunity, perhaps, to establish predictors of clinical response.

This work was conducted on the Clinical Research Unit (CRU) of Western Psychiatric Institute and Clinic. I would like to thank the staff of the CRU for their assistance. Supported in part by NIMH Grants MH 25452 and MH 30915.

The regulatory systems that govern sleep, appetite, motor activity, and sexual activity are regulated by the same hormones and neurotransmitters that probably determine mood. From the viewpoint of a clinician, interest focuses on the changes in these neuroregulatory systems. For example, nearly all depressed patients experience some sleep disturbance. Although the majority of sleep pattern changes favor insomnia, from 15% to 30% of all depressed individuals report hypersomnia. Therefore, because sleep disturbance is one of the earliest and most frequent (90%) symptoms of depression, it is important to characterize the type of sleep changes: whether patients are sleeping more or less than they usually do, having trouble getting to sleep, maintaining their sleep, or getting a restful night's sleep. Recent changes in appetite and weight are equally important; usually appetite is decreased, but, in a considerable percentage of cases, weight increases despite the fact that the depressed patient reports that eating is not pleasurable and that he or she does not experience "hunger." Changes in motor activity are also common features of depression. Most individuals report motor retardation, some report agitation, and a few report both agitation and retardation. Finally, recent changes in sexual interest and activity represent areas in which dysfunction can be determined qualitatively.

This chapter will review the value of psychobiological measures as they relate to diagnosis and treatment in affective disorders. The study of EEG sleep in depression has afforded us an opportunity to examine, along with other biological parameters, notions of how aberrations in neurochemical pathways and circadian rhythms may be responsible for the proposed various disturbances in depression. To ascertain the impact of sleep research in the last decade, one needs to examine how the findings from sleep research have improved our ability to diagnose affective disorders and predict treatment outcome.

To date, four features of EEG sleep patterns have been established as the most frequently observed abnormalities of depressed patients (Table 1).[2,3] These are sleep continuity disturbances, a marked reduction in slow wave sleep, shortened rapid eye movement (REM) latency, and changes in REM activity (number of eye movements). Most, if not all, depressed

Table 1 EEG Sleep Features in Depression

1. Sleep continuity decrease

2. Slow wave sleep (stage 3 & 4) decrease

3. Shortened REM latency

4. Increased REM activity (first half of the night)

patients show some changes in sleep continuity from that exhibited during sleep among normals or among depressed patients in remission. Previous research has stressed the importance of the sleep discontinuity in 80–85% of all depressed patients, with the remaining 15–20% showing features of hypersomnia.[2] The reduction of delta sleep (stages 3 and 4, slow wave sleep), however, does not appear to be specific for depressive states, but rather is prominent in many chronic psychiatric and medical states.

The two REM sleep measures receiving the greatest amount of attention have been the shortened REM latency and the shift of REM sleep time and intensity of the rapid eye movements to the earlier portion of the night.[4,5] A key feature reported in depression has been the presence of increased REM activity in the beginning of the night. REM sleep time is usually described as the number of minutes of REM sleep during the entire night's sleep; but the number and type of rapid eye movements indicate wide individual variability. In many depressed patients, especially those older than 40 years, not only does their first REM period occur very early in the night, but the first REM period appears to be associated with a higher density of REM activity than is seen in age-matched normal controls or in other types of patient samples.

On the basis of EEG sleep measures, depressed patients have been separated from normals. Perhaps more importantly, they have been significantly separated from patients with psychiatric disorders other than depression, such as general anxiety disorders.[6] Indeed, whether depression is labeled melancholia, primary depression (unipolar or bipolar), or endogenous depression, the discrimination of these patients from those suffering from nonendogenous depression or from secondary depressive disorders on the basis of sleep measures has been confirmed several times from different investigative groups. Both Rush et al. and Feinberg et al. have distinguished endogenous and nonendogenous disorders primarily using REM sleep measures.[7,8] Akiskal and his collaborators have used sleep measures—particularly REM latency—in outpatients to differentiate primary from secondary disorders in acute and chronic syndromes.[9] With respect to characterological depression, they have demonstrated that clinical responders have shorter REM latencies than nonresponders.[10] Because these findings are now generalizable to outpatients, the application of sleep measures represents an important diagnostic tool.

Other sleep investigations have dealt with the relationship of EEG sleep to the diagnostic "boundaries" of affective disorders. For example, two studies found that schizoaffective patients show shorter REM latency and sleep characteristics that are more consistent with a depressive disorder than a schizophrenic disorder.[11] One recent study demonstrated that borderline patients have REM latencies no different from affectively ill controls, but significantly different from nonaffective personality disorder controls.[12] Another boundary issue relates to the appropriate diagnosis of depressive disorders at both ends of the age spectrum—the adolescent or the elderly. Current studies indicate that adolescents, younger depressives (18–30 years old), and geriatric depressives often show the same EEG sleep changes as do middle-aged depressive patients. Finally, regarding the notion of medical-depressive disease, two separate independent studies have demonstrated that REM density is reduced in depressed patients with concurrent medical problems.[13]

An inverse relationship exists between clinical severity of depression and short REM latency; the application of a cutoff of 50 minutes for REM latency has demonstrated that 70–75% of patients diagnosed with primary depression are accurately identified.[6,13] Using an arbitrary cutoff of 50 minutes for REM latency, data from our 1976 study shows an 83% sensitivity and a 74% specificity.[14] These findings led us to question how age affected levels of sensitivity and specificity and whether a REM latency cutoff of 50 minutes was appropriate for all age groups. When the relationship of age and REM latency was examined in a sample of 87 depressed patients between 18 and 60 years a definite age trend was demonstrated for REM latency (Figure 1).[15] In fact, when this sample of 87 patients was used to generate specific centile estimates for REM latency in each age group by 5-year increments, it became clear that values obtained at one age range may not be comparable for another. Central estimates of REM latency ranged from 63.5 minutes in the youngest group to 23.9 minutes in the oldest.

The overall group of 87 patients was then separated into different subgroups for further analysis. The group of 67 nonpsychotic patients was compared to a group of 20 psychotic patients (Figure 2). In the younger group between ages 18 and 25, psychotic patients generally showed longer REM latencies than nonpsychotic patients. However, after the age of 40, psychotic patients demonstrated a decreased REM latency as compared to nonpsychotic patients. The age/REM latency correlations therefore showed a greater correlation coefficient in the psychotic population ($r = -.75$) than in the nonpsychotic population ($r = -.37$), even though both age/REM latency correlations are significant. Because the REM latency distribution is somewhat skewed, a joint estimate of the standard deviation for an entire age group or for a particular decade is unsatisfactory.* Such age-related curves could allow the construction of age correction factors, which may have even more value in their correlation with clinical

* In applying a suitable data transformation to remove skewness from the data set, we can improve the mean as a better estimate for central tendency by taking the initial square root of the REM latency, which then enables us to establish minutes from the joint estimate of standard deviation on the transformed measure.

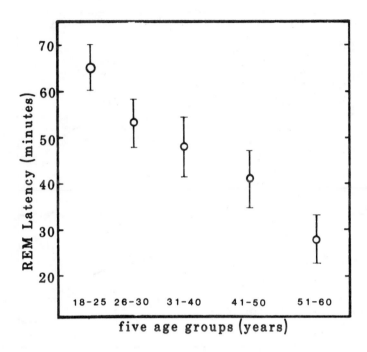

Figure 1   REM latency by age-group between 18 and 60 years (mean and standard deviation)
Note: n = 87.

diagnosis and outcome. It is interesting that sleep efficiency, reflecting wakefulness after the initial sleep onset, is age dependent, whereas sleep onset difficulty is not. The distinction has intriguing implications, since sleep onset difficulty in particular has been a key variable in predicting clinical treatment response. For the most part, there is some support for the speculation that EEG sleep in the majority of primary depressives mirrors "premature" aging, although better data are needed on REM latency in older normals. These age-corrected sleep measures will be very useful in the overall application of sleep measures for treatment response prediction. To summarize the possible methodological concerns about sex distribution, assuming control for the level of severity and age, there appear to be no major sex differences in the present state EEG sleep profile of a female or male depressed patient.

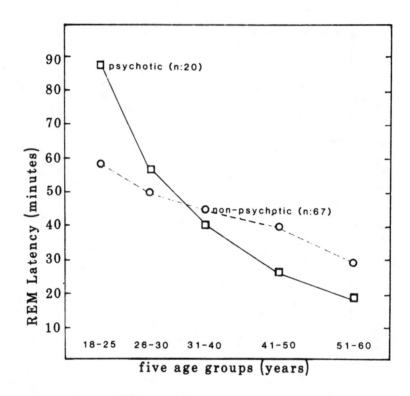

Figure 2 REM latency by age group and diagnosis
Note: n = 87.

The differential diagnosis of depression at any age can often be difficult, but this is particularly true of depression in the elderly. In line with increasing interest in depression among the elderly, particularly the differential diagnosis of depression versus pseudodementia, the EEG sleep characteristics were examined in a group of 18 depressed patients over the age of 60 who met Research Diagnostic Criteria (RDC) for a major depressive disorder.[16] The patients showed sleep features strikingly similar to those of patients with major depressive syndromes between the ages of 30 and 60: they had significantly reduced sleep continuity, shortened REM latency, and high REM density, suggesting that EEG sleep studies may be helpful in separating pseudodementia associated with depression from dementia in the elderly.

Whereas the number of hospitalized depressed younger adults has continued to increase, the characteristic sleep profile of a group of depressed patients in the second and third decades of life has now been examined, filling another gap in the age continuum. Preliminary findings regarding sleep characteristics in depressives between the ages of 18 and 30 suggest that sleep discontinuity and certain REM sleep parameters in the 34 patients studied differ from those reported in a more typical, older group of depressives.[17] We completed an investigation on 34 younger depressives (18–30 years old) and compared their sleep to an older group of 21 depressed patients (38–50 years old). All patients were drug-free for 2 weeks and hospitalized for treatment of a primary depression. As shown in Table 2, with respect to sleep differences, sleep efficiency was significantly lower among the older group ($p < .01$) as was the amount of delta sleep

Table 2 A Comparison of EEG Sleep in Young Depressives with Older Depressives

	Younger Depressives Age 18–30 years (n = 34) Mean + SEM	Older Depressives Age 38–50 years (n = 21) Mean + SEM	P
Sleep Continuity Measures			
Sleep latency (min.)	38.1 ± 3.6	44.3 ± 6.0	NS
Early morning awakening (min.)	7.8 ± 4.2	26.3 ± 7.5	.05
Awake (min.)	10.9 ± 2.7	33.5 ± 5.7	.001
Time spent asleep (TSA) (min.)	342.2 ± 7.5	303.8 ± 10.2	.01
Awake/TSA (%)	3.7 ± 1.0	13.0 ± 3.4	.01
TSA/total recording period (sleep efficiency) (%)	85.8 ± 1.7	74.7 ± 2.6	.001
Non-REM Sleep Measures			
Stage 1 sleep (%)	8.2 ± 0.6	10.1 ± 0.7	NS
Stage 2 sleep (%)	62.4 ± 1.5	63.4 ± 1.4	NS
Stage 3 sleep (%)	3.9 ± 0.9	0.3 ± 0.2	.001
Stage 4 sleep (%)	0.4 ± 0.3	0.0 ± 0.0	NS
Delta (stage 3 & 4) sleep (%)	4.4 ± 1.1	0.3 ± 0.2	.001
REM sleep in stage 2 (%)	1.3 ± 0.2	2.0 ± 0.5	NS
REM Sleep Measures			
REM latency (min.)	58.7 ± 3.6	44.4 ± 5.4	.05
REM sleep time (RT) (min.)	81.8 ± 4.1	73.3 ± 4.7	NS
REM sleep (%)	23.7 ± 1.1	24.2 ± 1.3	NS
REM activity (units)	105.9 ± 9.9	112.0 ± 16.3	NS
Average REM activity (RA/TSA)	0.31 ± 0.03	0.37 ± .05	NS
REM density (RA/RT)	1.24 ± 0.08	1.47 ± .12	NS
Number of REM periods	3.5 ± 0.1	3.5 ± .2	NS

(p < .001). It should be noted, however, that even in the younger group, 53% of the patients showed no stage 3 or stage 4 sleep and 82% showed no stage 4 sleep. REM sleep revealed only two significant differences between the two groups: REM latency, although clearly shortened in the younger depressives, was significantly shorter in the older group (p < .05); and REM density (RA/RT) in the first REM period was significantly greater in the older group (p < .01). Specifically, the data indicate that those sleep variables most "age sensitive" are a sleep efficiency measure reflecting the amount of sleep continuity after sleep onset (which is highest in the younger populations with a marked and dramatic decrease from age 31 on), REM latency, and REM density (REM activity/REM time), during the first REM period. REM density in the first REM period is lower in depressed patients under age 30, with a slight increase between 31 and 40 years, and a marked increase after age 40. Because the clinical picture of depression may vary depending upon age and developmental level, similar studies are needed in depressed children and adolescents. To date, few cases of EEG sleep have been published for this age group.[18,19]

Since there has been increasing interest in developing more homogenous groups for biological research studies as a method by which to validate biological correlates in the affective disorders, we sought to identify a subgroup of patients who would be most likely to demonstrate short REM latency. Our previous studies of nondelusional patients suggested this sleep abnormality would be most prominent in the primary endogenous (definite) subgroup as defined by RDC.[20] To aid in the identification of this group we included the additional criterion of at least one previous episode of depression. We then divided the group of 67 nonpsychotic patients into a subgroup of patients who met criteria for a definite endogenous, primary depression (at least two episodes) and a subgroup without this criterion. When the five age groups were reexamined (Figure 3) between the two subgroups, REM latency in the "pure" endogenous group was significantly reduced (p < .04) compared to the nonendogenous group; but just as important, REM latency seemed to be level within this group with little overall change over a 25-year age span (age 26–50). That is, REM latency varied only approximately 5 minutes from a mean of 44 minutes to 39 minutes over this age span. Clinical features separated by using this typology of endogenous recurrent subtype suggested that such endogenous patients showed high levels of agitation and anxiety, as well as a definite trend toward a poorer clinical response. Further investigations relating clinical response to tricyclic antidepressants in this particular subgroup of depressed patients are currently under way.

The examination of endogenous and other subtypes of depression in relation to objective sleep variables occupied our attention as we looked at a group of 115 nondelusional depressed patients. This group was diagnosed

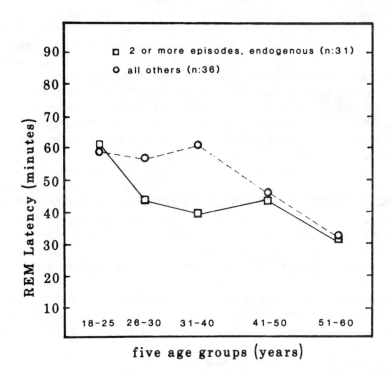

Figure 3 REM latency by age group and diagnosis in non-psychotics
Note: n = 67.

as having a definite RDC diagnosis of endogenous disorder. They were further broken down into a group of individuals who either were agitated, retarded—psychomotor retardation—or diagnosed as having both disorders. Here we were particularly interested in the differential contribution to sleep disturbance for such patients, with particular emphasis on REM latency, as well as some of the other variables that have been examined while looking at sleep disturbance in depression. For example, the mean REM latency in the entire group of nondelusional patients was 45.6 minutes. An endogenous patient with the age covaried subtracted only .3 minutes from the overall group mean REM latency. Similarly, psychomotor retardation subtracted only .6 minutes. However, adding the contribution of agitation significantly reduced mean REM latency to 40.6 minutes, so the major contribution to "reduced" REM latency in a group of nondelusional patients is the factor of agitation. Another technique is to examine the 115 patients by a three-way ANOVA, controlling for age and determining what contributions are made specifically by endogenosity, agitation, and retardation. The following was demonstrated: for overall sleep continuity disturbance, the major contribution is made by patients who are endogenous, particularly for sleep efficiency, sleep maintenance, and wakefulness. Endogeny has a strong relationship to REM intensity, both from overall nightly REM intensity and the REM activity and REM density of the first REM period. On the other hand, if one examines the contribution of agitation alone, the following emerges: the REM latency seems to be a major contribution emerging from agitation, as is the contribution of the stage 1 sleep (percent), and the amount of stage 2 REM (percent). Finally, reduced delta sleep appears most related to the contribution of agitation. With respect to retardation, the major finding was the significant inverse relationship to percent wakefulness. These results are consistent with the clinical data that agitation may be more negatively related to clinical response than either retardation, endogeny, or both.

While the evidence supporting the presence of REM sleep abnormalities in depressive episodes is well accepted, the data are based primarily on manual scoring techniques rather than automated procedures.[21] In a sense, these findings are comparable to a macroscopic view of sleep rather than a more microscopic examination. Some sleep laboratories have recently been applying automated REM techniques that count the actual number of rapid eye movements during the night.[22] Using an automated REM analyzer, two preliminary studies have demonstrated that actual REM count frequencies represent a useful measure in characterizing the sleep of depressed patients. The first report on three automated aspects of REM sleep (REM size, REM count frequency, and REM sleep time), in 35 drug-free depressed patients showed that while REM sleep time was not different in individual REM periods, the average size of a rapid eye movement increased as the night progressed.[22] However, in contrast to what has been reported in normal populations, REM count frequency in the depressed patients appeared to be higher during the first REM period, significantly decreased from the first to the second, and then remained constant throughout the remainder of the night.[23] In another group of 23 nonpsychotic patients with primary depression examined during a drug-free period and amitriptyline administration, the initial drug administration (50 mg amitriptyline for two nights) was associated with an immediate reduction in the number, average frequency, and average size of the rapid eye movement.[24] While the average REM size remained suppressed with continued drug administration (200 mg amitriptyline for two weeks), the average REM count frequency showed a rebound that was responsible for a partial recovery of the total number of REMs during the night.

Stimulated by these findings, we next studied in a more microscopic fashion the REM count frequency (or REM rhythm) contained within each individual REM period in a new group of 28 nonpsychotic depressed patients (Table 3). The clinical characteristics of the 28 patients, all primary unipolar nonpsychotic depressed inpatients, showed a mean age of 36.9 (12.9) with an initial Hamilton Depression Rating Scale (HDRS) of 37.1 (7.3). Twenty of the patients were females and the remaining 8 were males. Their median length of the current episode was 32 weeks, and the median number of previous episodes was 2. Twelve of these patients had a clear-cut clinical response at the end of 4 weeks of treatment (HDRS [sum of two raters] < 12), whereas 8 of the remaining 16 patients were partial responders (HDRS = 13–20), and the 8 final patients were definite nonresponders (HDRS > 20). When the baseline sleep data was examined in the 28 patients (Table 3), the sleep of these nonpsychotic depressed patients was similar to the sleep of the patients in previous examinations, demonstrating a sleep efficiency of 85% with several awakenings through-

Table 3 EEG Sleep Characteristics of 28 Primary, Nonpsychotic Unipolar Depressives

	Baseline
Sleep Continuity	
Total recording period (min.)	403.2 (22.9)
Sleep latency	29.0 (15.2)
Early morning awakening (min.)	15.7 (34.6)
Awake (min.)	17.3 (21.3)
Time spent asleep (min.)	341.4 (42.1)
Awake/time spent asleep (A/TSA)	5.9 (8.4)
Sleep efficiency (%)	84.9 (10.4)
Sleep maintenance (%)	91.6 (11.7)
Sleep Architecture	
Percent of stage 1	6.1 (3.9)
Percent of stage 2	62.9 (7.3)
Percent of delta	1.8 (3.9)
Percent of 1 REM	28.1 (4.9)
Percent of 2 REM	1.1 (1.1)
REM Measures	
REM latency (min.)	41.7 (19.5)
REM activity (units)	138.3 (52.4)
REM intensity (RA/TSA)	41.4 (17.9)
REM density (RA/RT)	146.2 (54.7)
Number of REM periods	3.6 (.8)

out the night. With respect to their sleep architecture, they showed a considerable decrease in delta sleep and a 28% increase in REM sleep. The group had a REM latency of almost 42 minutes and an average of 3.6 REM periods.

This recent effort to characterize the shape of each of the first three REM periods in a group of depressed patients demonstrates that during the baseline period prior to drug treatment, the first REM period has a rather flat profile, with no difference between the first- and second-half slopes (Figure 4). In contrast, the slopes of the second and third REM periods are downhill; thus, a gradual decrease in REM counts between the two halves of the REM period is featured. When the length of the REM period is examined, the first REM period maintains a level REM slope regardless of its length. The second REM period shows a downhill slope if the REM period is greater than 16 minutes. Likewise, the third REM period has a

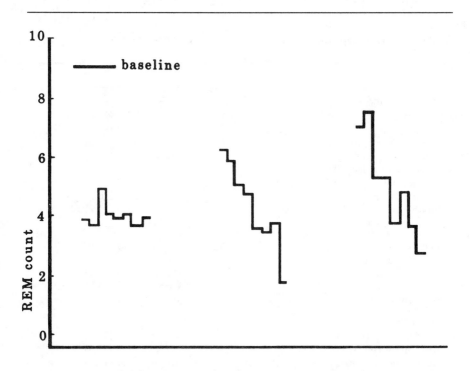

Figure 4 Average REM count by decile for 28 subjects (baseline) profile of sleep during first three REM periods

Table 4 Automated REM Activity

	Baseline	
	First Half[a]	Second Half[b]
Nonresponders	6.6(3.8)	6.2(3.8)
Partial Responders	4.2(2.8)	2.8(2.5)
Responders	<u>5.0(3.5)</u>	<u>3.3(2.8)</u>
Average	5.2(3.4)	3.9(3.0)

[a] Average REM activity during first half of the first three REM periods.
[b] Average REM activity during second half of the first three REM periods.

downhill slope (most of them were between 31 and 60 minutes, especially if the REM period was greater than 15 minutes). Indeed, the shapes of the second- and third-REM periods in the group of depressed patients is rather similar.

When the group of 28 patients is divided in terms of clinical response to drug treatment, the second half of the REM period is different in the nonresponders as compared to the partial and complete responders ($p < .05$, Table 4). This continued "high" rate of REM counts is particularly prominent in the first- and third-REM periods in the nonresponder group, especially in the second half of the REM period. Furthermore, the final Hamilton score correlated with the second half REM measure ($r = .46$, $p < .02$). These preliminary findings suggest that the characteristic shape of the REM period might eventually be used for identification of changes in REM architecture, for a more precise delineation of REM sleep abnormalities in depression, and also, perhaps, as a predictor of clinical response.

These results demonstrate that, even as late as 6 hours into the night (e.g., during a third REM period), significant differences among depressed patients are present among responder groups. The level of REM intensity shown by the nonresponders is pervasive throughout the REM period, rather than declining in REM count output as the REM period continues in length (Figure 5). Furthermore, it points out that the previous emphasis on the first hour or two of the night may be premature.

A preliminary analysis is available on a larger sample of the 74 patients treated with amitriptyline in a standardized manner. All patients were studied with automated REM activity during a drug-free interval and studied again while they were receiving 50 mg, 150 mg, and 200 mg of amitriptyline. When the clinical characteristics of the group were examined, 68 of the 74 often were unipolar, 53 were diagnosed definitely endogenous, 48 with a recurrent unipolar disease, and 6 were considered to

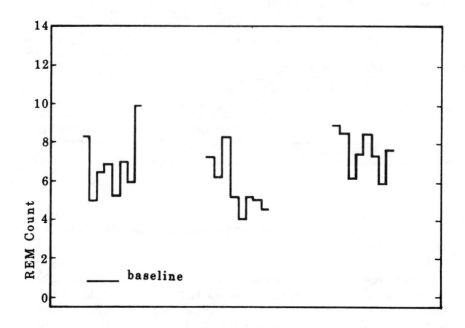

Figure 5 Average REM count by decile for eight non-responders profile of sleep during first three REM periods

be delusional depressives. The group's mean age was 37.3 (12.9) with an initial Hamilton Rating score of 37.2 (8.3). Forty-nine of the patients were females and 25 were males. The median length of their current episode was 30.5 weeks and the median number of previous episodes was 2.2. Twenty-two of the patients had a clear-cut clinical response at the end of 4 weeks of treatment (HDRS [sum of two raters] < 12), whereas 29 of the remaining 52 patients were partial responders (HDRS = 13-20) and the 23 final patients were definite nonresponders (HDRS ≥ 20). The baseline sleep of these 74 depressed patients included some difficulty falling asleep, with considerable intermittent wakefulness, and an overall sleep efficiency of 82.6% (Table 5). A somewhat elevated stage 1 percent was present in their sleep architecture, along with a considerable decrease in stage 3 and stage 4 sleep, as well as an increase in stage 2 REM with 1.1 percent. The overall REM latency was 44.8 minutes with an increase in REM activity (126.2 units) and REM density and an average of 3.5 REM periods. The initial analysis for these studies was not concerned with the within REM period distribution, but rather the all-night time period divided into sleep hours, or so-called hourly REM activity. In addition to reviewing hourly average activity we also examined the first half of the night versus the second half of the night. The major data analytic technique involved ANOVA with repeated measures.

An examination of the hourly REM activity count showed no significant effects for response groups and a barely significant effect at the .05 level between hourly distribution. When the interaction of hours and response was examined, however, the interaction was significant ($F = 2.28$; $p < 01$). This significant value was primarily due to the linear trend ($F = 4.95$; $p < .01$). The REM activity was then examined by halves of the night. When considering the overall sample of halves of the night alone, there were no significant effects. However, the interaction between response and halves was quite significant ($F = 6.04$; $p < .004$). An examination of this significant effect demonstrated that the interaction was largely because nonresponders had a decrease in their REM activity in the second half of the night, whereas responders and partial responders showed an increase in their REM activity in the second half of the night as compared to the first half (Table 6).

Table 5 EEG Sleep Measures in 74 Depressed Patients

	Baseline
Sleep Continuity	
Total recording (min.)	404.5 (21.3)
Sleep latency	37.5 (21.2)
Early morning awakening (min.)	12.3 (19.1)
Awake (min.)	20.8 (22.6)
Time spent asleep (min.)	333.8 (34.5)
Awake/time spent asleep (A/TSA × 100)	1.7 (8.7)
Sleep efficiency (%)	82.6 (8.7)
Sleep maintenance (%)	91.2 (8.4)
Sleep Architecture	
Percent of stage 1	7.3 (3.6)
Percent of stage 2	62.9 (7.3)
Percent of delta	1.7 (3.5)
Percent of stage 1 REM	26.7 (1.6)
Percent of stage 2 REM	1.1 (1.6)
REM Measures	
REM latency (min.)	44.8 (20.6)
REM activity (units)	126.2 (52.9)
REM intensity (RA/TSA)	37.9 (15.6)
REM density (RA/RT)	140.8 (48.4)
Number of REM periods	3.5 (.6)

Table 6 Automated REM Activity

	Baseline			
	Non-Responders (22)	Partial Responders (29)	Responders (23)	Total (74)
First half[a]	2.54 ± 1.67	1.56 ± 0.91	1.63 ± 1.10	1.87 ± 1.29
Second half[b]	1.91 ± 1.05	2.09 ± 1.21	1.94 ± 1.17	1.99 ± 1.14

[a] Average REM activity during first three hours of sleep.
[b] Average REM activity during second three hours of sleep.

The application of automated REM techniques has identified a number of new baseline REM measures that may be useful in predicting clinical response. Prior to this time, these variables had not been examined because the technical advances necessary in order to examine the sleep of depressed patients in a more microscopic fashion were lacking.

If diagnostic issues have represented one major advance, the other side of the coin, treatment response, has also shown a great deal of progress.[26] Several studies involving over 100 depressed patients have pointed out that the presence of a very short REM latency at baseline is a poor indicator of clinical response. Seventy percent of those depressed patients with an REM latency of 20 minutes or less were nonresponders to amitriptyline as compared to only 32% of depressed patients with an REM latency of greater than 20 minutes at baseline. If they are delusional, these patients may represent the groups who require electroconvulsive treatment (ECT). Based on such data, it appears that the delusional patients showing REM latency between 21 and 70 minutes respond to the combination of tricyclics and antipsychotic compounds. In our experience, if patients are nondelusional, patients with less than an 80% sleep efficiency may respond positively to tricyclic antidepressants, and those with greater than an 80–85% sleep efficiency often show the best clinical response to the administration of monoamine oxidase inhibitors. Finally, we would argue that the group of patients whose REM latency is greater than 70 minutes may in fact require psychotherapy or some other kind of psychosocial intervention. And, if such patients are delusional, they may require ECT as well as the use of antipsychotic compounds. One final point in the direction of the generalizability of such techniques is examining who ultimately required ECT, whether psychotic or nonpsychotic, on the basis of an amitriptyline protocol. The group least responsive to amitriptyline on the pharmacologic probe turned out to be the group that later required ECT. However, this does not mean that all tricyclic probes will necessarily operate in the same fashion. In order to better understand such clinical–sleep relationships, we need to examine what the long-term sleep effect may be; that is, what is responsible for the prolonged REM latency, 6 months, 1 year, or 2 years after taking medication in terms of signs of relapse.

However, baseline measures may not provide as much information as the application of a pharmacological probe in the early treatment period. In three separate studies, changes in sleep onset difficulty and the rapidity with which REM sleep suppression occurs were significantly related to clinical response.[26] One interpretation of these findings is that changes in lengthening REM latency represent a necessary but insufficient condition for clinical improvement. However, changes in REM sleep distribution are more significantly related to treatment responsiveness and may reflect the sufficient condition for clinical improvement. Further studies examining these questions are currently being pursued in several independent research settings.

Our approach with regard to EEG sleep abnormalities is based on the premise that many of the core symptoms of affective disorders such as sleep disturbance represent alterations in regulatory systems. These explorations for markers of vulnerability and assessment of the interdependencies among aspects of biological and psychological functioning will yield significant data that could advance our understanding of depressive disorders. These studies, therefore, could help us to establish a more accurate nomenclature of affective disorders, to determine with a greater precision choices of treatment, and to identify earlier signs of relapse or recurrence.

References

1. Kupfer DJ and Frank E. "Depression." In *Current Concepts.* Upjohn Company: Kalamazoo, MI, 1981.

2. Hawkins DR. Sleep and depression. *Psychiat Annals* 9:391–401, 1979.

3. Mendelson WB, Gillin JC, and Wyatt RJ. *Human Sleep and Its Disorders.* New York: Plenum Press, 1977.

4. Kupfer DJ and Foster FG. Interval between onset of sleep and rapid eye movement sleep as an indicator of depression. *Lancet* 11:684–86, 1972.

5. Kupfer DJ. REM latency: A psychobiologic marker for primary depressive disease. *Biol Psychiat* 11:159–74, 1976.

6. Gillin JC et al. Successful separation of depressed, normal and insomniac subjects by EEG sleep data. *Arch Gen Psychiat* 36:85N-90, 1979.

7. Rush AJ et al. Sleep EEG and dexamethasone suppression test findings in outpatients with unipolar major depressive disorders. *Biol Psych* 17:327–41, 1982.

8. Feinberg M et al. EEG studies of sleep in the diagnosis of depression. *Biol Psych* 17:305–16, 1982.

9. Akiskal HS et al. Differentiation of primary affective illness from situational, symptomatic and secondary depression. *Arch Gen Psychiat* 36:635–43, 1979.

10. Akiskal HS et al. Characterological depressions: Clinical and sleep EMG findings separating "subaffective dysthymias" from "character-spectrum disorders." *Arch Gen Psychiat* 37:777–83, 1980.

11. Kupfer DJ et al. EEG sleep and affective disorders: I schizoaffective disorders. *Psychiat Res* 1:173–78, 1979.

12. Akiskal HS. Subaffective disorders: Dysthymic, cyclothymic and bipolar II disorders in the "borderline" realm. *Psychiatric Clinics of North America* 4:25–46, 1981.

13. Kupfer DJ et al. The application of EEG sleep for the differential diagnosis of affective disorders. *Am J Psychiat* 135:69–74, 1978.

14. Coble PA, Foster FG, and Kupfer DJ. Electroencephalographic sleep diagnosis of primary depression. *Arch Gen Psychiat* 33:1124–27, 1976.

15. Ulrich RF, Shaw DH, and Kupfer DJ. The effects of aging on sleep. *Sleep* 3:131–41, 1980.

16. Kupfer DJ et al. Electroencephalographic sleep recordings and depression in the elderly. *J Am Geriat Soc* 26:53–57, 1978.

17. Coble PA et al. EEG sleep and clinical characteristics in young primary depressives. *Sleep Res* 10:165, 1980.

18. Kane J et al. EEG sleep in a child with severe depression. *Am J Psychiat* 134:813–14, 1977.

19. Kupfer DJ et al. Imipramine and EEG sleep in children with depressive symptoms. *Psychopharma* 60:117–23, 1979.

20. Spitzer RL, Endicott J, and Robins E. Research diagnostic criteria: Rationality and reliability. *Arch Gen Psychiat* 38:773–80, 1980.

21. McPartland RJ and Kupfer DJ. Rapid eye movement sleep cycle, clock time and sleep onset. *EEG Clin Neurophysiol* 45:178–85, 1978.

22. McPartland RJ et al. REM sleep in primary depression: A computerized analysis. *EEG Clin Neurophysiol* 44:513–17, 1978.

23. Aserinsky E. Rapid eye movement density and patterns in the sleep of normal young adults. *Psychophysiol* 8:361–76, 1971.

24. McPartland RJ et al. An automated analysis of REM sleep in primary depression. *Biol Psychiat* 14:767–76, 1979.

25. Kupfer DJ et al. Application of automated REM analysis in depression. *Arch Gen Psychiat* 39:569–73, 1982.

26. Kupfer DJ et al. "Recent Diagnostic and Treatment Advances in REM Sleep and Depression." In *Treatment of Depression: Old Controversies and New Approaches,* edited by Clayton P and Barrett J. New York: Raven Press, 1982. pp 31–52.

8

Faster Cholinergic REM Sleep Induction As a Possible Trait Marker of Affective Illness

Natraj Sitaram, M.D.

The notable similarity of the sleep of depressed patients and the effect of cholinergic stimulation upon sleep points to a possible biological marker for affective disorders.[1-6] Animal studies have suggested that cholinergic mechanisms specifically mediate the cycles of rapid eye movement (REM) and non-REM sleep (Figures 1 and 2). Local injections of carbachol or physostigmine into the brain stem of cats induce REM sleep.[7,8] Conversely, anticholinergic drugs and hemicholinium-3, an acetylcholine synthesis inhibitor, suppress REM sleep in animals.[7,9] Data from single cell recordings in head-restrained cats suggest that neurons within the fastigial tegmental gigantocellular field (FTG) may be the "executive" cells for REM sleep and that they interact reciprocally with locus coeruleus (LC) and raphe neurons (Figure 3). The FTG cells are cholinoceptive and possibly cholinergic too, as indicated by prolonged periods of REM sleep that can be induced by local administration of extremely small amounts of carbachol.[8] REM sleep in cats has been eliminated by means of bilateral FTG lesions.[10]

In earlier work we suggested a relationship between activation of central cholinergic neurons or supersensitive cholinergic receptors and the pathophysiology of sleep disturbance in depression.[11] Such a relationship is consistent with the hypothesis that an increased ratio of cholinergic to nonadrenergic activity underlies depression.[12]

We have compared patients whose primary affective disorder was in remission, with normal control subjects on the cholinergic REM-induction test. The method for sleep EEG recordings with simultaneous intravenous administration of drugs has been described.[13] Briefly, all-night recording of EEG, EOG (electrooculogram), and EMG (electromyogram) is begun at

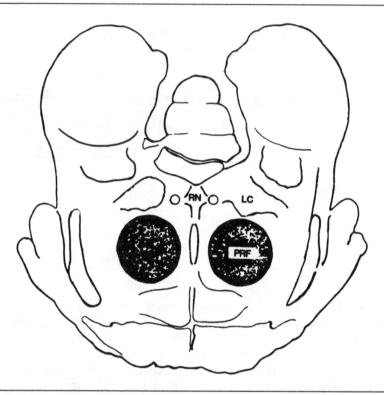

Figure 1 The anatomy of the pontine brain stem

Note: On this frontal section of the cat brain stem, the cells that are selectively activated during REM sleep (also called D-sleep) are in the paramedian reticular formation (PRF) (fastigial tegmental gigantocellular field), while the cells that are selectively inactivated lie more dorsally (in the region of the locus coeruleus [LC]) and medially (in the region of the raphe nuclei [RN]).

about 11:30 P.M. and the patients are awakened at 7:00 A.M. After a night of adaptation and a baseline (noninfusion), night subjects slept with an intravenous catheter throughout the night. The subject's vein is kept open with a slow drip of normal saline, which permits drug infusions at the appropriate times without waking the subject. On each night the subjects received two infusions: the first of methscopolamine (.3–.5 mg), a peripheral anticholinergic administered at the end of the first REM period; and a second infusion of either arecoline or placebo, randomized, about 25 minutes after the end of the first REM period. Pharmacological response was measured by the time from infusion to the onset of the second REM period (Inf-REM$_2$ latency).

The patients we selected for the trial were 15 normal volunteers; 17 patients with remitted primary affective disorder; 7 hospitalized patients with primary affective disorder; and 5 apparently normal volunteers, but who, upon screening with ·the Schedule for Affective Disorder and Schizophrenia-Lifetime Version[14] were found to have either a personal or family history of affective disorder. Of the 17 patients in remission, 9 had discontinued their medication 2–4 weeks prior to the test, 4 had been drug free for 4 months, and 4 had never received any somatic treatment. The hospitalized patients were maintained drug free for 2 weeks prior to the study.

Our results showed that arecoline induced REM sleep significantly more rapidly in remitted and in depressed patients than in normals (Figure 4). The values for the "normal" subjects with affective history was somewhat faster but not significantly different from those of normals.[13,15]

We designated "responders" as subjects with Inf-REM latency of 19.5 minutes or less and "nonresponders" as subjects with Inf-REM latency of

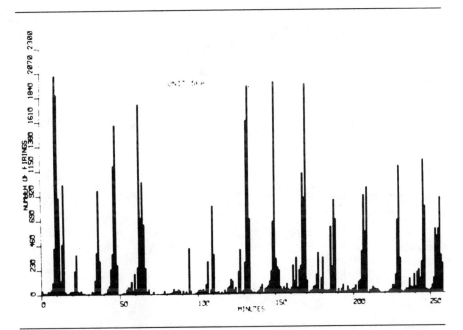

Figure 2 Discharge activity of FTG neuron 568 recorded over multiple sleep-waking cycles

Source: Reproduced with the permission of R. W. McCarley and Raven Press.

Note: Each discharge peak corresponds to a D-sleep (REM sleep) episode. Note the regular time course of activity: the peak in D, and abrupt drop after D ends (usually associated with waking), a gradual buildup of activity, and then an explosive increase that occurs just before D-sleep onset. The periodicity of discharge is evident even in this raw data sample using one minute bins. Small peaks correspond to abortive D-sleep episodes.

more than 19.5 minutes. Only 20% of the normal volunteers responded to arecoline (Table 1), compared to 82% of the remitted affectives ($p < .01$) (Fisher's exact probability test), 71% of depressed affectives ($p = .03$), and 80% of subjects with a personal or family history of affective disorders ($p = .03$). There were three false-positive arecoline responders in the normal group who had not differed in any way from the nonresponders on the initial interview, nor on any of the follow-up interviews.

Among the 5 normal volunteers with a strong affective component, 4 responded to arecoline, one had postpartum depression but no family

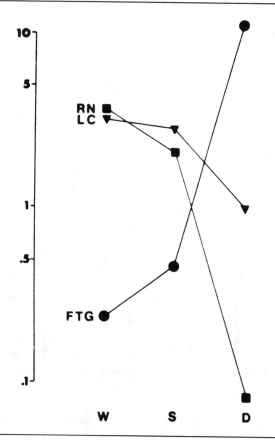

Figure 3 Pooled geometric mean discharge rates for populations of 34 giant cell field (FTG) neurons (circles), 21 locus coeruleus (LC) neurons (triangles), and 18 dorsal raphe nucleus (RN) neurons (squares) during waking (W), synchronized sleep (S), and desynchronized sleep (D)

Source: Reproduced with the permission of R. W. McCarley and Raven Press.

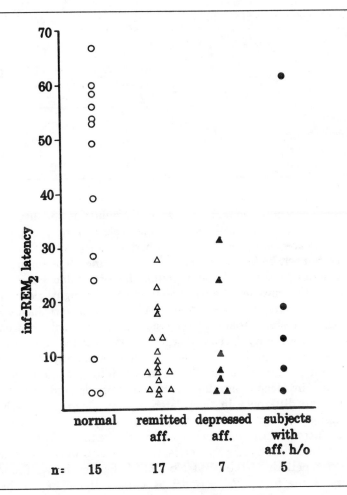

Figure 4 Arecoline REM-induction response
Note: The mean Inf-REM$_2$ + standard deviation for normals was 37.8 ± 23.2 minutes, for remitted affectives 11.6 ± 6.9 minutes (p <.01), *depressed* affectives 12.7 ± 7.2 minutes (p <.05), and subjects with affective history 2.18 ± 23.4 minutes ($p = ns$).

history of affective disorder and one had a depression secondary to major surgery for scoliosis. This latter volunteer experienced loss of interest in social activities and loss of energy for about 3 months, and her mother had been diagnosed as having unipolar depression with three suicide attempts. This patient had the shortest inf-REM$_2$ latency—only 3 minutes. A third subject had no personal history of depression but her mother had been hospitalized several times for depression and was a suicide. Another volunteer had no personal depressive history, but the father was hospital-

Table 1 Arecoline REM Induction as a Test of Affect Disorder

	Normals (N = 15)	Remitted Affectives (N = 17)	Depressed Affectives (N = 7)	"Normals" with Personal or Family History (N = 5)
Arecoline Responders	3	14	5	4
Arecoline Non-responders	12	3	2	1

ized for depression, the mother had a cyclothymic personality, and an aunt was reported to be an alcoholic. The sole subject in this group who did not respond to arecoline was a man who had volunteered as a normal control subject, but whose interview revealed two distinct depressions in the past, lasting about 3 weeks each, but no family history of depression.

Next we compared the baseline (noninfusion night) sleep EEG profile of remitted patients with normal volunteers. Hauri has shown that unipolar depressed patients in remission have a normal REM pattern, but their sleep continuity remains disturbed.[16] We wanted to investigate sleep patterns in remitted bipolar patients to see whether any of the characteristic sleep disturbances of the illness persist into remission. We found no difference in sleep continuity between normals and remitted bipolar patients; no difference in sleep latency, total sleep time, early morning awakening, intermittent awakening, delta sleep, or REM latency. There was an increase in REM percent among the remitted bipolar patients. In addition to overall sleep parameters, when we examined the breakdown of successive periods of the REM/Non-REM sleep cycle, we found that the density of the first REM period was statistically higher in the remitted bipolar patients (1.52 ± 0.41 units) as compared to normals (1.15 ± 0.3 units, $p < .05$). The duration and densities of the second and third REM periods were no different.[17]

At this point, we had two characteristics of remitted affective patients: (1) a *pharmacological* marker, namely, reduced latency to the second REM period in response to arecoline; and (2) a *physiological* one, namely, increased REM density in the first REM period. We found a significant correlation between sensitivity to arecoline and increased REM density in the first period among all 17 of our remitted affective patients ($r = .69$) as well as the 19 normals ($r = .52$) (Figure 5). In other words, higher REM_1 density predicts increased sensitivity to arecoline. There was, however, no correlation between $Inf-REM_2$ latency and REM latency; duration of the first REM period; duration of delta (stages 3 + 4) sleep; stage 1; stage 2; or awake/movement time prior to arecoline infusion. The strong and rather specific correlation between cholinergic sensitivity and the phasic component (REM density) of the first REM period may at first appear to be a fortuitous post-hoc finding. However, a review of the pertinent literature reveals a large body of data, suggesting that eye movements during sleep may indeed be controlled by cholinergic neurons in the pontine reticular formation and in the vestibular nuclei.[18] In addition, our data concerning the increased first REM density in remitted bipolar patients is in agreement with that of Schulz and Trojan.[19]

Some of the remitted affective patients and normal control subjects in the study reported in Table 1 also participated in a psychogenetics study by Drs. Nurnberger and Gershon, in which affective patients and normal controls were tested for sensitivity to IV amphetamine. Our test and the amphetamine challenge were about two months apart. Preliminary data indicate a significant negative correlation ($r = .76, p < .01, n = 10$) between the cholinergic REM induction and amphetamine-induced behavioral excitation response in these patients and subjects (J.I. Nurnberger et al.,

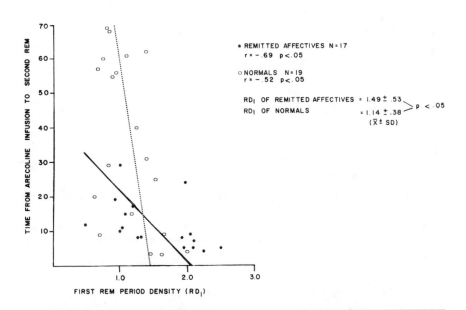

Figure 5 First REM period density correlates with arecoline response in normals and remitted affectives

unpublished data). Subjects who were supersensitive to cholinergic challenge were subsensitive to amphetamine-induced excitation. This suggests a balance between cholinergic and catecholaminergic sensitivity in humans.

The terms "super" and "subsensitivity" are used loosely, to indicate a physiological response consistent with a hypothesized increase or decrease of neurotransmitter activity; we performed no direct *in vivo* or *in vitro* binding studies. Nevertheless, our data derive from measuring a physiological endpoint, REM sleep, whose neurochemical underpinnings are well understood and whose dysregulation is central to the pathophysiology of depression. So far as it is possible to extrapolate information about receptor mechanisms from pharmacological challenges, our findings lead us to postulate a state-independent cholinergic hypersensitivity. We also found that anorexia nervosa patients with coexisting affective illness had a faster arecoline REM induction response than those without an affective component (N. Sitaram et al., unpublished data). Preliminary findings of enhanced cholinergic sensitivity in subjects with a family history of affective illness are also reported.

Finally, increased cholinergic sensitivity seems to correlate negatively with amphetamine-induced elation and excitation, which is consistent with reports that physostigmine attenuates the behavioral effects of amphetamine and methylphenidate in laboratory animals, reverses the methylphenidate-induced psychosis in schizophrenics, and has antimanic effects in manic patients.[12] Further studies in primary affective patients to elucidate the specific relationships between neurotransmitter receptor sensitives may well prove to identify important diagnostic and prognostic markers.

References

1. Kupfer DJ et al. The application of EEG sleep for the differential diagnosis of affective disorders. *Amer. J. Psychiatry* 135:69–74, 1978.

2. Vogel GW et al. Improvement of depression by REM sleep deprivation. *Arch. Gen. Psychiatry* 37:247–53, 1980.

3. Gillin JC et al. Successful separation of depressed, normal and insomniac subjects by EEG sleep data. *Arch. Gen. Psychiatry* 36:85–90, 1979.

4. Sitaram N et al. REM sleep induction by physostigmine infusion in normal volunteers. *Science* 191:1281–83, 1976.

5. Gillin JC, Sitaram N and Mendelson WB. Physostigmine alters onset but not duration of REM sleep in man. *Psychopharmacology* 58:111–14, 1978.

6. Sitaram N, Moore AM, and Gillin JC. The cholinergic induction of dreaming in man. *Arch. Gen. Psychiatry* 35:1239–43, 1978.

7. Jouvet M. Recherches sur les structures nerveuses et les mechanismes responsables des differentes phases due somneil physiologique. *Arch. Ital. Biol.* 13:285, 1962.

8. Amatruda TT et al. Sleep cycle control and cholinergic mechanisms: Differential effects of carbachol at pontine brain stem sites. *Brain Res* 98:501–15, 1975.

9. Domino EF and Stawinski M. Modification of the cat sleep cycle by hemicholinium-3, a cholinergic antisynthetic agent. *Res Commun Chem Path Pharmacol* 2:461–65, 1971.

10. Jones BE. Elimination of paradoxical sleep by lesions of the pontine gigantocellular tegmental field in the cat. *Neurosci. Letter* 13:285, 1979.

11. Gillin JC, Sitaram N, and Duncan WC Muscarinic supersensitivity: A possible model for the sleep disturbance of primary depression? *Psychiatr. Research* 1:17–22, 1979.

12. Janowsky DC, El-Yousef MK, and Davis JM. A cholinergic-adrenergic hypothesis of mania and depression. *Lancet* 2:632–35, 1972.

13. Sitaram N and Gillin JC. Development and use of pharmacological probes of the CNS in man. *Biol. Psychiatry* 15:925–55, 1980.

14. Endicott J and Spitzer RL. A diagnostic interview: The schedule for affective disorders and schizophrenia. *Arch. Gen. Psychiatry* 35:837–44, 1978.

15. Sitaram N et al. Faster REM sleep induction in remitted patients with primary affective illness. *Science* 208:200–2, 1980.

16. Hauri P et al. Sleep of depressed patients in remission. *Arch. Gen. Psychiatry* 31:386–91, 1974.

17. Sitaram N et al. Cholinergic regulation of mood and REM sleep: Potential model and marker of vulnerability to affective disorder. *Am J. Psychiatry* 139; 5, 571–76, 1982.

18. McCarley RW. "Mechanisms and Models of Behavioral State Control." In *The Reticular Formation Revisited,* edited by Hobson JA and Brazier MA. New York: Raven Press, 1980.

19. Schulz H and Trojan B. A comparison of eye movement density in normal subjects and in depressed patients before and after remission. *Sleep Res* 8:49, 1979.

The Diagnosis and Classification of Affective Disorders

Nancy C. Andreasen, M.D., Ph.D.

Major achievements have been made in the diagnosis and classification of affective disorders during the past 10 years. Whereas clinicians and researchers once despaired that adequate reliability could be achieved in evaluating symptoms or making diagnoses,[1-3] the development of structured interviews such as the Schedule for Affective Disorders and Schizophrenia (SADS) or Present State Exam (PSE) and the use of diagnostic criteria have demonstrated that psychiatrists can achieve a remarkably high level of agreement about the symptoms and illnesses from which their patients suffer.[4-12] Further, the *Third Diagnostic and Statistical Manual* of the American Psychiatric Association (*DSM-III*) has made some of these major advances part of the standard practice of most clinicians in the United States.[13]

Nevertheless, we should not be complacent and assume that all problems concerning diagnosis and classification have been resolved. Many important issues and controversies remain, particularly in the area of affective disorders.

It is useful to draw on the analogy of the remainder of medicine in order to highlight the problems in classification that persist. How are classifications of disease made in the rest of medicine? The standard approach is to subdivide diseases by organ system and then by types of derangements within the organ system. Applying this model to psychiatry, we can see how much confusion exists. What organ or organs are the province of psychiatry? Is it the brain? Or are psychiatrists concerned with both the brain and the various organs that it affects, ranging from the adrenals or thyroid through the gastrointestinal system to peripheral nerves and muscles? If it is the brain, then we must remind ourselves that the brain is not homogeneous as, for example, the liver is. Are we concerned with the entire brain or only a part of it, such as the cortex? We are only beginning to understand the relationships between various functional, anatomical, and neurochemical systems in the brain and how they may relate to psychiatry. Some psychiatrists may feel that the brain does not belong to us at all, but rather to neurology, and that the "psyche" alone is the concern of psychiatry. Others may argue that we should be concerned with the brain, the remainder of the body, and the environment in which they live.

One futuristic fantasy about classification in psychiatry might predict that some day textbooks of psychiatry will divide psychiatric diseases into those affecting the brain, those affecting other parts of the body, and those affecting interactions with the environment. At present, however, we certainly have no simple agreement about which of those areas, if any, is our proper domain. Further, whatever our domain, we have no definitive knowledge about the characteristic derangements occurring in it. Therefore, it is small wonder that there is so much controversy about the best approach to diagnosis and classification of the affective disorders.

The current approach to classification in psychiatry places its primary emphasis on clinical description rather than on diseases of specific organ systems. In practice, this means that disorders are classified into groups that share common clinical features, such as disorders of affect, disorders of thinking, or disorders of behavior. Thus, the affective disorders form a specific subset that shares a single common feature. They all involve an abnormality of mood or affect.

Research vs. Clinical Classifications

To understand some of the controversy concerning the diagnosis and classification of affective disorders, it is useful to explore some reasons behind it. Two reasons have already been mentioned. First, there is a philosophical controversy within our field concerning its proper area of concern. Second, at present we have no definitive knowledge concerning the causes of the disorders we are called upon to treat. A third reason is the tension that tends to exist between the needs of researchers and the needs of clinicians, and at times these needs even work at cross-purposes. These differences are summarized in Table 1.

Classifications designed to facilitate research have usually been developed in order to assist in the search for etiology. If that search places a major emphasis on biological correlates or causes, then the researcher usually needs to study very homogeneous groups. Otherwise positive results may be lost through the pooling of samples containing a great deal

Table 1 Research vs. Clinical Classifications

Research	Clinical
1. Homogeneous groups	1. Flexibility
2. Narrow definitions	2. Broad definitions
3. Many patients "undiagnosed"	3. Adequate coverage
4. Predictive validity	4. Predictive validity

of variance. Because biological research tends to be relatively costly, and therefore is often limited to relatively small samples, it is even more important that the groups be homogeneous. Homogeneous groups are usually achieved through the use of very narrow or restrictive definitions. If an investigator is primarily interested in research, then he can afford to have a system in which many patients are undiagnosed, since he is more interested in identifying pure samples than in classifying and treating every patient available. His ultimate goal is predictive validity: to be able to make a definitive statement about etiology, outcome, or response to treatment.

On the other hand, clinicians have very different needs. A clinician needs maximum flexibility rather than homogeneous groups. He must deal with patients as individuals and work with them in a broad context of symptoms and environment. Because clinicians must deal with large numbers of patients, they need adequate coverage in their diagnostic system so that each patient can be classified in some way. To achieve this flexibility and adequate coverage, they need relatively broad definitions of illnesses rather than narrow, restrictive ones. Nevertheless, the clinician and the researcher share one need in common. Both are eager to have a high degree of predictive validity.

Areas Of Consensus

While there is considerable controversy about the classification of affective disorders, nevertheless there are also important areas of consensus. General agreement has been reached in much of the psychiatric community concerning at least three things. First of all, both clinicians and researchers tend to agree that a distinction between bipolar and unipolar affective disorder is important and valid. This distinction has been supported by a wide variety of investigations, including genetic and family studies, neurophysiological studies, and neurochemical studies.[14-18] The two subtypes of affective disorder respond differentially to treatment and have a somewhat different outcome.[19-21] Although an occasional investigator has suggested that these two types of affective disorder may differ only in

137

severity,[22] most agree that they probably represent two distinct subtypes. The characteristics of these two subtypes will be discussed in more detail by Dr. Clayton in Chapter 13.

A second area of agreement is that affective disorders probably represent a heterogeneous cluster of disorders that have different causes and different clinical characteristics. In fact, as we shall see, much of the controversy concerning the diagnosis and classification of affective disorders turns on the best methods for further subtyping this heterogeneous grouping.

A third area of widespread agreement concerns the importance of biological factors in the affective disorders. While few think biological factors are the only cause of affective disorders or that they are the cause of all affective disorders, most agree that biological factors may contribute heavily to at least a subset of the affective disorders. The research in this area is discussed extensively in other chapters in this book.

Areas Of Debate

Although much consensus exists about the diagnosis and classification of affective disorders, there is also much debate. This debate has focused on three main areas. These include the limits of the concept, which methods of subtyping are most effective, and the relationship of phenomenology or "phenomenotype" to biological factors or "biotype."

Limits of the Concept

Clinicians and researchers are not yet in agreement as to how broad the category of affective disorders should be. During recent years, the concept of affective disorder has been broadened enormously at both ends. The nature of this broadening is illustrated in Table 2, which compares the *DSM-II* classification with *DSM-III*. In *DSM-II* the concept of affective disorders was limited largely to the more severe affective disorders, such as manic-depressive illness, psychotic depressive reaction, and involutional depression. Other milder affective illnesses such as depressive neurosis or cyclothymic personality were classified elsewhere and not included under the major concept of affective disorders. In *DSM-III*, all types of affective disorders have been brought together under a single heading and have been treated as a single concept. Thus, very mild conditions, or "subaffective disorders" as Akiskal refers to them in Chapter 15, are included in the concept. Furthermore, very severe disorders have also been included. Although the term schizoaffective disorder does not appear under the heading of Affective Disorders, many patients previously referred to as schizoaffective (and therefore classified as a type of schizophrenia in *DSM-*

Table 2   Affective Disorders: *DSM-II* vs. *DSM-III*

DSM-II	DSM-III
Psychoses	*Major Affective Disorders*
Manic-depressive	Bipolar
Manic	Manic
Depressed	Depressed
Circular	Mixed
Psychotic depressive reaction	Major depression
Involutional depression	Single episode
	Recurrent
Neuroses	Other specific affective disorders
	Dysthymic
Depressive	Cyclothymic
Personality Disorders	Atypical affective disorders
	Bipolar
Cyclothymic	Depression

II) are now diagnosed as having a major affective disorder with mood incongruent psychotic features.

The broadening of the concept of affective disorder has occurred for a variety of reasons. During the past 20 years, effective treatments such as lithium and tricyclic antidepressants have been developed. The availability of these treatments has led clinicians to search more carefully for evidence of affective disorders in their patients, since it is axiomatic in clinical medicine that one should search out and aggressively treat illnesses that are reversible or have a good prognosis. Whereas affective disorders have always had a better prognosis than schizophrenia, the recent development of effective treatments has further widened the differential between these two classes of disorders. Further, the drugs developed for the treatment of schizophrenia have recently been noted to have a variety of long-term adverse side effects such as tardive dyskinesia. This recognition has also led clinicians to tend to diagnose affective disorders preferentially.

While clinical pressures have led to a broadening of the concept, research pressures are beginning to recommend that the concept should be narrowed. As previously discussed, biological researchers in particular need to study narrowly defined homogeneous groups. If their samples are defined too broadly, then important findings may be lost because heterogenous disorders have been pooled. Using an excessively broad concept may also, however, be very risky for clinical work over the long run. For example, if the concept of depressive illness is made so broad that it includes simple unhappiness as well as "biological" depression, then many patients will be treated with somatic therapies such as tricyclics and will probably respond quite poorly. In addition to leading to confusing research on treatment and outcome, the inappropriate use of somatic therapy for simple unhappiness may lead to unnecessary side effects and decrease the credibility of clinicians because of poor predictive validity.

Diagnostic criteria were originally developed both to improve reliability and to define narrower concepts of illness. Three sets of criteria are currently in use in research and clinical work. These include the St. Louis Criteria, the Research Diagnostic Criteria (RDC), and the *DSM-III* Criteria. The St. Louis Criteria are the earliest and tend to be the most restrictive, but they also tend to have the least conceptual elegance because they *are* the earliest. The Research Diagnostic Criteria were developed as an offshoot of the St. Louis Criteria and represent a collaboration between Robins of St. Louis and Spitzer and Endicott of New York. The *DSM-III* Criteria were written as a result of collaboration between members of a subcommittee of the task force that wrote *DSM-III*. The specification of duration of symptoms is one primary method of narrowing or widening these criteria. The original St. Louis Criteria require 4 weeks of illness, the RDC 1 week, and *DSM-III* 2 weeks. The RDC and *DSM-III* provide additional criteria for defining various subtypes of affective disorder such as endogenous or psychotic. The RDC provides the broadest range of subtypes, a total of 10.

These various criteria have been used in research and clinical work for only a few years. Consequently, we are still trying to determine how effective they are in defining sufficiently narrow and homogeneous categories. During the past several years, some researchers have become concerned that the disorders defined by these criteria may still be too broad to be effective for biological research. As other discussions in this book indicate, researchers are beginning to restrict their work to narrower categories such as "endogenous" depression and are even beginning to seek methods for restricting the definition further.

Competing Sets of Subtypes

Although it seems clear that for some purposes narrower subtypes of depression must be defined, considerable disagreement exists concerning the best method for subtyping. At present a variety of competing systems is in existence. This discussion will focus primarily on subtypes of depression. Many of the competing methods for subtyping depression are summarized in Table 3. The most popular approach to subtyping, as Table 3 indicates, has been to develop simple dichotomies. Unfortunately, however, these dichotomies tend to be confusing because they are often similar but not equivalent, and differ by emphasizing various aspects of the disorder. For example, some approaches, such as mild *versus* severe, focus on the severity dimension. Others, such as chronic *versus* episodic or primary *versus* secondary, focus on course and chronology. Others, such as neurotic *versus* psychotic or agitated *versus* retarded, focus on cross-sectional symptoms. Some, such as biological *versus* characterological or familial *versus* spectrum, have etiological theories built in. The relationship between these subtypes is often unclear. For example, severe, psychotic, endogenous, and biological depression are often considered to be more or less synonymous, although frequently in actual practice they are not. Similar problems exist with an equation between mild, chronic, neurotic, and characterological depression.

Some of the controversy rests on underlying theoretical considerations and controversies. One such controversy is whether classification systems should be categorical or dimensional. The categorical approach to classification is used in most of medicine and conceptualizes illnesses as representing discrete disorders that differ from one another and from normality. A more dimensional approach is often suggested by investigators who apply more psychological or mathematical models. They conceptualize illnesses as consisting of a clustering of characteristics that are highly correlated with one another, that may overlap, and that may exist on a continuum with normality.

A related theoretical controversy is whether diagnostic systems should be hierarchical or overlapping. Hierarchical approaches to classification usually begin with a broad category and then develop further specific subtypes that are independent from one another. By and large, the *DSM-III* system and the St. Louis Criteria are hierarchical. The RDC are a blend of hierarchical and overlapping approaches. Some categories in the RDC, such as schizophrenia or mania, are mutually exclusive. On the other hand, most categories in the RDC may overlap with one another. Thus, a single patient may be diagnosed as having many different subtypes of depression, such as bipolar, endogenous, psychotic, secondary, and situational. Most hierarchical approaches would not permit this system of diagnosis.

At the present time, none of these theoretical approaches should be

Table 3 Subtypes of Depression

- Mild vs. severe
- Chronic vs. episodic
- Neurotic vs. psychotic
- Reactive vs. endogenous
- Primary vs. secondary
- Bipolar vs. unipolar
- Agitated vs. retarded
- Biological vs. characterological
- Familial vs. spectrum

considered preeminent. Investigators should select the theoretical approach appropriate to the kind of research questions that they are asking. Often dimensional and overlapping approaches are particularly useful for nosological research, which attempts to explore the relationship between various illnesses and various subtypes of illnesses. On the other hand, hierarchical and categorical approaches are often more useful in biologically oriented research, which seeks narrowly defined homogeneous categories.

If an hierarchical approach to classification is used, problems remain. At present, several different ways to subdivide affective disorders hierarchically are in use. These are summarized in Figures 1 through 3. The hierarchical schema appearing in Figure 1 probably represents a fairly accurate portrayal of how most clinicians and researchers actually think about the subtyping of affective disorder. In this hierarchical schema, the first subdivision is into bipolar and unipolar, because of the wide acceptance that this particular distinction enjoys. Bipolar disorders are

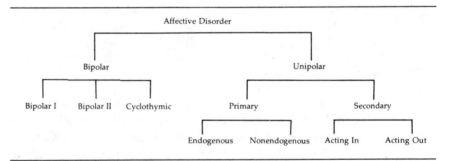

Figure 1   One hierarchical schema

further subdivided on the basis of severity into Bipolar I, Bipolar II, and cyclothymic disorder. The unipolar disorders are further subdivided into primary and secondary, depending on whether the patient has had an antecedent psychiatric diagnosis. If affective disorder is the patient's first illness and he is designated as primary, then the disorder is further subtyped into endogenous or nonendogenous on the basis of characteristic symptoms and severity. Secondary patients can often be classified on the basis of their antecedent diagnoses. If they have had diagnoses that represent a high degree of internalization, such as anxiety or phobic disorders, then they might be considered to represent an "acting-in group," while those who have antecedent diagnoses such as antisocial personality form an "acting-out group."

Alternate schema appear in Figures 2 and 3. Figure 2 portrays the schema used in *DSM-III*. In this system, the first main subdivision is into

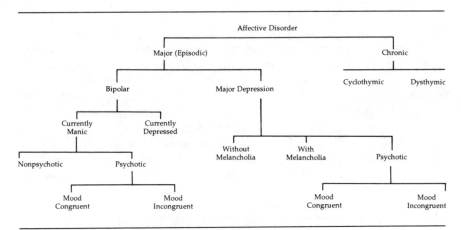

Figure 2   An alternate hierarchical schema (*DSM-III*)

major disorders, which tend to be episodic, and into chronic disorders. The major disorders are further subdivided on the basis of a history of mania. Those patients who are currently manic or have previously been manic are classified as bipolar, while those patients who have never experienced mania are classified as major depression. The bipolar disorders are further subdivided on the basis of current symptoms into currently depressed, currently manic, or currently mixed. If the current episode involves depression, then patients are further subclassified into those who are psychotic, those with melancholia, and those without melancholia. In this

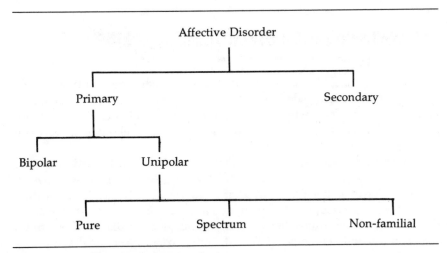

Figure 3   An alternate hierarchical schema

classification system "melancholia" is roughly synonymous with endogenous. Psychotic patients are further subdivided into those with mood congruent features and those with mood incongruent features. A similar subdivision occurs in the patients with mania, but of course without the distinction between those with and without melancholia. The chronic disorders are subdivided into those that are cyclothymic, representing mild forms of bipolar disorder, and those that are dysthymic, representing mild forms of unipolar disorder. It should be noted, however, that the *DSM-III* classification is not a pure hierarchy, since the major or episodic disorders and the chronic disorders may overlap with one another. That is, a patient may have both bipolar disorder and cyclothymic disorder if the cyclothymic disorder antedated the onset of full-blown mania.

While the schema of Figure 2 is a complicated one developed for clinical purposes primarily, the schema in Figure 3 is relatively simple and was developed primarily for research, particularly research in genetics. This hierarchy has been most persuasively argued in the work of Winokur, Woodruff, and others.[23-25] In this approach, the first subdivision is into primary and secondary. This approach places great emphasis on finding "pure" categories of affective disorder in order to explore genetic and other important biological correlates. Thus it is logical for the first subdivision to exclude secondary depressions, because they almost certainly represent a very heterogeneous and possibly different type of affective disorder. Thereafter the disorders are subdivided into bipolar and unipolar, and the unipolar disorders are further subdivided on the basis of family history into "pure" depressives (who have a family history of affective disorder), spectrum depressives (who have a family history of alcoholism or antisocial personality), and nonfamilial depressives (who have no family history of these illnesses).

The Relationship of "Phenomenotype" to "Biotype"

Genetic research often speaks of the relationship of genotype, or the specific characteristics defined in an individual's genetic makeup, to phenotype, or the characteristics manifested in the individual's appearance and behavior. Genetic researchers recognize that the relationship between genotype and phenotype is complex.

In research that explores the relationship between biological factors and clinical symptoms, it is useful to develop a similar pair of concepts, which I refer to as phenomenotype and biotype. The earliest classification systems were developed on phenomenotype alone, because that was all that was available to nosologists such as Kraepelin or Bleuler. Sometimes the term "phenomenology" is used to refer to cross-sectional symptoms only. These form an important component of the phenomenotype, but

Table 4 Definition by "Phenomenotype"

1. Onset
2. Course
3. Outcome
4. Types of symptoms
5. Severity of symptoms

should not be studied in isolation. A complete definition of phenomenotype should include the five types of variables listed in Table 4: onset, course, outcome, types of symptoms, and severity of symptoms. Onset may vary depending on whether it is slow, insidious, or acute; it is also important to observe the quality of a patient's premorbid adjustment. The course of a disorder may vary by being episodic or chronic with a variation in the amount of recurrence for those disorders that are episodic, and a variation in whether more episodic features are superimposed on chronic features. The outcome of a disorder may be good or involve some impairment and may reflect steady improvement or steady deterioration. The types of symptoms used to define a disorder will depend on the specific disorder. For example, in the case of depression, clinicians and researchers are often interested in defining characteristic general features as well as more specific features that define subtypes, such as vegetative symptoms or endogenous phenomenology. Severity of symptoms is another important aspect of diagnosis that has been ignored in much recent nosological research. In the future, researchers may find that they can make useful distinctions and improve the match between phenomenotype and biotype by changing their threshold for severity of symptoms.

The features that characterize the "biotype" are summarized in Table 5. These include familial data, neurochemical and neuroendocrine data, neurophysiological data, neuroanatomical data, and treatment response. A large amount of genetic research has examined the relationship of familial data to phenomenology and has provided much of the foundation for the distinction between bipolar and unipolar affective disorders. As many other chapters in this book attest, neurochemical and neuroendocrine correlates, such as the dexamethasone suppression test and high *versus* low

Table 5 Definition by "Biotype"

1. Familial data
2. Neurochemical and neuroendocrine data
3. Neurophysiological data
4. Neuroanatomical data
5. Treatment response

MHPG, have provided large amounts of information concerning the classification of affective disorders. Neurophysiological data, such as sleep EEG, has also been very useful. To date very little emphasis has been placed on neuroanatomical information, such as the role of hemispheric specialization or localization of abnormalities within the brain, but this area appears to be quite promising in the future. Response to treatment is another important technique for defining possible biological subtypes of depression.

Historically, most research in psychiatry has proceeded by identifying phenomenotypes. These phenomenotypes, such as endogenous depression, have then been used to search for biological correlates. (I think the term "biological correlates" is preferable to "biological markers" because it more accurately reflects our lack of certainty or knowledge.) However, an alternate strategy that might be even more powerful would be to begin with a feature or a group of features that define a biotype. This approach can be used to identify a group of individuals who are in some sense biologically homogeneous and therefore might reflect an important etiological factor. This type of approach has already been used in some genetic research and in CT scan research.[24-28] A highly pragmatic approach to pharmacological research would be to use treatment response as an independent variable and clinical phenomenology as a dependent variable. Using this approach, one might ultimately be able to identify the clinical features of those patients that would predict a good response to treatment.

In any case, much work remains to be done both conceptually and in the laboratory concerning the relationship between phenomenotype and biotype. We are as yet not at all clear about whether clinical symptoms alone, as defined by phenomenotype, can be used to identify a homogeneous group of patients or a specific disorder. We do not know whether groups identified by biological measures tend to have a characteristic set of symptoms. We are not sure how often phenomenotype and biotype agree. We have not done sufficient work to relate all the characteristic features that define biotype with one another, although recently, as indicated in this book, several research teams have tried to combine measures based on sleep EEG with those of the dexamethasone suppression test.

Summary and Conclusion

Enormous progress has been made to date on the diagnosis and classification of affective disorders. We have good standardized instruments for evaluation and reliable diagnostic systems. We have a standard system of classification developed for use in clinical work, *DSM-III*, that promises to yield a large amount of descriptive information that will also be useful in research. Furthermore, clinicians can communicate with one another with improved confidence and precision.

Much controversy remains, however, and much work remains to be done. We must begin with an initial recognition that different approaches to classification and diagnosis are needed in clinical *versus* research work. Consequently, even in research, different strategies for diagnosing and classifying should be used depending on the goals of the research. Nosologists or epidemiologists are more likely to examine broad overlapping categories than are biological researchers. In the future, nosologists can assist biological researchers by exploring with them whether additional power can be achieved through narrowing of criteria and the most efficient way to produce that narrowing. Finally, the exploration of the relationship between phenomenotype and biotype should be an important area during the coming decade, involving increased collaboration between biological and nosological researchers.

References

1. Kreitman N, Sainsbury P, and Morrissey J. The reliability of psychiatric assessment: An analysis. *Journal of Mental Science* 107:887–908, 1961.

2. Beck AT et al. Reliability of psychiatric diagnosis: II. A study of consistency of clinical judgments and ratings. *American Journal of Psychiatry* 119:351–57, 1962.

3. Sandifer MG, Pettus G, and Quade D. A study of psychiatric diagnosis. *Journal of Nervous and Mental Disease* 139:350–56, 1964.

4. Endicott J and Spitzer RL. A diagnostic interview: The Schedule for Affective Disorders and Schizophrenia. *Archives of General Psychiatry* 35:837–44, 1978.

5. Wing JK. "A Standard Form of Psychiatric Present State Examination and a Method for Standardizing the Classification of Symptoms." In *Psychiatric Epidemiology: An International Symposium*, edited by Hare EH and Wing JK. London: Oxford University Press, 1970. pp. 93–108.

6. Spitzer RL, Endicott J and Robins E. Research Diagnostic Criteria: Rationale and reliability. *Archives of General Psychiatry* 35:773–82, 1978.

7. Feighner JP et al. Diagnostic criteria for use in psychiatric research. *Archives of General Psychiatry* 26:57–63, 1972.

8. Andreasen NC et al. Reliability of lifetime diagnosis: A multi-center collaborative perspective. *Archives of General Psychiatry* 38:400–05. 1981.

9. Andreasen NC and Grove WM. The classification of depression: Traditional views vs mathematical approaches. *American Journal of Psychiatry* 139:45–52, 1982.

10. Helzer JE et al. Reliability of psychiatric diagnosis: II. The test-retest reliability of diagnostic classification. *Archives of General Psychiatry* 34:141–46, 1977.

11. Spitzer RL and Forman JBW. *DSM-III* field trials: I. Initial interrater diagnostic reliability. *American Journal of Psychiatry* 136:815–17, 1979.

12. Grove WM et al. Reliability studies of psychiatric diagnosis: Theory and practice. *Archives of General Psychiatry* 38:408–13, 1981.

13. American Psychiatric Association. *Diagnostic and Statistical Manual of Mental Disorders (DSM-III)*, 3rd ed. Washington, D.C.: American Psychiatric Association, 1980.

14. Winokur G, Clayton PJ and Reich T. *Manic-Depressive Illness.* St. Louis: C.V. Mosby Company, 1969.

15. Dunner DL, Gershon ES, and Goodwin FK. Heritable factors in the severity of affective illness. *Biological Psychiatry* 11:31–42, 1976.

16. Goodwin FK et al. "Biochemical and Pharmacological Differentiation of Affective Disorder: An Overview." In *Psychiatric Diagnosis: Exploration of Biological Predictors*, edited by Akiskal HD and Webb WL. New York and London: Spectrum Publications, 1978.

17. Brown WA, Johnstone R, and Mayfield B. The twenty-four hour dexamethasone suppression test in a clinical setting: Relationship to diagnosis, symptoms, and response to treatment. *American Journal of Psychiatry* 136:543–47, 1979.

18. Buchsbaum MS. "The Average Evoked Response Technique in the Differentiation of Bipolar, Unipolar and Schizophrenic Disorders." In *Psychiatric Diagnosis: Exploration of Biological Predictors*, edited by Akiskal HD and Webb WH. New York and London: Spectrum Publications, 1978.

19. Dunner DL, Stallone F, and Fieve RR. Lithium carbonate and affective disorders. *Archives of General Psychiatry* 33:117–20, 1976.

20. Angst J et al. The course of monopolar depression and bipolar psychoses. *Psychiatrika Neurologica et Neurochirurgia* 76:489–500, 1973.

21. Mendels J. Lithium in the treatment of depression. *American Journal of Psychiatry* 133:373–78, 1976.

22. Gershon ES et al. The inheritance of affective disorder: A review of data and hypotheses. *Behavior Genetics* 6:227–61, 1976.

23. Andreasen NC and Winokur G. Secondary depression: Familial, clinical, and research perspectives. *American Journal of Psychiatry* 136:62–66, 1979.

24. Andreasen NC and Winokur G. Newer experimental methods for classifying depression: A report from the Collaborative Study. *Archives of General Psychiatry* 36:447–52, 1979.

25. Winokur G. Unipolar depression: Is it divisible into autonomous subtypes? *Archives of General Psychiatry* 36:47–52, 1979.

26. Weinberger DR et al. Lateral cerebral ventricular enlargement in chronic schizophrenia. *Archives of General Psychiatry* 36:735–39, 1979.

27. Weinberger DR et al. Cerebral ventricular enlargement in chronic schizophrenia: Its association with poor response to treatment. *Archives of General Psychiatry* 37:11–13, 1980.

28. Andreasen NC et al. Ventricular enlargement in schizophrenia: Relationship to positive and negative symptoms. *American Journal of Psychiatry* 139:297–302, 1982.

10

Phenomenological Heterogeneity of Depressive Disorders

John Overall, Ph.D.

Major depressive disorder, as defined by explicit criteria in the new *Diagnostic and Statistical Manual* (*DSM-III*) of the American Psychiatric Association, is a diagnosis that encompasses several phenomenologically distinct syndromes. I propose that an additional *descriptive axis* is needed to complete the multiaxial system for the diagnosis of depression and other psychiatric disorders. Phenomenological classification is not intended to supplant careful diagnosis. Instead, phenomenological classification can extend diagnostic considerations in a meaningful way. Within the framework of a multiaxial conception of psychiatric disorders, the Axis I (major syndrome) classification defines the disease state which may or may not be superimposed on a more enduring Axis II (personality) disorder. What is lacking is an adequate picture of what the patient looks like at a given time or phase of his illness.

The fact that objective criteria for the diagnosis of depressive disorders have been provided is the basis for recognition that an additional axis is needed. Before the advent of objective criteria for establishing diagnoses, any work that suggested lack of clinically relevant homogeneity was inevitably greeted with skepticism that the diagnoses were not carefully or properly made. Only in the presence of explicit criteria can the advantages and shortcomings of diagnostic concepts be investigated scientifically.

Classification is the process of organizing or grouping individuals according to similarities and differences in relevant characteristics. Psychiatric symptom profile patterns tend to be complex and multidimensional. An appropriate classification scheme groups individuals so that those in each category or class can be considered alike for practical clinical purposes. Classification is important as a way of communicating and thinking about psychopathology; without it each individual would have to be considered unique. Each classification category is associated with a conceptual prototype, or concept of a typical patient, and each individual who is assigned to the category is recognized to be similar to the prototype for that category. The term "type" is used to indicate that an individual falls within bounds of similarity to a particular prototype, which permits him to be adequately described by reference to the conceptual prototype. A scientific approach to psychiatry requires generalizing from experience with similar individuals, and classification defines populations of individuals to whom such generalization is appropriate.

According to the dictionary definition, *phenomena* have two important attributes. Phenomena are events, happenings, or current states, as contrasted with the permanent essence of things; and in contrast to inferred, conjectured, or theorized conditions, they are also observable conditions capable of being perceived through the senses. Thus, phenomenological classification involves grouping of individuals based on similarities and differences in current observable manifestations of psychopathology. It provides a concise description of what the patient looks like, something not adequately conveyed by the major syndrome diagnosis of depressive disorder.

Objective Criteria for Establishing the Diagnosis

As I have emphasized, diagnosis is important and is not to be replaced by mere symptom description. That is why phenomenological classification has been proposed as a separate axis in the multiaxial classification scheme. This is not to say that the current *DSM III* criteria for establishing a diagnosis need be accepted without careful evaluation and eventual modification. As we will see, the *DSM III* criteria exclude a substantial proportion of dysphoric patients who are currently treated for depression. Little evidence is available to indicate that patients who meet the more narrow definitions of depression respond to specific forms of treatment any better or worse than patients who fail to meet the narrow criteria.

In considering a subclassification of depressive disorders along phenomenological or descriptive lines, a somewhat broader diagnostic net may prove desirable. Several objective criteria for establishing a diagnosis of depressive disorder have been proposed in the literature, and they differ in the breadth of the populations that are defined. To emphasize the fact that depressive disorders are phenomenologically heterogeneous, no matter how narrowly the diagnosis is defined, three objective sets of diagnostic criteria are reviewed briefly here.

Saint Louis Criteria

The landmark work that sets the stage for recent efforts to enhance the reliability of diagnostic practices in psychiatry comes from the Department of Psychiatry at Washington University in Saint Louis. Feighner et al. propose simple objective criteria for some 16 psychiatric diagnoses, including the diagnosis of primary depressive disorder.[1] These diagnostic criteria are reproduced in an excellent book written by Woodruff, Goodwin, and Guze, also in the Saint Louis group.[2]

The stated purpose of the Saint Louis Diagnostic Criteria is to objectively define homogeneous patient populations for research purposes. However, it is not necessary to include all patients for such a purpose. What is desired are pure groups whose diagnoses can be agreed upon by almost anyone. Hence, the Saint Louis Criteria are among the most restrictive, excluding large numbers of patients who otherwise would be diagnosed and treated for depression.

To satisfy the Saint Louis Criteria for definite primary depressive disorder, a patient must manifest dysphoric mood plus at least five of eight associated symptoms: (1) poor appetite or weight loss, (2) sleep difficulty, (3) loss of energy, (4) agitation or retardation, (5) loss of interest or decreased sex drive, (6) feelings of self-reproach or guilt, (7) diminished ability to think or concentrate, and (8) recurrent thoughts of death or suicide. The illness defined by these symptoms must have been present for at least one month, and there should be no history of other psychiatric conditions.

Our own research experience has revealed that about two-thirds of the patients who are diagnosed and treated for depression in our clinical setting fail to qualify for a diagnosis of primary depressive disorder according to the Saint Louis Criteria. Thus, those criteria will be of special interest with regard to phenomenological homogeneity of the highly selected patient population so defined.

New York Criteria

The Research Diagnostic Criteria (RDC) for major depressive disorder as defined by Spitzer, Endicott, and Robins[3] are quite similar to the Saint Louis Criteria, as suggested by the fact that Eli Robins coauthored both works. There are, however, some important differences that result in the New York RDC defining a somewhat broader population. Among the differences are additional inclusion criteria, reduced and more specific exclusion criteria, and shortened duration requirement. Note that the New York RDC for major depressive disorders were incorporated verbatim into the *DSM III*, so the results to be considered with regard to phenomenological classification apply equally to both.

To qualify for a diagnosis of major depressive disorder according to the New York Criteria, a patient must have *either* dysphoric mood or pervasive loss of interest or pleasure, plus five of eight associated symptoms which—except for the addition of "increased appetite or weight gain"—are identical to those in the Saint Louis Criteria. Because the New York Criteria are intended to define a population of major depressive disorders that is not necessarily the "primary" disorder, exclusion criteria are confined to few and very specific symptoms of schizophrenic thinking disorder; and only two weeks' duration of the illness defined by these symptoms is required. Because of the alternative manifestations that can be counted in satisfying the requirements for the diagnosis of major depressive disorders, the reduction in exclusion criteria, and the shortened duration requirement, the New York Criteria for major depressive disorders include a larger segment of the patient population. In our own experience, about one-third of the patients who are considered clinically to require treatment for symptoms of depression fail to satisfy these criteria.

Composite Checklist Criteria

In recognition of the restrictive nature of other research diagnostic criteria for depressive disorders, a Composite Diagnostic Checklist for Depression was constructed to include the specific items required by the Saint Louis Criteria, the New York Criteria (and thus by *DSM-III*), plus items taken from our own actuarial research.[4] The Composite Checklist (Figure 1), also includes items for recording primary *versus* secondary,[1] endogenous *versus* reactive,[6] and unipolar *versus* bipolar clinical histories.[5] Also included are family history and demographic items required to further subclassify unipolar depressive disorder into "pure depression" versus "depressive spectrum disease," according to criteria defined by Winokur.[7] Especially relevant for phenomenological classification is the fact that the Composite Checklist includes target symptoms identified with anxious, hostile, agitated, and retarded subtypes of depression.

Instructions for completing the checklist data form weight key symptoms if they are severe or if they are particularly characteristic of severe depression. For example, if a patient has "severe" dysphoric mood, "moderately severe" mood should be checked as well. If a patient has "early awakening or middle insomnia," he also has "sleep difficulties." If a patient has "pervasive loss of interest," he also has "loss of interest."

Actuarial scoring of the Composite Diagnostic Checklist for Depression has the aim of confirming a diagnosis of depressive disorder for a larger proportion of the patient population for whom reduction of depressive symptoms is perceived clinically to be a primary therapeutic goal. Because the Composite Checklist includes the specific items required

Composite Diagnostic Checklist for Depression

Name of Subject _____   Date _____

Name of Interviewer _____

Check all items that are present

A. Dysphoric mood
☐ Moderately severe
☐ Severe
☐ Distinct quality-different from grief
☐ Worse in morning
☐ Unresponsive to environmental changes

B. Associated symptoms
☐ Looks sad, tearful, or depressed
☐ Decreased appetite or weight loss
☐ Increased appetite or weight gain
☐ Difficulty falling asleep
☐ Early awakening or middle insomnia
☐ Hypersomnia
☐ Excessive somatic concern
☐ Pessimistic
☐ Loss of energy
☐ Psychomotor retardation
☐ Psychomotor agitation
☐ Clinging dependency
☐ Anxiety
☐ Demandingness
☐ Blame projection
☐ Self-pity
☐ Resentful, irritable, angry or complaining
☐ Feelings of guilt or self-reproach
☐ Brooding about unpleasant events
☐ Loss of interest or pleasure
☐ Pervasive loss of interest
☐ Preoccupation with feelings of inadequacy
☐ Decreased sex drive
☐ Increased sex drive
☐ Diminished ability to concentrate
☐ Diminished ability to think
☐ Thoughts of death or suicide
☐ Delusions with definite depression theme
☐ Hallucinations with definite depression theme

C. Duration of depressive symptoms
☐ Less than two weeks

☐ Two to four weeks
☐ More than four weeks
☐ More than six months

D. Course of illness
☐ First episode
☐ Chronic state
☐ Recurrent unipolar
☐ Bipolar (previous manic)
☐ Bipolar (previous hypomanic)

E. Depressive Spectrum History
☐ Family history of depression predominantly female relatives
☐ Family history of alcoholism or sociopathy in male relatives
☐ Depression about equally prevalent in relatives of both sexes
☐ No significant alcoholism in family history
☐ No significant sociopathy in family history
☐ No significant depression in family history
☐ Probable schizophrenia in family history

F. Demographic characteristics
☐ Female
☐ Present age 40 or older
☐ Onset of first episode before ages 40
☐ Married or divorces
☐ Two or more children
☐ Skilled, sales or clerical worker, or housewife
☐ High school graduate
☐ College graduate
☐ Moderate religious attitude
☐ Abstain alcohol
☐ Frequent or heavy alcohol use
☐ No previous hospitalization
☐ Lower-middle or middle S.E.S. class
☐ Complaint of marital problems
☐ Severe discord in childhood home

G. Symptoms suggestive of schizophrenia

☐ Thought broadcasting, insertion, or withdrawal
☐ Delusions of being controlled
☐ Any recurrent delusion or hallucination (except typical of depression)
☐ Preoccupation with any non-affective delusion or hallucination
☐ Auditory hallucination in which voice keeps up running commentary or two voices converse with each other
☐ Any non-affective hallucinations throughout the day for several days or intermittantly for a week
☐ Formal though disorder
☐ Period of one month during present illness in which delusions or hallucinations present without prominent dysphoric mood

H. Pre-existing psychiatric condition (other than mania or depression), such as schizophrenia, alcoholism, drug dependence, personality disorder, or organic brain syndrome

☐ No
☐ Probable
☐ Definite
Type

I. Organic etiology
☐ No
☐ Yes
Type

J. Precipitating factors
☐ None apparent
☐ Probable
☐ Definite

K. Phenomenological type
☐ Anxious depression
☐ Agitated depression
☐ Retarded depression
☐ Hostile depression

L. Endogenous depression
☐ No
☐ Probable
☐ Definite

Figure 1 Composite diagnostic checklist for depression

155

to confirm a diagnosis of depression according to the Saint Louis or New York Research Diagnostic Criteria, patients who meet those narrower criteria usually are included in the broader population defined by the actuarial scoring of the composit data form.

To qualify for a diagnosis of depressive disorder according to the Composite Checklist Criteria, a patient must have (a) at least eight items from Sections A and B, including dysphoric mood and at least one of the following: anxiety, psychomotor retardation, psychomotor agitation, or resentfulness and related symptoms; (b) at least four of the demographic items from Section F; and (c) none of the items from Section G. Like the Saint Louis Criteria, the Composite Checklist requires the presence of at least moderately severe dysphoric mood, not required by the New York Criteria. Like the New York Criteria, the Composite Checklist excludes only those patients who have specific symptoms of thinking disorder, although the exclusion criteria are broadened to include any recurrent delusion or hallucination (except typical of depression). Experience has confirmed that less than one-fourth of patients who are treated clinically with the aim of reducing symptoms of depression fail to satisfy the Composite Checklist Criteria.

Phenomenological Classification

Over the past two decades, several groups of investigators have employed empirical methods to identify naturally occurring subtypes within the broader population of depressive disorders. Grinker et al. factor analyzed large collections of descriptive data from different sources.[8] They reported four distinct, recurrent patterns in the resulting factor scores for clinically depressed patients. The patterns distinguished retarded, anxious, agitated, and angry types of depressed patients. Some 10 years later, Paykel applied hierarchical cluster analysis methodology to data from a structured research interview.[9] He also concluded that the population of clinically depressed patients consists of four distinct syndromes. Out of a British tradition, he was concerned with the distinction between "neurotic" and "psychotic" depression, so the names assigned his empirical groupings were guided by that interest, although he also described a hostile type of depression.

Our own work in the phenomenological classification of depressive disorders has been based on the application of cluster analysis and related numerical taxonomy methods to Brief Psychiatric Rating Scale (BPRS) profiles for clinically diagnosed depressive disorders and to BPRS profiles for large samples of patients from the general psychiatric population. The first analysis involved depressed patients who were subjects in a clinical trial of an antidepressant drug.[10] This analysis resulted in the identification of three homogeneous subgroups with distinctly different BPRS profile patterns. They were given the names "anxious depression, hostile depression, and retarded depression." Subsequently, in a series of 2,000 patients from a combined French and American sample, the anxious, hostile, and retarded depression types were identified again, and agitated depression was confirmed as a fourth distinct constellation.[11] Mean profiles for the four subtypes of depressive disorders as defined in that analysis are presented in Figure 2.

Recently, a large data bank containing BPRS profiles for patients in clinical trials of neuroleptic, antidepressant, or anxiolytic drugs was obtained through the courtesy of Dr. Jerome Levine of the National Institute of Mental Health. Because all of the patients were specifically selected for controlled clinical drug trials, this source of data was considered important for refining phenomenological classification concepts and procedures for use in clinical psychopharmacology research. The pretreatment (baseline) BPRS profiles for 2,623 patients from this source were analyzed. An "iterative reclassification" method of profile analysis was used to modify the prototype profiles for the phenomenological types to make them maximally representative of the cluster configuration in the psychopharmacology data bank. The mean BPRS profiles for the four

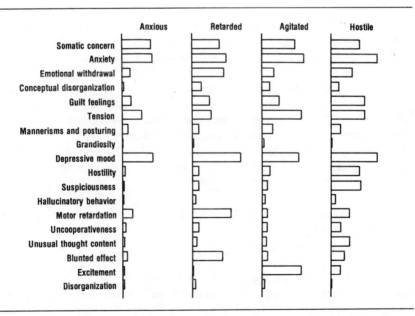

Figure 2 Mean BPRS profiles for four depression types identified by cluster analysis in a combined French and American sample of 2,000 patients

phenomenological types resulting from these analyses are presented in Figure 3. Some sampling variability is apparent when one compares the results shown in Figures 2 and 3; however, the profile patterns clearly support the classification concepts of anxious, agitated, retarded, and hostile depression in each case.

Decision Rules for Phenomenological Classification of Individuals

Given the BPRS profile for an individual it is possible to calculate a numerical index of similarity to the prototype profile for each phenomenological type. The individual can then be assigned to the phenomenological class in which his profile is most similar to the prototype pattern. Mean profiles for the four depression subtypes (Figures 2 and 3) can serve as the prototype patterns to which the individual BPRS profiles are compared.

Several different numerical indices of profile similarity have been proposed in the literature. In general, they are of two major types: vector product indices of profile similarity and distance function indices of profile dissimilarity. The simple d^2 distance is defined as the sum of squared differences between corresponding elements in two profiles.[12]

$$d^2 = \Sigma \, (x_i - p_i)^2$$

where x_i and p_i are the ith elements in the individual and prototype profiles, respectively, and summation is across all elements in the profiles.

Vector product indices of profile similarity are defined as the sum of cross-products between corresponding elements in two profiles. It is often considered useful to effect certain transformations or rescaling of the profiles before calculating the vector product. The index of multivariate profile similarity that we have used most often in assigning individuals to phenomenological types is the so-called normalize vector product index. The prototype profiles are first rescaled by dividing each element by the square root of the sum of squares of all elements in the profile.

$$\hat{p}_i = p_i / \sqrt{\Sigma \, p^2} \ .$$

The elements of the individual's BPRS profile can be rescaled (normalized) in a similar fashion.

$$\hat{x}_i = x_i / \sqrt{\Sigma \, x^2} \ .$$

The normalized vector product is then calculated as the sum of cross-products between corresponding elements in the two normalized profiles.

$$V = \Sigma \, \hat{x}_i \, p_i \ .$$

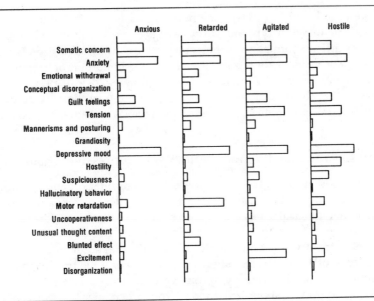

Figure 3 Mean BPRS profiles for four depression types defined by iterative reclassification of patients in the psychopharmacology data bank

Note that the vector product indices are sensitive to the location of the zero point on the scales. The normalized vector product is calculated from BPRS ratings that have been scored on a 0–6 scale of severity. "Not present" is a meaningful zero point on a scale of symptom severity, and a meaningful zero point is necessary for comparison of vector products.

Another index that can be used to assign individuals to phenomenological types is the classification function. Neither the simple d^2 distances nor the vector product similarity indices, as defined above, take into account the correlations among elements within the profiles. Classification functions are weighted combinations of the BPRS symptom ratings, where the weights have been calculated to maximize the discrimination of each group from all others. In concept, the classification functions are similar to simple discriminant functions.

$$C = \Sigma \ w_i \ x_i$$

where w_i is the weighting coefficient applied to the i [th] element in the individual's BPRS profile. A different set of weighting coefficients defines the classification function for each phenomenological type. To classify an individual among the four depression subtypes, the four classification function scores are calculated and the individual is assigned to the phenomenological type for which the composite score is greatest.

159

These and other objective methods for assigning individuals among the phenomenological types recently have been reviewed.[13] In Overall and Hollister's article, normalized prototype profiles and classification function weighting coefficients are represented. Here it is important only to indicate how individuals can be assigned to phenomenological types and to emphasize that the procedures are as objective and operationally defined as are the criteria for establishing a research diagnosis of depressive disorders.

Diagnosis and the Phenomenology of Depressive Disorders

Whether it is meaningful or necessary to consider phenomenological classification in the diagnosis of depressive disorders depends on whether the phenomenological types are all true depressive disorders. The empirical cluster analysis work that led to delineation of the different symptom profile patterns was done on samples of patients diagnosed without the aid of *DSM III* or other objectively specified criteria. From the time of the initial description of the different symptom patterns to the present, there has remained a question about whether all four phenomenological types are represented among true depressive disorders. A related question concerns whether phenomenological classification is not already implied in careful and correct diagnosis of major depressive disorders.

The literature on depression suggests that agitated and retarded types are more likely to be considered real depressive disorders, whereas the anxious and hostile types are likely to be considered atypical, minor, borderline, or neurotic. This view is strengthened by the fact that psychomotor agitation and retardation are listed in *DSM-III* among the criteria for "major depressive episode." Symptoms of irritability and excessive anger (hostility) are listed among the criteria for dysthymic disorder, which is equated with the older concept of depressive neurosis, and anxiety is not included among the criteria for any type of depressive disorder. Thus, if agitated and retarded subtypes are major depressive disorders, the hostile subtype is dysthymic disorder, and the anxious type belongs in neither category, one would have to conclude that phenomenological classification is already implied in a careful *DSM-III* diagnosis. As we will see, that is not the case.

Overall and Zisook have reported on application of rigorous research diagnostic criteria and phenomenological classification to a sample of 161 patients who received a clinical diagnosis of depression in a university hospital outpatient clinic.[14] Each patient was interviewed by one of two master's level psychologists who were specially trained and experienced in recording diagnostic criteria data on the Composite Diagnostic Checklist for Depression (Figure 1) and completing symptom ratings on the BPRS. From the information recorded on those data forms, determination was made concerning whether or not each patient satisfied the Saint Louis Criteria for research diagnosis of primary depressive disorder, the New York Criteria for major depressive disorder, and the Composite Checklist Criteria. The similarity of the patient profiles to the prototype profiles (Figure 2) was evaluated using the normalized vector product index described earlier. Of the 161 patients, 149 were found to have BPRS profiles similar enough to one of the prototype patterns to justify phenomenological classification.

As expected, the numbers of clinically depressed patients that met the alternative research diagnostic criteria differed substantially. Considering only the 149 patients who were classified according to phenomenological type, 81% satisfied the Composite Checklist Criteria for Depression and 61% satisfied the Saint Louis Criteria. Frequencies of the four phenomenological types among patients who did satisfy each of the diagnostic criteria are shown in Table 1. Two questions are important with regard to these results. The first concerns whether the diagnosis of depressive disorder subsumes several phenomenologically distinct syndromes. The answer is clearly positive. Not only were all four phenomenological types well represented in the total clinically diagnosed sample, but they were equally well represented in the selected samples defined by Research Diagnostic Criteria. In fact, the representation of the four phenomenological types was most uniform in the sample selected by the narrow Saint Louis Criteria. The Composite Checklist Criteria evidenced a slight tendency to select against the anxious and hostile subtypes, but all four types were still well represented.

Numerous larger data sets have previously been subjected to phenomenological classification. The problem has been that the criteria for diagnosis of depressive disorders were not explicitly specified. Thus, the possibility has existed that the apparent heterogeneity has resulted from misdiagnosis of large numbers of patients. The results shown in Table 1 clearly confirm that depressive disorders are heterogeneous in symptom profile patterns, no matter how rigorously one attempts to define the diagnosis.

Table 1 Frequencies of Four Phenomenological Types Among Patients Who Satisfied Various Diagnostic Criteria

Criteria	Anxious	Agitated	Retarded	Hostile
Clinical Dx	49	45	37	18
Composite Checklist	33	41	33	13
New York	26	29	23	13
Saint Louis	13	16	13	12

Implications of Phenomenological Heterogeneity

The relevance of phenomenological classification for research in clinical psychopharmacology has been suggested in a number of studies.[15] Psychiatrists tend to prescribe different drugs to patients in the different phenomenological categories. Tricyclic antidepressants are most uniformly prescribed for retarded depressions. Anxious depressions tend to be treated with the more sedative type antidepressants, such as doxepin or amitriptyline, or low potency neuroleptics. Placebo response has been reported to occur with approximately twice the relative frequency in anxious depressions as compared with agitated or retarded depressions. Because phenomenological classification is not implied in careful clinical diagnosis, the addition of a phenomenological axis to the multiaxial diagnostic scheme seems justified.

References

1. Feighner JP et al. Diagnostic criteria for use in psychiatric research. *Archives of General Psychiatry* 26:57–63, 1972.

2. Woodruff RA, Jr, Goodwin DW, and Guze SB. *Psychiatric Diagnosis*. London: Oxford University Press, 1974.

3. Spitzer RL, Endicott J, and Robins E. Research Diagnostic Criteria (RDC). *Psychopharmacology Bulletin* 11:22–24, 1975.

4. Overall JE. "Criteria for Selection of Subjects for Research in Biological Psychiatry." In *Handbook of Biological Psychiatry, Part VI: Practical Applications of Psychotropic Drugs and Other Biological Treatments* edited by van Praag H et al. New York: Marcel Decker, 1981.

5. Perris C. The separation of bipolar recurrent depressive psychoses. *Behavioral Neuropsychiatry* 1:14–24, 1969.

6. Mendels J and Cochrane C. The nosology of depression: The endogenous-reactive concept. *American Journal of Psychiatry* 124(Suppl.):1–11, 1968.

7. Winokur G. Types of depressive illness. *British Journal of Psychiatry*, 120:265–66, 1972.

8. Grinker RR et al. *The Phenomena of Depression*. New York: Hoeber, 1961.

9. Paykel ES. Classifications of depressed patients: A cluster analysis derived grouping. *British Journal of Psychiatry* 118:175–88, 1971.

10. Overall JE et al. Nosology of depression and differential response to drugs. *Journal of the American Medical Association* 195:946–948, 1966.

11. Overall JE. "The Brief Psychiatric Rating Scale in Psychopharmacology Research." In *Psychological Measurement in Psychopharmacology: Modern Problems in Pharmacopsychiatry*. Basel: Karger, 1974.

12. Cronbach LJ and Gleser GC. Assessing similarities between profiles. *Psychological Bulletin* 50:456–73, 1953.

13. Overall JE and Hollister LE. Decision rules for phenomenological classification of psychiatric patients. *Journal of Consulting and Clinical Psychology* 50:535–45, 1982.

14. Overall JE and Zisook S. Diagnosis and the phenomenology of psychiatric disorders. *Journal of Consulting and Clinical Psychology* 48:626–34, 1980.

15. Overall JE and Hollister LE. Phenomenological classification of depressive disorders. *Consulting and Clinical Psychology* 36:372–77, 1980.

11

Retardation: A Basic Emotional Response?

Daniel Widlöcher, M.D.

Historical Survey

Psychomotor retardation, through its major expression, stupor, played an important role in the characterization of melancholy during the nineteenth century.[1] Psychologists, paying attention to sadness as a basic emotion, distinguished active from passive (depressive) emotion and considered retardation a fundamental characteristic of depressive mood. The determining role of psychomotor retardation in the mechanism of depression was later abandoned for three reasons. First, psychiatrists began concentrating on the classification of depressive conditions. Second, under the influence of Meyer, Janet, and Freud, psychologists were more interested in psychological mechanisms (aggression, loss of object, narcissism) than in depressive response by itself. The third reason is the success of the mood disorder theory and the particular attention paid to psychic pain as the primary trouble. In spite of the differences between the three points of view, the result was that retardation has been viewed, generally, as one symptom among many, and often as a "by-product" of the mood disturbance.

Discovery of antidepressive drugs did not modify this position because of the global effect of drugs on depressive symptomatology. Similarly, rating scales measure the intensity of symptoms, rather than differentiate dimensions. Retardation is characterized as motor retardation on most scales, its mental expression usually scattered in different items (fatigue, loss of interest, failure of concentration, etc.). The differential scales that use retardation for discriminating purposes generally specify motor retardation. In many classifications, retarded depression is opposed to other clinical forms. In the continuing controversy about unipolarity or bipolarity of depressive illness, retardation is generally considered as mainly correlated with endogenous, psychotic, primary, or major depression.[2] But the role of retardation is not explicitly discussed with reference to the empirical data. Nor is the weight of the retardation factor considered in the various items that describe the impairment of thought activities.

Multivariate analysis clearly indicates that retardation is, along with self-blame, the most common symptom of depression, yet many authors still consider mood disturbance as the core symptom. Data collected by self-evaluation and by objective rating scales demonstrate that retardation is a dimension which explains a larger part of variance than mood disturbance.[3,4] Retardation seems to be, along with loss of appetite and early awakening, one of the best predictors of therapeutic positive result.[3,5] Szabadi et al. emphasized the value of a simple speech speed test as predictor of the therapeutic effect.[6] Those studies need further confirmation, but the assumption of a central role of retardation in depressive syndrome is worth considering. Clinical evidence suggesting that retardation is central to depression includes Spitz's work: Anaclitic depression in infants, related to early separation, is clinically characterized by loss of motility and inhibition of activity.[7] Young monkeys separated from their mothers respond with immobilization, a reaction that imipramine antagonizes.[8,9] Immobilization is also one of the main features of the "despair model" used in rodents as a pharmacological test for antidepressive drugs.[10,11] In some non-western human societies, it is suggested that retardation could be a more reliable sign than mood disturbance.[12]

Psychomotor Retardation as an Independent Variable

It can be assumed that retardation is a relatively independent variable and more closely related to the depressive syndrome and antidepressive drugs' efficiency than sadness, pessimistic ideas, etc. A broader assumption may be that retardation is the specific emotional response which defines the core of depression. Retardation is a general characteristic that modifies all the actions of the individual, including motility, mental activity, and speech. All of these behavioral traits vary according to the circumstances and the time of day, but are closely related and subject to an eventual dissociation, as we shall see, between motor and psychic activity.

Retardation is perceived by the subject as an inhibition, a lack of interest, and/or a fatigue that rest does not relieve. It very likely contributes to the feeling that time freezes without any perception of future, an experience that phenomenologists have described for a long time. Costello viewed retardation as a loss of incitation to action and a suppression of the effects of usual reinforcements.[13] Depressive retardation is the exact opposite of motor excitation with the impulsivity, flight of ideas, and logorrhea of mania.

From another viewpoint, retardation is a basic emotional response, phylogenetically determined, characterized by normal withdrawal from experiences of situations that cannot be dealt with by fight or flight.[14] We have to distinguish a normal retardation that accompanies all painful experience and is self-limiting, from a pathological retardation, spontaneously irreversible, which provokes the depressive illness. Biological and psychological factors create retardation response. From an etiological and nosological viewpoint, influence of both series of factors differ. But if we consider mechanisms, they are complementary: Retardation as a response, appropriate or not, is dependent on psychic stimuli which actualize it and neurophysiological mechanisms which generate it.

Retardation is correlated with sadness but less closely than with all the traits which make it up. Two different psychological relationships explain this correlation. Sadness, as a subjective expression of painful experience (from internal neurotic or external reactive sources) is linked with retardation response. In this case, psychic pain and retardation are consequences of the primary experience, but retardation is generally felt by itself as a painful and depreciative experience, and often, the two processes are mutually reinforcing.

Some objections may be raised in regard to this theory. The first one, and probably the most significant, is related to the constancy of retardation in depressive states. Agitated and retarded depressions have been contrasted. However, this distinction is usually dependent upon the presence or absence of motor retardation, and does not take into account psychic retardation. It has also been maintained that retardation is almost always a sign of major depressive illness. If retardation is closely related to intensity of depression, however, the correlation with major clinical illness is understandable and more to be expected than with reactive and neurotic depressions. We wonder if, in these later clinical categories, painful emotions and true minor reactive depressions are not mixed. It would be useful to discriminate more accurately between the two conditions; discrimination could explain the discrepancies of outcomes issued from diagnostic and therapeutic studies.

Relations between anxiety and retardation raise very similar difficulties. It has been clearly shown that retardation was, along with early awakening, a better discriminating item than depressive mood to differentiate anxiety and depressive states.[15] Nevertheless, anxiolytic drugs have a positive effect on retardation in depressive conditions.[16]

Finally, it can be argued that we put into the retardation response some traits which have been interpreted as independent symptoms or dependent on depressed mood itself, and/or any organic impairment. Indeed, multivariate analysis indicates that only a part of the variance is explained by a main factor and that other factors also play a role. But, in terms of psychological explanation, different causes may have the same final effect upon behavior. In gathering these traits in the field of retardation, that is, as direct expression of the freezing of activity, it is not ruled out that they can be partly independent and be expressions of sadness or organic impairment. Lack of interest, for instance, is not only a subjective expression of psychic retardation, but it also may be a consequence of intrapunitive attitudes or pessimistic ideas. One of the advantages of multivariate analysis is to take into account this kind of multidetermination instead of a too rigid nosologic classification. The basic question is, therefore, to decide if retardation results from a broad configuration of partly related behavioral traits, or if it constitutes a unique and central characteristic which defines the depressive syndrome.

Measure of Retardation

Until now, measure of retardation has been carried out mainly by factor analysis and statistical inference. Sets of items, well related to this dimension, have evolved in this way. Lorr et al. have isolated from the IMPS a set of nine items that may be used as a retardation rating scale.[17] Motor retardation has been tentatively measured through some simple tests: a definite motor task,[18,19] whole motility in the course of a fixed time interval,[20,21] and speech delivery.[6] All of these studies clearly demonstrate that retardation is strongly related to depression as a whole, but only motor and speech retardation are considered. It has not been demonstrated whether motor, speech, and mental retardation or cognitive slowing are related in some way to a unique factor, partly independent of other symptoms. Therefore it seems necessary to add to these different tools a specific rating scale, specially built for measuring retardation and taking in account, as far as possible, the balance between motor and mental retardation.

A first version of our retardation rating scale (Appendix A) included 26 items which corresponded to different behavioral characteristics supposedly related to retardation, plus one item measuring retardation as a whole, and one negative item describing anxious agitation. According to usual methodology, inpatients, treated with clomipramine or salbutamol were rated on the 0, 15th and 28th days of treatment, by two independent raters, and the mean between the two scores was kept.[22] Correlation between raters was very high. Principal component analysis indicated that Factor I accounts for 48% of variance and that all items participate in this factor, except the negative item (anxious agitation) and "fluctuation of

Appendix A First Version

1. Gait
2. Stride
3. Slowness of movements
4. Paucity of movements
5. Motor initiative
6. Face—Mimetic
7. Posture
8. Restlessness associated with anxiety
9. Verbal flow
10. Articulation of speech
11. Voice intensity
12. Monotonous voice
13. Brevity of responses
14. Answers beyond the theme of the question
15. Syntax
16. Variety of spontaneously evoked themes
17. Physical fatigue
18. Lack of interest
19. Activities
20. Memory
21. Concentration
22. Subjective evaluation of present time
23. Subjective evaluation of past time
24. Adaptation to the interview situation
25. Fluctuation of retardation in the interview time
26. General appreciation

retardation in the interview time." Factor II accounts for only 8% of variance and mainly consists of ideational items ("brevity of responses," "answers beyond the theme of the question," "variety of spontaneously evoked themes," and "subjective evaluation of past time"). Factor III is negatively related to the other factors; it represents anxious agitation and accounts for 5% of variance.

In a second version of 27 items (Appendix B), less valid and redundant items were excluded, and as we wonder whether or not the low value of

Appendix B Second Version

1. Gait—Stride
2. Motor initiative
3. Sterile agitation
4. Slowness and paucity of movements (Limbs)
5. Slowness and paucity of movements (Trunk)
6. Slowness and paucity of movements (Head and Neck) Mimetic
7. Verbal flow
8. Voice intensity
9. Monotonous voice
10. Pauses during interview
11. Brevity of responses
12. Adapted answers
13. Answers beyond the theme of the question
14. Syntax
15. Variety of spontaneously evoked themes
16. Richness of associations
17. Subjective experience of rumination
18. Fatigability
19. Activities
20. Subjective evaluation of present time
21. Perception of future
22. Subjective evaluation of past time
23. Memory
24. Concentration
25. Temporal disorientation
26. Description of present environment
27. General appreciation

Factor II was due to an imbalance, additional mental items were tentatively included for reinforcing Factor II. The new version was administered using the same methodology to 38 depressed patients.[23] Principal component analysis, despite the changes, shows a Factor I, taking in account 47% of variance and strongly correlated with the general item and all the other items except "anxious agitation," "construction of phrases," "memory," and "temporal disorientation." Factor II is not "reinforced" and takes in account only 7% of variance, opposing subjective mental items to others; a Factor III takes in account 5% of variance and seems related only to speech items.

So it seemed that the retardation rating scale investigated a psychological entity which corresponded to one single factor accounting by itself for almost 50% of the variance. The close correlation of almost all the items with global retardation and the Factor I stresses the unity of the syndrome. A third and final version (Table 1) with substantially fewer items (14) has been applied to many outpatients and inpatients. Validity, sensitivity, and reliability were tested in a sample of 142 inpatients,* quite representative of a population of depressive patients (Table 2). Comparisons were made between scores of the Hamilton Depression Rating Scale (HDRS) and the Retardation Rating Scale (RRS), and between these two scales and a score of global clinical evaluation of severity at day 0 and of improvement at days 8 and 28.

Role of Retardation in Depressive Illness

On one side, an alternative theory is proposed as an explanation of the phenomenology of depression, on the other side, a rating scale has been constructed for the evaluation of what the theory suggests to be the core of the symptomatology. The question is whether the rating scale can be used for testing some definite hypothesis in agreement with the general assumption.

If motor retardation and cognitive slowing, or mental retardation, play

---

* Another study on 84 outpatients produced similar results.[24] Means and standard deviations (Table 3) show that variables are well centered and their spreading indicates a good sensitivity of the scale. Principal component analysis (Table 4) shows the existence of a dominating Factor I, which expresses nearly 60% of the variance and confirms the validity of the scale as measuring a unique dimension. Factor II (9.16% of the variance) is correlated positively with motor items and negatively with mental items. Factor III (6.27% of the variance) is correlated positively with mental objective items and negatively with mental subjective items. Correlation between raters is high and concordance (Kendall's w coefficient) is good.[25] Individual variations are generally smaller than standard deviation of the observed variables, indicating a fair fidelity. Therefore, the metric qualities of the scale seem confirmed, and it can be assumed that we have a useful instrument for studying the role of retardation in depressive illness.

Table 1 Salpetriere Retardation Rating Scale

	Score (0 to 4):
1. Gait	_____
2. Movement	_____
3. Mimetic	_____
4. Language	_____
5. Voice	_____
6. Brevity	_____
7. Variety	_____
8. Richness	_____
9. Ruminations	_____
10. Fatigability	_____
11. Interest	_____
12. Time	_____
13. Memory	_____
14. Concentration	_____

Each item should be scored from *0* to *4* according to the following general model:

0 = normal

1 = doubt concerning the pathological character of the observed phenomenon

2 = pathologic nature of what is observed is definite but mild signs are evident to any rater

3 = severe

Is there an extrinsic factor (organic, iatrogenic . . .)
affectating the retardation?   *Yes* _____ *No* _____

If *yes*, state which: _____

If *yes*, indicate whether this factor is: *Major* _____ *Minor* _____

Translation: Michael Stone, M.D.

1. **Gait, stride** (within a standard distance)

   0 Normal.

   1 Mild slowing (retardation of movement), but of an uncertain pathological nature.

   2 Any *one* of the following attributes is observed:
      (a) a lack of suppleness to the stride, or to the swing of the arms
      (b) the patient drags his feet
      (c) stride of normal amplitude, but slowed down
      (d) slowed stride with small steps.

   3 More than one of the signs in No. 2 are noted

   4 The patient must be supported in order to walk.

2. **Slowness and paucity of movements** (of limbs, trunk)

   0 Movements are appropriate, normal in amplitude, supple and rhythmic; the trunk is nestled (wedged) comfortably in the chair, the shoulders relaxed.

   1 There may be a mild degree of cramping to the movements, not readily noticeable.

   2 A certain fixity (tightness of the body) is unmistakably present.

   3 The patient moves his limbs only rarely, in a slowed-down manner, with an awkwardness of gesture and below-normal amplitude of movement

171

Table 1 Salpetriere Retardation Rating Scale (Continued)

-or- the proximal portions of the arms are fixed, and only the hands move. The trunk is immobile, either plastered against the back of the chair or with the shoulders drooping.

4 The patient refuses to get out of bed, or lies completely fixed in his chair. No trunkal movements at all, and no mobility to the head/trunk axis.

3. **Slowness and paucity of movements of the head and neck** (mimetic)
   0 The head moves freely, resting flexibly on the body with the gaze either exploring the room or fixed on the examiner or on other objects of interest—in an appropriate fashion. Movements of the mouth are of a normal amplitude.
   1 There may be some reduction of mobility, not easily confirmed.
   2 Reduction of mobility is definite but mild. The gaze, while often fixed is still capable of shifting; there is a monotonous quality, though still with some expressiveness, to the facial gestures.
   3 The patient does not move his head. He does not explore the room and usually stares toward the floor, seldom looking at the examiner. He articulates poorly, barely moving his mouth; he never smiles; the expression is unchanging.
   4 The face is completely immobile and painfully inexpressive.

4. **Language and verbal flow**
   0 Flow of speech appears normal.
   1 Barely perceptible slowing of speech.
   2 A definite slowing of speech that nevertheless does not interfere with conversation.
   3 The subject speaks only upon the most forceful urging by the examiner.
   4 Stereotyped responses.

5. **Modulation of the voice** (intensity and modulation of speech)
   0 Appears normal.
   1 Barely perceptible waning.
   2 Voice is weak and monotonous; listener must place his ear closer.
   3 Speech is barely audible; listener must request certain phrases to be repeated
   4 Speech is inaudible.

6. **Brevity of responses**
   0 The subject has no difficulty in making responses of appropriate length.
   1 Responses appear to be somewhat briefer than would be expected.
   2 Responses are brief but not to the point of compromising the course of the conversation (. . . interfering with dialogue).
   3 Subject very laconic. Responses are restricted to just one or two (to just a few) words.
   4 Only monosyllabic responses.

7. **Variety of themes** (topics) **spontaneously approached**
   0 Association of ideas proceeds smoothly; there is a richness and variety to the themes (topics) broached by the subjects.
   1 Conversational themes (topics) are relatively rich and varied but the patient may have some difficulty in making a quick transition from one idea to another.

Table 1   Salpetriere Retardation Rating Scale (Continued)

Score (0 to 4):

    2 There is a rarity and impoverishment to new themes (topics) spontane-
ously brought up by the patient.

    3 No spontaneous offer of new themes (topics) along with a tendency to
• rumination of certain ideas.

    4 No elaboration. Conversation is meagre, monotonous; exploration of
topics is resisted.

8. **Richness of associations to topics proposed by the examiner** (viz.: occupa-
tion, family)

    0 Associations are made easily (and readily).

    1 Themes (topics) are relatively rich and varied, but the patient may have
difficulty in moving from one idea to the next.

    2 New topics rarely brought up and show little variety of theme.

    3 No new spontaneously offered topics; tendency toward rumination.

    4 Extremely meagre conversation.

9. **Subjective experience of ruminations**

    0 The patient has the impression that he can think freely, without encum-
berment, now, just as before.

    1 (some uncertainty between 0 and 2).

    2 The patient has the impression that his thoughts dwell on two or three
themes which recur over and over, adversely affecting his current life and
invading his internal world.

    3 The patient has the feeling that his spontaneous thoughts tend always to
collect around a single and painful preoccupation.

    4 The patient experiences a total incapacity to free himself from his painful
ruminations.

10. **Fatigability**

    0 Fatigue is not mentioned spontaneously nor after direct questioning.

    1 Fatigue is not mentioned spontaneously, but evidence for it does emerge
in the course of the interview.

    2 The patient is distressed by fatigability in his everyday life (eating, wash-
ing, dressing, climbing stairs . . .).

    3 Fatigability is such that the patient must curb some of his activities.

    4 Near-total reduction of activities owing to sense of an overwhelming fa-
tigue.

11. **Interest in habitual activities**

    0 Despite being in the hospital, or in treatment the patient retains his usual
interests.

    1 The patient blames a certain measure of loss of interest to being in the
hospital or some other pretext.

    2 The cessation of certain activities (television, newspaper, knitting . . .) is
attributed to a general lack of interest rather than (or as much as to)
fatigue.

    3 Loss of interest is very extensive, affecting also the patient's future.

    4 Total loss of interest.

12. **Patient's perception of the flow of time**

    0 The same as usual.

    1 The present time passes slowly but this relates to inactivity, to being in the
hospital . . .

Table 1 Salpetriere Retardation Rating Scale (Continued)

Score (0 to 4):

2 The perceived passage of time seems slower but this does not emerge except upon specific questioning.
3 The patient indicates spontaneously or quite readily a slowing in the (apparent) passage of time in response to a direct question.
4 Passage of present time is suspended (viz.: painful perception of an infinite "present").

13. Memory
0 The subject states he has no memory difficulty; the examiner detects no evidence of memory deficit.
1 A difficulty in memory is alluded to by the patient, but this is not easily objectified.
2 Memory deficit can be confirmed (viz., difficulty recalling what was served for breakfast), but is not very troublesome to the patient.
3 The memory difficulty is described as a handicap (can't find certain things; forgets who visited him and when . . .).
4 Veritable amnesia.

14. Concentration
0 Normal.
1 The patient believes his concentration is normal, but certain tasks requiring this capacity seem difficult to carry out.
2 The patient admits to problems with certain tasks because of trouble concentrating (reading, doing calculations, professional tasks . . .).
3 A serious difficulty in concentration, interfering even with ordinary pursuits such as reading a newspaper, watching the television . . .
4 Trouble concentrating affects even the interview.

15. General appreciation of retardation
0 None.
1 Questionable.
2 Definite.
3 Moderate.
4 Very serious.

a central role, it can be assumed that the retardation score is a reliable tool for evaluating intensity of the illness. When we compare scores issued from clinical observation, the HDRS, and the RRS, we observe a significative correlation (given size of the sample), particularly between HDRS and RRS scores (Figure 1).

There have been objections that some items included in the scale (especially mental objective and subjective items) could be correlated because they are dependent upon a general factor of depression. This factor would include other signs of depressive illness that we consider as partially independent of retardation. A principal component analysis has been done on all variables from the Hamilton and Retardation scales. The question was whether all the retardation items "remained together," more closely related to each other than to other symptoms. A Factor I was found which

Table 2 Population

Sex		.Women	Men	
	n	98	44	
	%	69	31	

Age		20–40 (years)	40–60 (years)	60–80 (years)
	n	45	59	38
	%	31.68	41.54	26.75

Previous Episodes		Present	Absent	Unknown
	n	85	48	9
	%	59.85	33.8	6.33

Diagnosis			n	%
	Primary Affective Disorders	Bipolar	24	16.9
		Unipolar	34	23.94
		Delusive Depr.	18	12.67
		First onset	30	25.35
	Secondary Affective Disorders (except Schizophrenia)		36	25.35

Table 3 Salpêtrière Retardation Rating Scale: Means and Standard Deviations

Items	1	2	3	4	5	6	7	8	9	10	11	12	13	14
Mean	1.836	1.929	1.843	1.393	1.550	1.257	2.014	1.936	2.321	2.757	2.500	2.000	1.907	2.336
Standard Deviation	1.050	1.064	1.108	1.023	0.992	1.095	1.119	1.127	0.962	1.003	0.809	1.200	0.988	0.853

Note: Global Score: M = 28.6; SD = 11.1.

Table 4   Retardation Scale: Principal Component Analysis

Factors	% Variance	% Cumulated
F.1	59.7	59.7
F.2	9.16	68.86
F.3	6.27	75.1

	Correlations Variables-Factors		
	F.1	*F.2*	*F.3*
1	0.78	0.36	−0.18
2	0.84	0.3	−0.15
3	0.87	0.27	−0.1
4	0.83	0.37	−0.02
5	0.82	0.34	0.01
6	0.83	0.19	0.23
7	0.84	−0.08	0.39
8	0.83	−0.11	0.35
9	0.74	−0.33	0.2
10	0.58	−0.25	−0.39
11	0.7	−0.27	−0.27
12	0.63	−0.41	0.27
13	0.71	−0.31	−0.24
14	0.72	−0.41	−0.26

explains about 35% of variance and contains all the items of the Retardation Rating Scale. Those items are not closely related to any other factor. This result confirms the unity of the syndrome measured by the items of the scale. Moreover, "retardation," "work and activities," and "mood" are the only items of the Hamilton Depression Rating Scale which are also strongly related to this factor, and to it only. Factor II (10% of the variance) seems dependent upon anxiety (3 items of the HDRS: "restlessness associated with anxiety," "psychic anxiety," and "somatic anxiety") and negatively correlated with the motor and speech retardation items of the retardation scale.

Table 5   Correlations Between Initial Scores of HDRS (H 1) and Initial Scores of RRS (R 1), Improvement Score of HDRS (ΔH) Improvement Score of RRS (ΔR)

Comparison	Pearson's Coefficient *r*	Level of Significance *p*
H.1 − R.1	.68	.01
ΔH − ΔR	.79	.01
ΔH − R.1	.56	.01

The more important implication of the theory is that retardation as a behavioral pattern would be very closely related to the neurophysiological alteration on which antidepressive drugs (or at least some of them) have a positive effect. Because retardation is often considered a good predictive factor of therapeutic results, it was worthwhile to consider data issued from the RRS that could be used for testing this assumption.

Initial scores of retardation show a good correlation with therapeutic result (Table 5). However, it is well known that most severe conditions are those which improve best and we had to exclude this bias. For this reason, the study was reanalyzed, selecting patients who were considered as treatment successes according to two criteria. The first criterion was global clinical judgment based on an improvement of at least 7 points on a scale of 10. The second criterion was based on the HDRS score (final score less than 10 points and improvement ≥ 10 between day 0 and day 28). Agreement between the two criteria was approximately 80%, and disagreement was confined to patients with low initial scores. Seventy-five percent of patients were responders according to each criterion. It was expected that in the group with a lower score of retardation, positive results would be less frequent, if in this group there were patients with a slight retardation

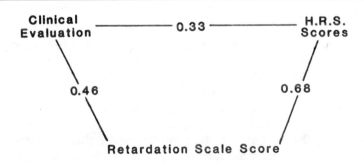

Figure 1 Correlations between initial scores

and patients without any retardation (supposed not to be responders to antidepressive drugs). Results according to HDRS criteria confirm the assumption, but with the clinical judgment criterion no differences between high and low retardation scores were seen (Table 6). It has been argued that weight of anxiety and psychic pain is perhaps heavier with clinical judgment than with Hamilton criteria and some nonspecific improvements are perhaps mixed with release of true depressive syndromes.

Table 6 Relations Between Retardation Initial Score and Responses to Treatment (Number of Patients)

Retardation Score	According to Clinical Criterion Improvement ≥ 7 or 10	
	Failure	Success
< 16	2	17
< 30	13	34
< 40	10	37
> 40	4	16

Retardation Score	According to HDRS Criteria H 3 < 10 − H ≥ 10	
	Failure	Success
< 16	12	8
< 30	16	37
< 40	7	42
> 40	3	17

Evidence supporting this explanation is found when therapeutic success according to Hamilton criteria and scores of motor, mental objective, and mental subjective retardation are compared. By comparing the means of these scores with the HDRS scores, using a Fisher test, objective and subjective mental scores are highly related and motor items to a lesser extent are related to therapeutic success. Such a result could be explained by the assumption that motor retardation interferes with anxious agitation. So we need further inquiries about relationship between motor retardation and anxious agitation.

Table 7 Correlations Between Presence or Absence of Restlessness Associated with Anxiety and Speech motor (6 Items), Mental Objective (6 Items) and Subjective (3 Items) Scores Means

Restlessness / Retardation Scores	Speech and motor	Mental Subjective	Mental Objective
+	6.8	13.4	3.9
−	9.7	13.9	3.9

When motor and mental subjective and objective score means are compared with presence or absence of agitation, as indicated by the HDRS item (Table 7), we see that the presence of anxious agitation is related to the motor score and not to mental subjective and objective scores. This fact supports strongly the assumption of an interference between motor retardation and anxious agitation, while cognitive slowing seems independent of anxiety, and is one reason why a scale that deals with cognitive slowing as much as motor retardation could be useful.

Conclusion

Retardation as a behavioral pattern is the primary disorder in a depressive condition, and is supported by many observations and statistical assumptions as convincing as arguments in favor of the mood disorder theory. But this alternative assumption has not been taken seriously because retardation has been limited too often to its motor expression, and cognitive slowing has been mixed with grief and sadness rather than related to motor retardation.

Construction of a scale measuring the entire freezing of mental and behavioral actions was imperative and empirical results indicate a strong correlation between both sides of retardation. However, when it is a matter of predicting therapeutic success, cognitive slowing seems a better sign than motor retardation. This may be due to interference between anxious agitation and depressive retardation. Separating agitated depression from retarded depression is perhaps only justified in regard of this late distinction and because the anxious agitation obliterates motor retardation. In any case, cognitive slowing seems a constant dimension of depression and, probably, its core.

References

1. Dumas G. *Les Etats Intellectuels dans la Mélancolie,* Thèse. F. Alcan, ed, p. 142 1895.

2. Nelson JC and Charney DS. The symptoms of major depressive illness. *Am. J. Psychiatry* 138, 1981.

3. Pichot P, Piret J, and Clyde DJ. Analyse de la symptomatologie depressive subjective. *Revue de Psychologie Appliquee* 2:105 1966.

4. Mendels J and Cochrane C. The nosology of depression. The endogenous reactive concept of major depressive illness. *Am. J. Psychiatry* 124:1–11, 1968.

5. Bielski RJ and Friedel R. Prediction of tricyclic antidepressant response. *Arch. Gen. Psychiat.* 33:1479, 1976.

6. Szabadi E, Bradshaw M, and Besson JAO. Elongation of pause time in speech: A simple objective measure of motor retardation in depression. *Brit. J. Psychiat.* 129:592–97, 1974.

7. Spitz RA. "Hospitalism. An inquiry into the Genesis of Psychiatric Conditions in Early Childhood." In *Psychoanalytic Study of the Child*, Vol. I, 1945.

8. Harlow HF and Suomi SJ. *Production and Alleviation of Depressive Behaviors in Monkeys in Psychopathology: Experimental Models.* San Francisco: W. H. Freeman and Co, 1977.

9. Hrdina PD and Von Kulmiz. *Separation Induced Behavioral Disorders in Infra-human Primates: An Animal Model of Depression?* Depressive disorders. Symposium Hoechst 13, 1977.

10. Porsolt RD et al. Behavioral despair in rats: A new model sensitive to antidepressant treatments. *European J. Pharmacol.* 47:379–91, 1978.

11. Porsolt RD, Bertin A, and Jaffre M. Behavioral despair in mice: a primary screening test for antidepressants. *Arch. Int. Pharmcodyn. Ther.* 229:327–36, 1977.

12. Zeldine G. et al. A propos de l'Echelle d'Evaluation en psychiatrie transculturelle. *L'Encéphale* 1:133–45, 1975.

13. Costello CG. *Anxiety and Depression (The Adaptative Emotions).* London: Univ. Press Montreal, 1976.

14. Engel GL. Anxiety and depression withdrawal: The primary affects of unpleasure. *Int. J. Psychoanal.* 43:82–97, 1962.

15. Gurney C et al. Studies in the classification of affective disorders. The relationship between anxiety states and depressive illnesses. II. *Brit. J. Psychiat.* 121:162–66, 1972.

16. Pichot P *Étude comparative de l'action de l'amitryptiline et de l'association amitryptiline-chlordiazepoxide,* edited by Pragues O et al. Advances in Neuropsychopharmacology Proceedings of the 7th C.I.N.P. 11–15 July 1980. North Holland Pub.

17. Lorr M, Klett CJ, and McNair M. *Syndromes of Psychosis.* Oxford: Pergamon Press, 1963.

18. Blackburn IM. Mental and psychomotor speed in depression and mania. *British J. Psychol.* 126:329–35, 1975.

19. Weckowicz TE et al. Speed in test performance in depressed patients. *J. Abnormal Psychology* 87 (5):578–82, 1978.

20. Weiss B et al. Psychomotor activity speed and biogenic amines metabolites in depression. *Biological Psychiatry.* 9:45–54, 1974.

21. Kupfer DJ et al. Psychomotor activity in affective states. *Arch Gen Psychiatry* 30:765–68, 1974.

22. Frechette D. *Le Ralentissement Psychomoteur Dans la Dépression: Contribution à Son Evaluation Quantitative.* Thèse pour le Doctorat d'Etat en Médecine. Paris, 1978.

23. Jouvent R et al. Le ralentissement psychomoteur dans les états dépressifs: Construction d'une échelle d'evaluation quantitative. *L'Encéphale* 6:41–58, 1980.

24. Jouvent R et al. Analyse multifactorielle de l'Echelle de Ralentissement Dépressif utilisee chez les déprimés ambulatories. *Psychologie Médicale*, 13 B, 1981.

25. Fermanian J. *Contribution à la méthodologie des essais thérapeutiques en psychiatrie: Etudes des problèmes théoriques et pratiques posés par l'utilisation des échelles d'évaluation.* Thèse pour le Doctorat d'Etat en Biologie Humaine, Paris, 1979.

Recent Genetic Studies of Bipolar and Unipolar Depression

David L. Dunner, M.D.

Classifying depressed patients into bipolar and unipolar subtypes was first proposed in 1962 by Leonhard et al., based on the clinical differentiation of depressed patients with and without mania.[1] Family history studies noted that patients with bipolar illness had more psychosis and suicide among their relatives than patients with unipolar illness. Since 1962, several studies in Europe and the United States have refined and extended this original observation. More importantly, a model for investigation in psychiatry has been developed to the point that genetic data are important for validating clinical diagnosis in psychiatry, particularly among the affective disorders.

This chapter will review data supporting evidence for genetic factors in the etiology of affective disorders, the development of methodology for genetic studies, and the resulting classification systems. We will highlight data from three recently completed large American studies of the genetics of bipolar and unipolar depression. We will review the current status of biological markers for affective disorders and finally present some areas of interest for future research.

Evidence for Genetic Factors

Several lines of evidence suggest that some forms of depression may have an etiology on a genetic basis. In order for a genetic etiology to be proven, several factors should be evident. First of all, the disorder should cluster within families; patients with the illness should have relatives who also demonstrate the illness. Second, studies of twins should show that the illness is more prevalent among monozygotic than dizygotic twins. A third line of evidence would come from adoption studies. Adoption studies are designed to differentiate environmental from genetic factors. Data from such studies should reveal that subjects who have a biological parent with illness but who were raised in a foster home develop the illness nevertheless; whereas subjects whose biological parents do not have the illness but who were raised in a home where there is affective disorder, do not develop affective disorder in excess of controls. Fourth, the illness could be shown to be linked to a gene of known Mendelian transmission.

Affective disorders, particularly manic-depressive illness, are familial. The evidence that bipolar illness clusters in families was reported by Leonhard et al.[1] Perris and Angst both suggested that affectively ill relatives of bipolar patients tended to have bipolar and not unipolar disorders, whereas affectively ill relatives of unipolar patients tended to have unipolar illness and not bipolar illness.[2,3] In the 1960s the Washington University group published a series of familial studies in manic-depressive illness, particularly bipolar disorders.[4,5] These studies showed a high familial risk for affective disorder in relatives of manic patients. Second, a very comprehensive family study of affective disorder suggested that manic-depressive illness may be linked to a gene transmitted on the X-chromosome.[5] Subsequent studies in the late 1960s from the National Institute of Mental Health (NIMH) also showed a differential familial loading for relatives of patients with bipolar compared with unipolar disorders.[6] Relatives of bipolar patients had elevated morbid risks for bipolar illness, unipolar illness, and suicide, compared to relatives with unipolar patients.

Few twin studies of affective disorder appear in the literature of the last 10 years or so. Kallmann's study is still considered the definitive work, showing very high concordance rates for bipolar illness in monozygotic compared to dizygotic twins.[7]

The adoption technique, utilized in the Danish studies of schizophrenia, has been tried in studies of bipolar illness. Data from adoptees in Iowa indicated that primary affective illness may have a familial factor.[8] Another study of adoptees from manic-depressives also supports the concept of a genetic factor in the etiology of affective disorders.[9]

In the search for genetic linkage of affective disorders, the studies of Winokur et al. pointed toward a genetic factor on the X-chromosome.[5] Attempts to extend and replicate these findings have resulted in considerable controversy. Mendlewicz and coworkers showed linkage of bipolar affective disorder with two markers on the X-chromosome, color blindness, and XG blood type.[10,11] Gershon et al. were unable to replicate these findings and subsequently criticized the data from the Mendlewicz studies on methodological grounds.[12,13]

184

In summary, the separation of bipolar affective disorder as a distinct subtype has resulted in a clearer definition of the genetic factors that may be involved in the etiology of affective disorders. Most studies attempting to assess genetic factors in affective illness that have separately considered bipolar patients have resulted in positive results. The relatives of bipolar patients show a higher genetic loading and particularly more bipolar illness than relatives of other affectively ill patients. Clearly, unipolar illness as presently defined is a much more heterogeneous collection of disorders than bipolar disorder. Attempts to find subtypes of unipolar disorder using a genetic classification have not been particularly successful. However, Winokur's group separated unipolar patients into women with an early age of onset (depressive spectrum disease) whose relatives showed depression and alcoholism, and depressed men with a late age of onset (pure depressive disease) whose relatives showed depression only.[14]

Methodology for Family Studies

The renewed interest in the genetics of bipolar and unipolar depression in the late 1960s and the interest in defining these disorders led to several family studies in the 1970s. The simplest method, the so-called family history method, was to ask patients about illness in their relatives. This tends to underestimate illness in relatives. An interview (Schedule for Affective Disorders and Schizophrenia—SADS) developed early in the 1970s was used to document illness in relatives.[15] Interviewing relatives directly (the "family study" method) led to greater precision regarding the diagnosis of illness in relatives. In a refinement of this technique, relatives are interviewed blind to the proband diagnosis in order to decrease investigator bias. Most of the recent genetic studies conducted in the United States employed a blind family study method, wherein relatives were interviewed with a standardized instrument with the interviewer unaware whether the person being interviewed was the patient, relative, or a control.

Classification of Affective Disorder

Early genetic studies supporting the separation of bipolar from unipolar patients were based on studying families of patients who had been hospitalized for affective disorders. For the most part, patients considered bipolar manic-depressive had been hospitalized for at least one manic episode, whereas patients considered unipolar had at least one episode of depression. In the Perris study, three episodes of depression were required for a patient to be called unipolar.[2] In 1970 we proposed a classification for affective disorder.[6] Knowing that some depressions occur in the course of other psychiatric disorders and thus might be viewed as complications of these primary disorders, we required that patients have a primary affective disorder according to the criteria of Feighner et al.[16] In reviewing the patients in our sample it was apparent that two groups of patients had manic symptoms. One group of patients had manic symptoms resulting in hospitalization specifically for mania; these patients were termed Bipolar I. These patients were congruent with prior American and European genetic studies of affective disorders by Perris, Angst, and Winokur.[2,3,5] However, there remained a group of patients who had manic symptoms that did not result in hospitalization specifically for mania. These patients had depressions requiring hospitalization and hypomania; we classified them separately from other unipolar and bipolar patients and termed them Bipolar II. It is likely that many other studies of affective disorders had included such Bipolar II patients as unipolar.

We later extended this classification to include subjects who had never been hospitalized for affective disorder but who had received outpatient treatment.[17] Thus our classification system proposed that bipolar patients might be separable into four types: Bipolar I, subjects who have been hospitalized specifically for mania; Bipolar II, subjects with depression and hypomania who had been hospitalized specifically for depression; Bipolar Other, those who had depression and hypomania and who had received outpatient treatment for affective disorder; and a group we term Cyclothymic Personality, referring to subjects who had bipolar affective symptoms but who had not been treated. For Unipolar patients we required at least one depressive episode that met criteria for primary affective disorder and that resulted in either hospitalization or treatment for depression.

The group termed Bipolar I seems to be relatively homogeneous when data from clinical, biological, pharmacological, and genetic studies are evaluated.[18] Bipolar II patients tend to have the clinical appearance of unipolar patients but tend to be pharmacologically and biologically similar to Bipolar I patients. The Bipolar Other group seems to be congruent with Akiskal's cyclothymic patients.[19] Subsequent studies suggest that Bipolar I subjects may well be indistinguishable from Bipolar II subjects.[20] In our classification system the group termed Cyclothymic Personality was reserved for diagnosing relatives of subjects in our genetic studies.

The classification system is not entirely congruent with *DSM III.* The bipolar affective disorder of *DSM III* would include most Bipolar I patients, some Bipolar II patients, and some patients whom we term Bipolar Other. Approximately a third of patients we classified as Bipolar I had mood incongruent delusions and would be Atypical Bipolar disorder or Atypical Psychosis in *DSM III.*[21] Furthermore, although the term Atypical Bipolar disorder specifically mentions Bipolar II illness, many Bipolar II patients will meet *DSM III* criteria for bipolar affective disorder. The group classified as Cyclothymic disorder in *DSM III* is seemingly not congruent with our Bipolor Other or Akiskal's Cyclothymic disorder in that such patients meet criteria for more severe disorders in the *DSM III* nomenclature.[19] The group we considered Unipolar disorder meets the *DSM III* criteria for major affective disorder. However, major affective disorder in *DSM III* includes both primary and secondary depressions and thus represents a population of depressed patients of greater heterogeneity than we had proposed and studied. *DSM III* will be the standard for diagnosis of the 1980s, but the clinical and genetic studies of the 1970s used slightly different concepts of affective subtypes.

Recent Family Studies of Bipolar and Unipolar Depression

Three large American studies of the genetics of affective disorders have been recently reported. The New York study was a prospective investigation of approximately 400 patients who met criteria for Bipolar I, Bipolar II, and Unipolar disorders.[22] Diagnosis of the probands was confirmed by SADS–L interviews of about 90% of the living relatives available for interview. Diagnosis of relatives was blind to proband diagnosis and confined to data from the SADS–L. Morbid risks, calculated according to the method of Strömgren, used ages at risk from the New York clinic population. Data regarding ages at risk are presented for first degree relatives age 18 and older. These data were available for approximately 2,000 first degree relatives.

The NIMH sample was also a prospective study consisting of 171 probands separated into Bipolar I, Bipolar II, and Unipolar types.[23] Eleven patients termed schizoaffective were also included. Probands had been hospitalized on the research wards of the NIMH and relatives of these subjects were given a structured interview. Data were available for approximately 1,000 first degree relatives.

The Iowa study was a retrospectively obtained sample of 100 bipolar patients, 225 unipolar patients, and 160 surgical controls.[24] Patients had been hospitalized at the Iowa Psychopathic Hospital 30 to 40 years ago. Approximately 1,600 first degree relatives of these subjects were evaluated blind to proband diagnosis using a structured interview similar to the SADS. In contrast to the New York and NIMH samples, most of the relatives of the Iowa sample who were actually interviewed were siblings and children because the probands' parents were for the most part deceased. Furthermore, the Iowa group did not separate probands into Bipolar I and Bipolar II types, although it could be assumed that most of their bipolar probands were Bipolar I.

Results of these studies are summarized in Table 1. In general, the risk for a first degree relative to have an affective disorder is approximately 15–

Table 1 Morbid Risk of Affective Disorder in Relatives of Bipolar and Unipolar Patients

	Patient Diagnosis	Relative Diagnosis		
		Bipolar I	Bipolar II	Unipolar
New York	BPI	2.8	4.6	6.4
	BPII	.8	6.0	10.6
	UP	.2	3.0	8.4
NIMH	BPI	3.5	3.3	10.8
	BPII	2.1	3.7	13.6
	UP	1.2	1.2	13.2
Iowa	BPI	5.3		12.4
	UP	3.0		15.2

Note: Data are morbid risk (%). Morbid risks were calculated by dividing the number of ill subjects by the total number of subjects after the latter were corrected for age of risk for the various disorders.

20%. Second, there is a general consistency in these three studies in that an increased morbid risk for mania (Bipolar I illness) is shown for relatives of Bipolar I patients as compared to relatives of Unipolar patients. Third, the risk for Unipolar illness exceeds that for bipolar illness in relatives of bipolar patients. Additionally, relatives of bipolar patients generally have about the same rate of unipolar illness as relatives of unipolar patients.

The Iowa study did not provide a separate comparison of relatives of Bipolar II subjects. In the New York and NIMH data, relatives of Bipolar II patients tend to have an excess of bipolar illness (types I and II) compared to relatives of unipolar patients. This rate of bipolar illness approximates the combined rate of bipolar illness for relatives of Bipolar I patients.

Certain methodological differences in these studies should be noted. The New York study was entirely prospective and was based on an outpatient sample who came to three outpatient research centers. Criteria for determining that a relative was ill required that the relative have treatment or hospitalization for psychiatric illness. The NIMH sample was derived from an inpatient population. Criteria for illness in relatives included illness causing social disability in addition to treatment and hospitalization. This may explain why the rates for affective illness in the NIMH sample are slightly higher than the New York sample. For the Iowa sample, the probands were obtained retrospectively and the data reported were for those relatives actually interviewed or for whom medical charts were available to indicate psychiatric disorder. Thus, whereas the data in the New York and NIMH samples are for all relatives, the data for the Iowa sample pertain to only approximately 40% of the total number of relatives because many were deceased.

In spite of these methodological differences, the three studies provide a strong data base for an understanding of the genetic contributions to bipolar and unipolar affective disorder. Approximately 400 bipolar probands were studied and the data reflect an analysis of approximately 3,000 first degree relatives. These data clearly demonstrate an increased morbid risk for mania among relatives of manic depressive patients.

Attempts to analyze the genetic data from the New York sample for chromosomal linkage using a Mendelian model were not positive. It should be noted that the hypothesis for an X-linked dominant gene as a major genetic factor in bipolar disorder was not supported by data from the New York sample. Furthermore, the data from these three studies do not clearly support a specific mode of inheritance for bipolar illness.

Biological Markers

Research into biological factors associated with affective illness in the 1970s was largely concentrated on attempts to relate biological factors, such as the activities of blood enzymes or concentrations of catecholamine metabolites in cerebrospinal fluid and urine, to depression. The search for biological markers for a genetic disorder should be predicated on the notion of discovering trait rather than state associations. Thus the marker should be present in the well state as well as in the ill state and should be clustered in ill relatives of subjects with the disorder and observed less frequently among well relatives of patients or among controls. Recent reviews indicate that in general there is no satisfactory marker for bipolar and unipolar affective disorders at this time.[18,25] Attempts to demonstrate such markers have been extensive over the past 10 years and have produced a strategy for studying relatives of subjects with affective disorder. Not only are standardized interviews used to establish diagnosis, but also blood tests or provocative tests are made to determine if a biological marker is associated with vulnerability to the illness. Some markers that have been studied and found not to be satisfactorily related to affective disorders include the activities of catecholamine metabolizing enzymes, such as monoamine oxidase and catechol-O-methyltransferase. More recently, cholinergic supersensitivity has been suggested as a possible trait marker for affective illness.[26] Further studies of this system in affectively ill patients are awaited with interest.

Suggested Areas for Future Research

A very pertinent research area for the 1980s is the so-called high risk study wherein children of subjects who have a familial psychiatric disease are studied in order to determine the antecedents of the illness. The characteristics required for a high risk study include that the disease be familial, such as bipolar manic-depressive illness, and that the proband diagnosis be satisfactory so that the adult probands can be classified in a relatively homogeneous way. The disorder should become clinically evident early in life so that one might have the opportunity of following children into the age of risk. This is particularly true of bipolar disorder, where at least half of the patients have been hospitalized by the age of 30. A high risk study is dependent on a thoughtful assessment of relevant markers to the illness.

The identification of a trait marker for affective disorder is a goal for research in the 1980s. Bipolar affective disorder is a suitable clinical substrate for such research.

References

1. Leonhard KI, Korff I, and Schultz H. Die temperamente in den familien der monopoluren und bipolaren phasischen psychosen. *Psychiat Neurol* 143:416–34, 1962.

2. Perris C. A study of bipolar (manic-depressive) and unipolar recurrent depressive psychoses. *Acta Psychiat Scand* 42(Suppl 194):1–188, 1966.

3. Angst J. "Zuratiologie und Nosologie Endogener Depressiver Psychosen." In *Monographien aus dem Gesamtgebeite der Neurologie und Psychiatrie.* Berlin: Springer-Verlag, 1966, No. 112.

4. Clayton PJ, Pitts FN Jr., and Winokur G. Affective disorder: IV Mania. *Compr Psychiatry* 6:313–22, 1965.

5. Winokur G, Clayton J, and Reich T. *Manic Depressive Illness.* St. Louis: C.V. Mosby Co., 1969.

6. Dunner DL, Gershon ES, and Goodwin FK. Heritable factors in the severity of affective illness. *Biol Psychiat* 11:31–42, 1976.

7. Kallmann FJ. "Genetic Principles in Manic-depressive Psychosis." In *Proceedings of the American Psychopathological Association,* edited by Zubin J and Hoch P. New York: Grune and Stratton, 1954.

8. Cadoret RJ. Evidence for genetic inheritance of primary affective disorder in adoptees. *Amer J Psychiat* 135:463–66 1978.

9. Mendlewicz J and Rainer JD. Adoption study supporting genetic transmission in manic depressive illness. *Nature,* London. 268:327–29, 1977.

10. Mendlewicz J, Fleiss JL, and Fieve RR. Evidence for X-linkage in the transmission of manic-depressive illness. *JAMA* 222:1624–27, 1972.

11. Mendlewicz J and Fleiss JL. Linkage studies with X-chromosome markers in bipolar (manic-depressive) and unipolar (depressive) illness. *Biol Psychiat* 9:261–64.

12. Gershon ES et al. Color blindness not closely linked to bipolar illness: Report of a new pedigree series. *Arch Gen Psychiat* 36:1423–30, 1979.

13. Gershon ES. Nonreplication of linkage to X-chromosome markers in bipolar illness. *Arch Gen Psychiat* 37:1200, 1980.

14. Baker M et al. Depressive disease: Classification and clinical characteristics. *Compr Psychiatry* 12:354–65, 1971.

15. Endicott J and Spitzer RL. A diagnostic interview: The schedule for affective disorders and schizophrenia. *Arch Gen Psychiat* 35:837–44, 1978.

16. Feighner JP et al. Diagnostic criteria for use in psychiatric research. *Arch Gen Psychiat* 26:57–63, 1972.

17. Fieve RR and Dunner DL. "Unipolar and Bipolar Affective States." In *The Nature and Treatment of Depression,* edited by Flack FF and Draghi SC. New York: John Wiley & Sons, 1975. pp. 145–66.

18. Dunner DL. "Unipolar and Bipolar Depression: Recent Findings from Clinical and Biological Studies." In *The Psychobiology of Affective Disorders,* edited by Mendels J and Amsterdam JD. Basel: S. Karger, 1980. pp. 11–24.

19. Akiskal HS et al. Cyclothymic disorder: validating criteria for inclusion in the bipolar affective group. *Amer J Psychiat* 135:1227–33, 1977.

20. Dunner DL et al. Classification of bipolar affective disorder subtypes. *Compr Psychiat,* in press.

21. Rosenthal NE et al. Toward the validation of RDC schizoaffective disorder. *Arch Gen Psychiat* 37:704–810, 1980.

22. Dunner DL, Go R, and Fieve RR. A family study of patients with bipolar II illness (Bipolar depression with hypomania). Presented at the annual meeting, American College of Neuropsychopharmacology, San Juan, Puerto Rico, Dec. 1980 (Abstracts p. 25).

23. Gershon ES et al. Clinical, biological and linkage data in affective disorders pedigrees. Presented at the annual meeting, American College of Neuropsychopharmacology, San Juan, Puerto Rico, Dec. 1980 (Abstracts p. 26).

24. Tsuang MT, Winokur G, and Crowe RR. Morbidity risks of schizophrenia and affective disorders among first degree relatives of patients with schizophrenia, mania, depression and surgical conditions. *Brit J Psychiat* 137:497–504, 1980.

25. Gershon ES. "The Search for Genetic Markers in Affective Disorders." In *Psychopharmacology: A Generation of Progress,* edited by Lipton MA, DiMascio A, and Killam KF. New York: Raven Press, 1978. pp. 1197–1212.

26. Sitaram N et al. Faster cholinergic REM sleep induction in euthymic patients with primary affective illness. *Science* 208:200–2, 1980.

The Prevalence and Course of the Affective Disorders

Paula J. Clayton, M.D.

The affective disorders are disorders of mood. In the past, numerous names have been used to characterize these disorders. They include reactive depression, neurotic depression, psychotic depression, endogenous depression, agitated and retarded depression, depressive spectrum disorders, primary and secondary depression, manic depressive disease, and involutional melancholia. In the *Diagnostic and Statistical Manual* 3rd ed. (*DSM III*) the term affective disorder was adopted and the one separation that currently remains, although it is tentative, is the separation of the affective disorders into unipolar and bipolar.

Unipolar affective disorder (monopolar affective disorder) refers to patients who have depressions only. Bipolar affective disorder refers to patients who have episodes both of mania and depression or episodes of mania only. The new *DSM III* divides the patients into major depressive disorder (comparable to unipolar affective disorder) and bipolar affective disorder (comprising patients with both poles of the illness and mania only). To date, there are no data to suggest that unipolar mania differs from bipolar disorder. Originally, it was felt to be rare, comprising about 2%–5% of the patients who have episodes of mania. Nurenberger et al. recently reported that 16% of a group of Bipolar I patients had never been hospitalized or treated for depression.[1] Abrams et al. reported that 18% of patients hospitalized for affective disorder (not necessarily bipolar) were unipolar manics.[2]

The *DSM III* also includes a less severe but more chronic affective

This research was supported in part by U.S. Public Health Service Grant MH-25430.

disorders category under which is listed cyclothymic disorder and dys-thymic disorder. Atypical affective disorders can also be coded. There is no depressive neurosis. On the other axes, personality disorders, physical illness, stressors, and level of functioning can be coded.

Because there are clinical, genetic, and perhaps treatment differences between the two major affective disorders, it is reasonable to review them separately. However, it may be that in the future, these disorders will be considered, as Kraepelin did, as one.[3] Major depressive disorder tends to begin later, to be more heavily female, to be less frequent, to necessitate less frequent hospitalizations, to be more likely to be chronic, to be less familial, and rarely to include a family history of mania.

Major Depressive Disorder

Epidemiology

The true prevalence of this disorder is unknown. In the population studies which have been done throughout the world, there is a marked difference in case definitions and case ascertainment. Weissman and Myers found that the lifetime prevalence in a United States population for a definite major depressive disorder was 18% (12.3% in males and 25.8% in females).[4] In a recent review, Boyd and Weissman reported that in the two studies from the United States using treated and untreated community studied subjects with structured interviews and consistent criteria, the lifetime prevalence was between 8%–12% for men and 20%–26% for women.[5] However, the range of prevalence for all studies was more varied, being 2%–12% for men and 5%–26% for women. All studies show that unipolar depression whether designated in the community, in a general practitioner's office, in a private psychiatrist's office, in a general psychiatric clinic, or in an inpatient setting, is two times as common in women as in men. The age of onset is broad, ranging from 15 to 70 years, with the average age of onset in the early 40s. Childhood depression and depression in later life are popular concepts but remain rare.

Unipolar affective disorder is a recurring illness. The more recent, carefully done, follow-up studies of hospital populations show that between 5% and 15% of cases have only one episode.[6,7] A follow-up of an outpatient maintenance therapy study indicated that only 20% of these less severe patients had a single episode.[8] Earlier reports from hospital populations indicated there were more people with single episodes. However, in these early studies it was not clear how many people died by suicide or other causes after the first episode, how many had their onset very late in life and therefore did not live long enough to have a second episode, and how many people had a single episode which became chronic.

Recurrence is an important aspect of this disorder to consider because the issue is not only the treatment of the presenting episode but also the consideration of a patient for prophylactic treatment.

The duration of an episode of depression varies from study to study, but the average duration varies between 4 and 8 months.[9] Recent reports have indicated depressions are of even longer duration. Dr. Kupfer reported in Chapter 7 that the average duration of his depressed inpatients was 42 weeks.

The usual course reported in the literature is one of recurrences of solitary depressions separated by several interval-free years, although there are some people who have annual depressions in a specific season of the year. Recent studies have shown that far more patients are intermittently symptomatic.

The number of episodes an individual has may be limited. The mean number of episodes in unipolar depression is 5 to 6.[6,7] The best predictor of course, however, is previous course; that is, if a patient has had three episodes in the past two years, it is very likely that she or he will have a similar course after the current episode. There is some indication that the relapse rate is higher and more frequent as age increases and this may be related specifically to women.

Somewhere between 10% and 20% of all patients so diagnosed will have a chronic course.[10,11] Again, this may be more frequently seen in those with older ages of onset. In an acute treatment study of cognitive therapy *versus* imipramine therapy in outpatients, 25% of these treated patients were chronically symptomatic for 1 year.[12] The average age of the patients was 33 years but older age and previous episodes were related to symptomatic status. Another outpatient treatment study reported similar results with about 21% mostly or chronically depressed.[13] Thus, even (or perhaps specifically) outpatient depressive illness outcome is not as favorable as had previously been thought.

Genetics

Studies have shown that about 25% of patients with unipolar affective disorder have a parent or other first degree relative with an affective disorder.[9] When studied by interviews as opposed to taking family histories, almost one-third of patients are found to come from families in which two generations suffer from an affective disorder. Twin studies and adoption studies suggest that the increased family prevalence may be in large part genetic. Mania is relatively rare, as is schizophrenia. Alcoholism is common, especially in those cultures where heavy drinking is common. The question of assortative mating is controversial.

Treatment

Tricyclic antidepressants have been found to be superior to place-bos.[14,15] Newer data indicate that cognitive behavior therapy and interpersonal psychotherapy (IPT) are as good as pharmacotherapy in the treatment of depressed outpatients.[12,13,16] The exciting aspect of these therapies yet to be tested is the question of whether they could be prophylactic; that is, can the patient learn techniques of dealing with depression that would either prevent it from recurring, or if it did recur, that he or she could apply to interrupt the course? In addition, electroshock therapy is an effective treatment for depression.[17] In some studies it has been shown to be more effective than antidepressants, particularly with the psychotically depressed patient. In no study was it shown to be less effective. Electroshock therapy may reduce the mortality, both by suicide and from other causes, in patients with affective disorder.[18] Additionally, antidepressants are as good as lithium, if not better, in the prophylactic treatment of recurrent depressive disorder.[19]

Complications

An increased mortality is associated with affective disorders. In large part this is accounted for by the increased rate of suicides in these disorders, but there is also an increased mortality from other causes. Without dividing patients by polarity, a summary of the relationship between suicide and primary affective disorders showed that suicide risk among patients with these disorders was more than 30 times greater than that of the general population.[20] Approximately 15% of all deaths of patients with affective disorder was accounted for by suicide. Although the disease itself is more common in women, suicide is more common in men. The risk of suicide as compared to other causes of death is increased early in the course of the illness.[20,21]

Suicide attempts are increasing in all countries, but suicide rates vary from country to country. In the United States, the suicide rate is increasing in the young and may continue to rise as they get older.[22]

Bipolar Affective Disorder

Epidemiology

Weissman and Myers reported a lifetime prevalence of Bipolar I and II affective disorder to be 1.2.[4] This means that although it is far less frequent than unipolar affective disorder, it is as common as schizophrenia. Boyd and Weissman, looking at lifetime risk of Bipolar I disorder, found the rate to be between .2% and .9%.[5] In a completely different way of estimating prevalence based on the use of lithium carbonate, Eastwood et al. found a rate of bipolar affective disorder to be 1 and 2 per 1,000 of the population, which is very similar to the previously reported results.[23]

Follow-up studies of depressed inpatients have shown that about 13%–15% of patients develop a mania.[24] Even in the Perris study, where he required that the patients entering the study have three previous episodes of depression, 13% became bipolar.[25] In most studies from inpatient settings, the ratio of unipolar to bipolar patients is reported to be 10 : 1; however, Krauthammer and Klerman estimated that the ratio with certain depressives excluded to be more like 4 : 1.[26] This figure may change as psychiatrists become more astute in diagnosing more subtle cases of bipolar affective disorder. Akiskal et al., in a 4-year follow-up of neurotic depressive inpatients and outpatients, found that 22% were unipolar and 18% were bipolar.[27] In looking at a total population of Amish, Egeland et al. found that the unipolar to bipolar ratio was almost 1 : 1.[28]

Even in bipolar illness, there is a probable slight preponderance of women over men. There is one report that in the early age group, if the disease starts as mania, the sex of the patient is more likely to be male and if the disease starts as depression, the patient is more likely to be female. This would increase the percentage of men identified in small series as bipolar, leaving younger patients as women who had not yet manifested their bipolarity.

Bipolar illness is a disease of much earlier onset and much more limited risk. The onset is usually from the teens through the 50s, with 30 years as the average median age of onset. Numerous studies have indicated that in the teenage years there are more cases of bipolar affective disorder than schizophrenia. In three studies, 91%, 90%, and 89% of the bipolar patients were ill by the time they were 50 years old. Some indication exists that becoming ill with mania after the age of 50 is more deleterious and has a more chronic course. Literature on late onset bipolarity is confusing because many of the patients discussed had episodes of depression which began before the age of 50 but did not become manic until after. The age of onset of the entire illness, however, would be considered before 50.

Bipolar illness is definitely a recurrent illness. In one series of 393 patients, virtually every patient had a recurrence.[6,7] In a second hospitalized series, only 7% were without recurrence.[29] A third series showed no patients without relapse.[10] There is no comparable series from an outpatient clinic, and recent data indicate that these patients can avoid hospitalization.[5]

Bipolar patients have more episodes than unipolar, the median being around 8.[6,7] The mean duration of the episode of bipolar affective disorder is shorter, usually about 4 months, with the episode of depression lasting longer than the episode of mania. As with unipolar affective disorder, the duration of episodes does not change remarkably with increasing number of episodes. Initially, the interval between episodes decreases but it seems to bottom out in a set pattern with a cycle every 6 to 9 months. As with unipolar illness, the best way to predict a patient's course is by his previous course. In bipolar illness, too, there is a hint that there may be extinction of the repetitive pattern with a certain number of episodes. This needs further investigation, but it may mean that although the short-term course is malignant, the long-term outlook may be better.

The question of chronicity in bipolar affective disorder is still unanswered because it is difficult to define chronicity. If chronicity is judged by either the presence of symptoms, social decline, or both, it is estimated that about one-third of bipolar patients have a chronic course.[24] However, chronic mania is rare. Given the prevalence, early onset, and chronicity, many patients previously thought to be schizophrenic should be diagnosed as bipolar.

Genetics

Affective disorder, be it mania or depression, is more common in the relatives of patients with bipolar affective disorder than in unipolar patients. Significantly more bipolars than unipolars have an affected parent or two generations of illness.[9] Twin and adoption studies support the notion of a genetic component. Between 4% and 10% of bipolar patients had a relative with mania, and genetic markers have been proposed. To date, no firm statement can be made about the association between bipolar illness and X-chromosome transmission or between bipolar illness and the human leukocyte androgen.[30,31] Here, too, the question of assortative mating is controversial.

Treatment

The treatment of bipolar affective disorder is similar to the treatment of unipolar affective disorder. Depression can be treated in exactly the same way. Mania can be treated with lithium, phenothiazines, lithium and phenothiazines in combination, perhaps Tegretol and electroshock therapy.[24,32] The efficacy of lithium in the treatment of acute mania is now well accepted. Prophylactic use of lithium is also well established. It should be remembered, however, that in all studies, only about 50% of bipolar patients remain free from relapse for 3 years.[24]

Complications

The risk of suicide in bipolar affective disorder is also high. Suicide may be as common in women as in men with this disorder, but it appears that there is a trend, even in bipolars, for the suicide to occur less frequently as the disease continues.[21] Some studies have shown that there are marital disruptions, school interruptions, and job loss after the onset of this illness, although other studies did not replicate these findings. These complications, which may depend on the adequate stabilization of the disease, can also include alcohol abuse, and possibly a decrease in fertility.[33]

References

1. Nurnberger J Jr. et al. Unipolar mania: A distinct clinical entity? *Am J Psychiatry* 136:1420–23, 1979.

2. Abrams R et al. Unipolar mania revisited. *Journal of Affective Disorders* 1:59–68, 1979.

3. Kraepelin E. *Manic-Depressive Insanity and Paranoia.* Edinburgh: E & S Livingstone, 1921.

4. Weissman MM and Myers JK. Affective disorders in a United States urban community: The use of research diagnostic criteria in an epidemiological survey. *Arch Gen Psychiatry* 35:1304–11, 1978.

5. Boyd J and Weissman M. Epidemiology of affective disorders. *Arch Gen Psychiatry* 38:1039–46, 1981.

6. Angst J et al. The course of monopolar depression and bipolar psychoses. *Psychiat Neurol Neurochir* 76:489–500, 1973.

7. Grof P, Angst J, and Haines T. "The Clinical Course of Depression: Practical Issues." In *Classification and Prediction of Outcome of Depression*, edited by Angst J. Stuttgart, New York: F.K. Schattauer Verlag, 1973.

8. Weissman MM. Personal communication, 1978.

9. Winokur G. "Mania, Depression: Family Studies, Genetics, and Relation to Treatment." In *Psychopharmacology: A Generation of Progress*, edited by Lipton MA, DiMascio A, and Killam K. New York: Raven Press, 1978.

10. Murphy GE et al. Variability of the clinical course of primary affective disorder. *Arch Gen Psychiatry* 30:757–61, 1974.

11. Robins E and Guze SB. "Classification of Affective Disorders: The Primary-Secondary, the Endogenous-Reactive, and the Neurotic-Psychotic Concepts." In *Recent Advances in the Psychobiology of the Depressive Illnesses.* Proceedings of a Workshop Sponsored by the NIMH, edited by Williams TA, Katz MM, and Sheild JA Jr. Washington, DC: U.S. Government Printing Office, 1972.

12. Kovacs M et al. Depressed outpatients treated with cognitive therapy or pharmacotherapy. *Arch Gen Psychiatry* 38:33–39, 1981.

13. Weissman MM et al. Depressed outpatients. Results one year after treatment with drugs and/or interpersonal psychotherapy. *Arch Gen Psychiatry* 38:51–55, 1981.

14. Biggs JT and Ziegler VE. "Tricyclic Antidepressants in Outpatient Therapy." In *Current Psychiatric Therapies, Vol. 17*, edited by Masserman JH. New York: Grune & Stratton, 1977.

15. Davis JM. Overview: Maintenance therapy in psychiatry: II. Affective disorders. *Am J Psychiatry* 133:1–13, 1976.

16. Rush AJ et al. Comparative efficacy of cognitive therapy and pharmacotherapy in the treatment of depressed outpatients. *Cognitive Ther Res* 1:17–37, 1977.

17. Fink M. Efficacy and safety of induced seizures (EST) in man. *Compr Psychiatry* 19:1–18, 1978.

18. Avery D and Winokur G. The efficacy of electroconvulsive therapy and antidepressants in depression. *Biol Psychiatry* 12:507–23, 1977.

19. Prien R. "Lithium and the Long-Term Maintenance Treatment of Recurrent Depression: A Continuing Controversy." In *Treatment of Depression: Old Controversies and New Approaches*, edited by Clayton PJ and Barrett J. New York: Raven Press, in press.

20. Guze SB and Robins E. Suicide and primary affective disorders. *Br J Psychiatry* 117:437–38, 1970.

21. Tsuang MT. Suicide in schizophrenics, manics, depressives, and surgical controls. *Arch Gen Psychiatry* 35:153–55, 1978.

22. Murphy G and Wetzel R. Suicide risk by birth cohort in the United States, 1949–1974. *Arch Gen Psychiatry* 37:519–23, 1980.

23. Eastwood R, Stiasny S, and Tice S. Estimates of the prevalence of bipolar affective disorder. Methods based on treatment with lithium. *Acta Psychiat Scand* 63:83–90, 1981.

24. Clayton PJ. The epidemiology of bipolar affective disorder. *Compr Psychiatry* 22:31–43, 1981.

25. Perris C. A study of bipolar (manic-depressive) and unipolar recurrent depressive psychoses. *Acta Psychiat Scand* 42 (suppl 194) 1966.

26. Krauthammer C and Klerman GL. "The epidemiology of Mania." In *Manic Illness*, edited by Shopsin B. New York: Raven Press, 1979.

27. Akiskal H et al. The nosological status of neurotic depression. *Arch Gen Psychiatry* 35:756–66, 1978.

28. Egeland J and Hostetter A. Amish study: I. Affective disorders among the Amish, 1976–1980. *Am J Psychiatry* 140:56–61, 1983.

29. Bratfos O and Haug JO. The course of manic-depressive psychosis. *Acta Psychiat Scand* 44:89–112, 1968.

30. Nurnberger JI and Gershon ES. "Genetics." In *Handbook of Affective Disorders*, edited by Paykel ES. London: Churchill Livingstone, 1982.

31. Weitkamp MD et al. Depressive disorders and HLA: A gene on chromosome 6 that can affect behavior. *New England Journal of Medicine* 305:1301–6, 1981.

32. Juhl RP, Tsuang MT, and Perry PJ. Concomitant administration of haloperidol and lithium carbonate in acute mania. *Dis Nerv Syst* 38:675–76, 1977.

33. Baron M, Risch N, and Mendlewicz J. Differential fertility in bipolar affective illness. *Journal of Affective Disorders* 4:103–12, 1982.

14

Later Life Depression—Clinical and Therapeutic Aspects

Jose L. Ayuso-Gutierrez, M.D.

Introduction

Later life depressions do not really constitute a special nosological category and only differ from other depressions in time of onset. These affective disorders respond to the same principles as depressions that present at other stages of life and that can be treated with the customary therapy with similar results. By convention and most frequent acceptance in epidemiological geriatric studies, the lower age limit of this group has been fixed at 65. Moreover, by using strictly chronological terms to define later life depression, we avoid establishing any etiological connection with hypothetical involutive mechanisms. Nonetheless, in spite of the nosological identity with other depressions, later life depressions offer certain idiosyncrasies in the following aspects: epidemiology, etiopathogenesis, symptoms, and therapy.

Epidemiology

Depression is one of the most important psychiatric disorders of later life, having a greater numerical significance than the psychopathological disorders associated with structural changes in the brain tissue. According to Ban, 10% of the general population over 65 suffers from depression.[1] Gurland et al. report that the point prevalence rate of depression of a clinical level of importance amounts to about 13% of the elderly population of New York City.[2] There may be cases of masked depression that are overlooked in these statistics; although afflicted with substantial depressive symptomatology in the form of physiologic symptoms, a subject may not describe a typical depressive affection and would not be identified in these surveys. Aside from these purely quantitative distinctions, later life depressions are marked by a greater risk of suicide and a more prolonged evolution.

The clinical histories of 100 patients over 65 years of age who were hospitalized with the diagnosis of primary major depressive disorder in the Hospital Clinico of Madrid were analyzed with respect to age of onset: before (senile or early form) or after 65; and form, unipolar and bipolar. No attempt was made to select the histories; the study was based on the first 100 patients with these characteristics who were admitted to the hospital after the study began. The results are listed in Table 1.

The absolute predominance of unipolar depression in the elderly is notable with a ratio of 32 unipolar forms to every bipolar form; in other age groups hospitalized for depression there were 3 unipolar forms for every bipolar form. Note that the majority of our elderly subjects with symptoms of unipolar major depressive disorder (58.7%) gave no history of previous depressive episodes. Likewise, the senile onset of bipolar depression is exceptional (in our sample there was no case), an observation that coincides with other studies.[3,4]

Etiopathogenesis

What reasons account for the high frequency of depression in the aged? From a multifactorial perspective, the higher prevalence of depression in the aged can be attributed to two factors: increased vulnerability and higher incidence of precipitant psychosocial situations.

The elderly person's greater vulnerability to environmental noxa is possibly conditioned by biological factors such as increased monoamine oxidase activity;[5] decreased norepinephrine levels in brain;[6] or loss of

Table 1 Distribution of the Depressions in Hospitalized Patients Over 65 Years

Type of Depression	Onset of Illness Before 65		Onset of Illness After 65	
Unipolar	Women	26	Women	40
Depression	Men	14	Men	17
	Total	40		57
Bipolar	Women	0	—	
Depression	Men	3	—	
	Total	3	—	

Note: N = 100.

Table 2 The Incidence of Precipitants in Later Life Depressions (In Percentages)

Psychosocial Precipitants	<65 Years N = 100	>65 Years Late Onset N = 57
Death in the family	0	14
Change of residence	2	7
Change in the family structure	5	5.2
Illness within the family group	2	7
Economic-work problems	9	7
Family problems	6	7
Total	24	47.2

Note: d.f. = 5; Chi-square = 13.7911; p < .025.

adrenergic neurons or of their terminations, leading to decreased amine storage and synthesis.[7]

The elderly are also subject to a higher incidence of precipitant psychosocial situations. Grief, uprooting, and changes in the family structure are situations encountered most frequently in old age and are situations that predispose people to the development of depressive illness.[8]

We have compared the incidence of psychosocial factors in 57 elderly inpatients admitted consecutively to the hospital with late onset depression to 100 cases of persons under 65, also admitted consecutively, but not in selected groups.[9] The evaluation of psychosocial factors was based on information obtained from interviewing the patient and his family. The average age of the senile depressed group was 68.2 years and the average age of the control group was 43.3 years.

Table 2 relates the incidence of psychosocial precipitants in both groups. The overall incidence of harmful life events was found to be unequally distributed between the two samples. In the elderly group, 47.2% of the cases presented evidence of a psychosocial precipitant circumstance; in the younger group, stressful life events could only be verified in 24% of the cases. The difference between the groups is statistically significant. The most frequent stressful life event prior to depression in the aged is the death of the spouse and subsequent widowhood.

Symptomatic Characteristics

From the clinical point of view, the pathoplastic conditioning of advanced age is amply reflected in the entire depressive spectrum. Basically, the symptomatology of later life depressions consists of the following:

- More frequent agitation.
- More frequent paranoid symptoms.
- More frequent somatization of anxiety and hypochondriac complaints.
- Decreased presence of guilt feelings.
- Rarity of psychomotor retardation.
- Relative frequency of hallucinations, generally auditory and conditioned by isolation.
- Relative frequency of delusions of economic ruin.
- Greater risk of suicide.

The diagnosis of depression in the elderly presents specific problems not encountered in younger patients and caused by the greater clinical variability of the depressive syndromes. It is helpful to recall several more or less atypical depressive syndromes that can offer difficulties in the diagnosis of this affective disorder in the aged subject (Table 3).

Therapeutic Measures

Psychotherapy

Any therapeutical approach to old age depression should be complemented with supportive psychotherapy to minimize the impact of environmental factors and to help the patient cope with his difficulties. The object of such intervention is to provide support, to help resolve conflicts and mobilize defenses, and to obtain the patient's cooperation in the therapeutic program. The doctor should keep in mind the advisability of providing the following information:

- An explanation of the temporal character and favorable prognosis of the depressive disease.
- An explanation of the relationship between the somatic and psychic symptoms and the basic affective disorder.
- Information on the effects of the medication, especially its prolonged period of latency and the side effects related to its therapeutic activity.
- Instruction to family members on the care and management of the patient with special attention to the risk of suicide. They should be encouraged to make opportune changes in the patient's surroundings.
- Stimulation of the patient's self-esteem, with emphasis on his achievements and positive attainments in life.

Pharmacotherapy

The mainstay of depression pharmacotherapy is the tricyclic drugs and the new generation of antidepressants. Most evidence confirms that these

Table 3 Special Clinical Forms of Later Life Depression

Clinical Form	Principal Clinical Characteristics
Hypochondriac Depression	• Preoccupation with bodily functions plays a prominent role • Frequently associated with objective organic factors • Prevalence of hysteriform elements
Masked Depression	• Somatic symptoms uppermost, obscuring underlying depression
Pseudodemential Depression	• Prevalence of confusion and apathy • Onset frequently rapid • Previous intellectual level generally low
Paranoid Depression	• Social isolation and sensory deficits are frequently the cause of different degrees of paranoia in the depressed elderly
Nihilistic Delusional Depression	• Ideas of corporal negation

drugs are as effective in the elderly as they are in younger people. Nonetheless, the success of pharmacotherapy depends largely on scrupulous attention to certain guidelines:

1. Use the minimum effective dose. In general, only one-third to one-half of the usual dose is required to attain therapeutic blood levels: 50—100 mg/day of imipramine or amitriptyline, or the equivalent dose of other drugs.
2. Use the least number of drugs possible. Patients need not be routinely given sleep medications or antianxiety agents.
3. Keep in mind that the therapeutic effect of these drugs appears later in older patients.
4. Side effects, especially anticholinergic and cardiovascular effects that may mimic symptoms of dementia or of a worsening of depression, must be carefully monitored.
5. Daily dosage should be divided to avoid the peak effect of a single dose.
6. Avoid parenteral administration because the effects produced are excessively rapid and the elderly patient's adaptability is limited.

These measures are dictated to a great extent by the pharmacokinetic and pharmacodynamic modifications that accompany aging. The tricyclics reach higher plasma levels in patients older than 65 than in younger depressed patients.[10] Even at equivalent plasma levels, the aged patient may have an increased amount of free drug available because of the reduction in plasma proteins and consequent decreased protein binding that occur with aging.[11] Because drug elimination is slower in the elderly, it takes longer to reach steady state equilibrium, and the onset of drug effects may be very delayed.[12] Because of the higher plasma levels obtained, the decreased cholinergic functioning of the central nervous system, and the changes in certain organ systems that accompany advancing age, anticholinergic side effects are more frequent and troublesome in older as compared to younger subjects.[7]

Considering the increased susceptibility of elderly patients to antidepressant side effects, the best compounds are those that have the minimum anticholinergic and cardiovascular effects. Among the tricyclic drugs, these effects are least pronounced in the group of secondary amines (desipramine, nortriptyline), and are even less marked in the new generation of antidepressant drugs (mianserin, nomiphensine, viloxazine).

The problem posed by the interaction of the antidepressants with other frequently associated medications merits special attention. These medications include the neuroleptics, antianxiety agents, barbiturates, and antihypertensives (Table 4). For example, neuroleptics and antidepressants are not infrequently combined in cases where the predominant symptoms are of agitation or delirium. Recently compiled evidence indicates that the neuroleptics inhibit the hepatic enzymes determining the protracted destruction of the tricyclic component and its subsequent elevation in plasma.[13–15] According to these findings, this use of various drugs can contribute to an increase in the risk of adverse reactions in the elderly.

There are no indications that antianxiety agents significantly alter the metabolism of the tricyclics.[15] However, they should only be used in the aged patient with discretion since confusional states are occasionally observed after the combined administration of tricyclics and benzodiazepam.[16] This combination frequently produces excessive sedation and ataxia in the aged patient.

Barbiturates should be excluded from any therapeutic program, not only because they increase the risk of toxicity but because they noticeably decrease the plasma levels of the antidepressants.

Special attention is required in the treatment of patients who are hypertensive as well as depressed. The use of centrally active antihypertensives, such as reserpine, should be avoided because of their manifest depressogenic activity. On the other hand, the peripherally active antihypertensives such as bethanidine and guanethidine are blocked by the tricyclics, which compete for the adrenergic receptors. In view of these drawbacks, if the depression is sufficiently grave, electroshock may be the most appropriate treatment. Where electroshock is contraindicated, it is recommended that the hypertension be treated with diuretics.

Table 4 Interactions Between Tricyclic Antidepressants and Other Drugs

Drug	Effect
Neuroleptics	Increased blood levels
Antianxiety Agents	No evidence of changes in blood levels
Barbiturates	Decreased blood levels
Antihypertensives	Hypotensive effect diminished

Unfortunately, a large percentage of the persons who suffer from later life depression do not respond to conventional psychopharmacologic treatments and require other therapeutic measures. In these cases, the alternative therapies should be considered. For example, the combination of sleep deprivation + antidepressant drugs, substantially amplifies clinical response.[17]

Monoamine oxidase inhibitors (MAOIs) may be considered if the tricyclics are ineffective and if proper dietary compliance can be assured. There is evidence that MAOIs are particularly efficacious in older patients, perhaps because of enhanced MAO activity with advancing age.[12]

Finally, electroconvulsive shock therapy is safe and significantly more effective than tricyclics in patients older than 50 years of age.[18]

References

1. Ban TA. The treatment of depressed geriatric patients. *Am J Psychotherapy* 32:93–104, 1978.

2. Gurland B et al. "The Epidemiology of Depression and Dementia in the Elderly: The Use of Multiple Indicators of These Conditions." In *Psychopathology of the aged*, edited by Cole JO and Barrett JE. New York: Raven Press, 1980.

3. Winokur G, Clayton PJ, and Reich T. *Manic Depressive Illness*. St. Louis: The Mosby Company, 1969.

4. Landoni G and Ciompi L. Études statistiques sur l'age de prédilection des troubles dépressifs. *Evolut Psychiat* 38:583, 1971.

5. Samorajski T. "Age-Related Changes in Brain Biogenic Amines." In *Aging Volume I: Clinical, Morphological and Neurochemical Aspects in the Aging Central Nervous System*, edited by Brody H, Harman D and Ordy JM. New York: Raven Press, 1975.

6. Robinson DS et al. Monoamine metabolism in human brain. *Arch Gen Psychiatry* 34:89–92, 1977.

7. Jarvik LF and Kakkar PR. "Aging and Response to Antidepressants." In *Clinical Pharmacology and the Aged Patient*, edited by Jarvik LF, Greenblatt DJ, and Harman D. New York: Raven Press, 1981.

8. Tellenbach H. *La Melancolia*, Madrid: Ediciones Morata, 1976.

9. Ayuso-Gutiérrez JL, Mateo-Martin I, and Fuentenebro de Diego F. Análisis etiopatogénico y clínico de las depresiones en la tercera edad. *Acta Psiquiátrica y Psicólogica de América Latina* 25:187, 1979.

10. Nies A et al. Relationship between age and tricyclic antidepressant plasma levels. *Am J Psychiat* 134:790–93, 1977.

11. Bender AD. Pharmacodynamic principles of drug therapy in the aged. *J Am Geriatric Soc* 22:296–303, 1974.

12. Robinson DS. "Age-Related Factors Affecting Antidepressant Drug Metabolism and Clinical Response." In *Geriatric Psychopharmacology*, edited by Nandy K. New York: Elsevier North Holland, 1979.

13. Gram LF and Overo KF. Drug interaction: Inhibitory effects of neuroleptics on metabolism of tricyclic antidepressants in man. *British Medical Journal* 1:463–65, 1972.

14. Rafaelsen OJ and Gram LF. "Interaction Between Antidepressants and Other Groups of Psychopharmaca." In *Classification and Prediction of Outcome of Depression*, edited by Angst J. Stuttgart: Schattauer Varlag, 1974.

15. Olivier-Martin R. "Pharmacocinetique des Antidépresseurs Tricycliques." In *Colloque sur la Depression*, edited by Vencovsky E. Paris: Expansion Scientifique, 1978.

16. Martin EW. *Hazards of Medication*. Philadelphia: Lippincott, 1971.

17. Richard J and Droz P. *Les Dépressions Tardives*. Basel: Ciba-Geigy, 1978.

18. Avery D and Winokur G. The efficacy of electroconvulsive therapy and antidepressants in depression. *Biol Psychiatry* 12:507–23, 1976.

15

Dysthymic and Cyclothymic Disorders: A Paradigm for High-Risk Research in Psychiatry

Hagop Souren Akiskal, M.D.

Introduction

Current epidemiologic estimates place the lifetime risk for manic-depressive illness at 1.2%.[1] This figure is obtained with the use of the Schedule for Affective Disorders and Schizophrenia, which is most rigorous in the definition of the "typical" or syndromal forms of these disorders.[2] However, Kraepelin and other authors in the "classic" descriptive tradition have observed cyclothymic and related temperamental deviations that do not reach the clinical threshold of severity required for the diagnosis of bipolar psychosis.[3-10] Until recently, little clinical attention was paid to this larger universe of "bipolar oscillations."

Three related developments have changed this picture during the last few years. First, the advent of lithium treatment has led to a reconsideration of the clinical boundaries of both psychotic and nonpsychotic affective illness, with the hope of increasing the pool of patients who may benefit from this salt.[11-17] Second, psychiatrists have moved into community settings, where frequent encounters with milder affective conditions have created the need for diagnostic rubrics like dysthymia and cyclothymia. Third, the focus of psychiatric research is shifting from patients with major disorders to individuals at risk. In the area of affective illness, the emphasis is on (1) identifying biological or clinical markers of vulnerability to aid in the detection of persons at risk before the illness is manifested or

The writing of this review was in part supported by the Department of Mental Health and Mental Retardation, State of Tennessee, and USPHS MH 05931 from the National Institute of Mental Health. Christy Wright provided editorial assistance.

in its early stages, and (2) applying pharmacologic and psychotherapeutic modalities to prevent clinical and social complications.

The term "subaffective disorder" is used here to refer to these milder and early expressions of the major affective disorders.[18,19] Because subaffective conditions were first described in the biological kin of hospitalized manic depressives, they are often considered genetically attenuated forms of bipolar illness.[20] In cyclothymia, depressive and hypomanic oscillations alternate; dysthymia denotes intermittently depressive mood swings. These oscillations are typically of short duration (a few days), of subsyndromal severity (falling short of the symptomatic picture of the full-blown illness), and recur at irregular intervals over long periods of time. In this chapter, recent research findings on the identification, clinical description, course, family history, and other external validating strategies of these subaffective disorders will be summarized.

Identification of Subaffective Disorders

High-Risk Family Approach

The classic method of identifying subaffective disorders is to study the biological kin of hopsitalized manic-depressive probands. Using this approach, Kraepelin pioneered in delineating the milder forms of the affective psychoses, which he termed "manic," "cyclothymic," "depressive," and "irritable" temperaments.[3] In his words:

> There are certain temperaments which may be regarded as rudiments of manic-depressive insanity. They may throughout the whole of life exist as peculiar forms of psychic personality without further development; but they may also become the point of departure for a morbid process which develops under peculiar conditions and runs its course in isolated attacks.[3]

Thus, Kraepelin postulated a continuum between affective temperaments and the affective psychoses. This view was most cogently expressed by Kretschmer, who hypothesized that the "endogenous psychoses are nothing more than marked accentuations of normal types of temperament."[4] Kretschmer introduced the term "cycloid" to refer to the entire domain of affective temperaments, which varied enormously between depressive and hypomanic poles.

More recent research tends to limit polarity of temperament to polarity of illness.[21-23] In other words, depressive temperaments are said to occur in families of unipolar probands, and cyclothymia in families of bipolar probands. However, Gershon et al. linked cyclothymia, but not chronic minor depression, to *both* unipolar and bipolar disorders.[24] In line with these observations, Angst and colleagues demonstrated both cyclothymic *and* subdepressive temperaments in families of bipolar probands.[25]

Thus, while the *existence* of subaffective temperamental disorders has been established, there is still some uncertainty regarding the specificity of temperament to affective subtype.

The high-risk family paradigm is a powerful tool in identifying the most "typical" subaffective precursors of the major affective disorders. However, it is limited to the most familial-genetic forms of temperament and thereby excludes the larger universe of temperamental deviations in the general population.

High-Risk Biochemical Approach

In the ideal, this strategy identifies high-risk populations by examining all noncase individuals with a known trait biological marker for a given disease (e.g., normal glucose tolerance test in diabetes mellitus). Unfortunately, no such universal trait marker exists for major affective disorders.[26] However, Murphy and associates at NIMH have reported low platelet monoamine oxidase (MAO) activity in a subgroup of patients with bipolar disorders;[27] and Schooler et al. and Buchsbaum et al. have extended this line of work in imaginative attempts to define the clinical correlates of low platelet MAO activity in noncase college students.[28,29] The significant correlations included sensation-seeking, high leisure activity, high ego strength, and positive affects, as well as suicidal and certain antisocial behaviors. Further, the family history of this group tended to be positive for similar behaviors. Structured psychiatric evaluations were not conducted in these studies, so the low-MAO group cannot be characterized diagnostically. But the hypothesis that such subjects are at risk for major affective episodes, especially mania, is quite plausible. Future research is needed to clarify whether low MAO activity identifies specific vulnerability to bipolar disorder or a general susceptibility to bipolar, schizophrenic, and antisocial disorders.

Lithium-Responsive "Personality" Disorders

Although pharmacologic response is not a standard method of delineating psychiatric disorders, it may be useful in identifying phenotypic boundaries.[30-32] Current evidence indicates that lithium salts, compared with neuroleptic agents, have a more specific range of clinical effectiveness, largely limited to disorders characterized by phasic shifts in mood and activity.[33] The principal indications include cyclic (Bipolar I), predominantly depressive (Bipolar II), and some reccurent "unipolar" (probably those with bipolar family history) forms of the major affective disorders.

The question is whether the nonpsychotic end of the bipolar spectrum can be enlarged to include certain lithium-responsive "personality" disorders. These include "emotionally unstable character disorder";[34] the "bipolar—other" group, those hospitalized neither for depression nor for mania;[35] and certain "impulsive," aggressive, "irritable-hyperactive," histrionic and obsessional, and substance abusing personalities.[36-43] Although researchers in this area have utilized imaginative pharmacologic approaches to patients resistant to standard psychiatric treatment, their investigations have not led to operational clinical characterization of the disorders at the mild end of the affective spectrum. Nevertheless, such research has demonstrated the possible "masking" of mild affective disorder by characterologic attributes. In evaluating these studies, it must be kept in mind that lithium may exert an "anti-aggressive" effect independent of its influence in attenuating affective oscillations. Finally, in some distinctly subaffective conditions such as the "bipolar—other" group studied by Peselow et al., it may be impossible to demonstrate a clearcut beneficial effect of lithium because of noncompliance (i.e., patient drop out because they miss their short-lived "highs").[35]

In summary, the results obtained with Peselow's approach, while compatible with the existence of a spectrum of mild and intermittently chronic affective disorders, have not, to date, identified the core characteristics of these disorders.

High-Risk Behavioral Approach

In the behavioral high-risk paradigm, the research clinician screens a given population for evidence of subsyndromal manifestations of bipolar affective disorder; that is, signs and symptoms which are milder and shorter in duration than the usual clinical threshold for diagnosing bipolar disorders.[44,45] One can screen a random epidemiologic sample, an outpatient psychiatric sample, or a noncase population believed to be high risk.

The major advantage of defining high-risk groups by behavioral criteria is the inclusion of all phenotypes and phenocopies of a given disorder. As a result, the boundary between "normal" and "ill" is difficult to define. Nevertheless, by not limiting study to bipolar families, this approach permits a more rigorous testing of the hypothesis that affective temperaments are genetically based.[44]

Validating the Diagnosis of Cyclothymic Disorder

Clinical Description

Cyclothymic cases in our study were identified in semistructured diagnostic interviews of 500 chronic psychiatric outpatients who had no histories of psychiatric hospitalization.[44] Of this group, 96 patients had experienced frequent ups and downs over a period of at least 2 years, as specified in the first edition of the Research Diagnostic Criteria for cyclothymic personality.[46] Fifty of these subjects did not give convincing evidence for behavioral change in a biphasic direction and were therefore considered a "pseudocyclothymic" group. The remaining 46 patients—who had *behavioral* manifestations of a biphasic disorder with irregular brief cycles, but who fell short of the full syndromal or duration criteria for Feighner depression or mania—were considered "true" cyclothymics.[47]

Most cyclothymic subjects were in their mid-20s at index evaluation, but many had had psychiatric problems dating back to their late teens. Their clinical presentations were usually "nonaffective"; that is, repeated romantic or conjugal failure, episodic promiscuity, uneven work records, geographic instability, dilettantism, and substance abuse. These patients had received psychotherapeutic and psychopharmacologic treatment for "personality disorders," which were most commonly variations on the theme of borderline, hysterical and sociopathic conditions.

Operational criteria for cyclothymia were proposed based on the clinical characteristics of these 46 cases (Table 1). Onset in adolescence, biphasic manifestations with behavioral evidence of mood change, short cycles (3–10 days), and an irregularly intermittent course emerged as the most important diagnostic features. The most critical factor is the demonstration that mood swings, especially those in the hypomanic direction, are accompanied by objectively observable behavioral changes.

Our cyclothymic cases could be classified into three overlapping clinical subtypes:

1. **Predominately depressed cyclothymia.** In approximately half of our sample, depressed periods dominated the clinical picture, interspersed with "even," "irritable," and occasional "high" periods. In this group, the cyclothymic oscillation was often complicated by *major* depressive episodes—hence their resemblance to Bipolar II disorder as defined by Fieve and Dunner.[48]

2. **"Pure" cyclothymia.** In this pattern, which accounted for 40% of the sample, depression and hypomania alternated with about equal frequency. For example, an optimistic, overconfident, people-seeking phase would give way to self-absorption, self-doubt, pessimism, a sense of futility, emptiness, and suicidal ideation.

3. **Hyperthymic disorder.** In this subtype, which constituted less than 10% of the sample, hypomanic periods dominated, with decreased need for sleep, expansive behavior, and a generally "wild" lifestyle. However, occasional irritable periods and rare depressive dips marred these subjects' overall joyful dispositions. These individuals were enterprising, ambitious, and driven; many were socially and vocation-

Table 1   Clinical Characteristics of Cyclothymic Disorder[44]

General
1. Onset in teens or early adulthood.
2. Clinical presentation as a personality disorder (patient may not be aware of "moods" per se unless adroitly questioned).
3. Short cycles—usually days—which are recurrent in an irregular fashion, with infrequent euthymic periods.
4. Usually does not attain full syndrome of depression and hypomania during any one cycle, but entire range of affective manifestations occur at various times.
5. Abrupt "endogenous" shifts; i.e., often wakes up depressed.

Behavioral Manifestations
1. Irritable-angry-explosive outbursts that alienate loved ones.
2. Episodic promiscuity; repeated conjugal or romantic failure.
3. Frequent shifts in line of work, study, interest, or future plans.
4. Resort to alcohol and drug abuse as a means of self-treatment.
5. Episodic financial extravagence.

Biphasic Course
1. Hypersomnia alternating with decreased need for sleep (intermittent insomnia can also occur).
2. Shaky self-esteem which alternates between lack of self-confidence and naive or grandiose overconfidence.
3. Periods of mental confusion and apathy, alternating with periods of sharpened and creative thinking.
4. Marked unevenness in quantity and quality of productivity, often associated with unusual working hours.
5. Uninhibited people-seeking (which may lead to hypersexuality) alternating with introverted self-absorption.

ally successful. They complained of intermittent insomnia dating back to their early teens, and it was in their 40s and 50s that they became "worn out" and presented for treatment.[20]

Irritable periods occurred in all these subtypes, and dominated the clinical picture in 7 patients, who had very short-lived (hours to days) periods of unpredictable, explosive outbursts of anger with no special provocation. These patients tended to be younger, had more disturbed interpersonal behavior, were more likely to abuse alcohol as well as sedative-hypnotic drugs, had the most flagrant antisocial records, and resembled the "emotionally unstable personality" described by Rifkin and associates.[49]

Depue and associates have recently applied the behavioral high-risk paradigm to a noncase population of 930 undergraduate college students in Albany.[45] Of these, 126 subjects were designated as a subsyndromal bipolar group on the basis of a self-report inventory. These subjects were in their late teens, and only 13% had received outpatient treatment related to their psychiatric status. However, interpersonal, academic and civic disturbances were frequent findings. They typically had short mood cycles (2–6 days) of depression and hypomania and, like the patients in the Tennessee studies, conformed to three subtypes. Thus, Depue and colleagues documented the prevalence of cyclothymia in a largely untreated population of probands who were an average of 10 years younger than the Tennessee cohort. Their sample displayed less interpersonal, academic, and civic dysfunction, but pursued the type of course we had described. These comparisons have public health implications because they suggest that serious psychosocial complications appear as cyclothymic individuals develop from adolescence to early adulthood.

The presence of prominent personality disturbances in cyclothymic patients creates differential diagnostic problems. Waters has argued that cyclothymia, unlike personality disorders, is experienced by the sufferer as an ego-dystonic disturbance.[50] We do not believe that this criterion is useful in distinguishing cyclothymia from personality disorders. Indeed, personality consequences of cyclothymia are often so prominent that the condition appears ego-syntonic. For this reason it is necessary to validate phenomenologically or psychometrically defined cyclothymic diagnoses by external validating criteria for bipolar disorder. The following illustrates how we have used prospective follow-up and family history to achieve this goal.

Prospective Course

Cyclothymic disorder is differentiated from manic-depressive illness by the following criteria: (1) the full range of clinical disturbances is not manifest, and it often falls short of the full syndromal criteria for manic and major depressive disorders; (2) thus, psychotic manifestations in the form of delusions and hallucinations are extremely unusual; (3) the cycles are typically brief, lasting days, rarely weeks; (4) "low" and "high" cycles usually alternate each other in an irregular pattern, and intervening "even" or "well" periods are relatively uncommon.

These characteristics are in part selection artifacts. The universe of bipolar patients is composed of an extreme variety of overlapping patterns. We attempted to limit selection of cases to patients who had never been hospitalized for an affective episode and who failed to meet the full complement of the St. Louis Criteria for bipolar affective disorder.[47] Fieve and Dunner classify such bipolar patients under a residual category of "bipolar other" as distinguished from Bipolar I and II groups.[48] The Bipolar II group includes patients who satisfy the criteria for a major depressive episode (usually hospitalized for such), but who have not come to clinical attention for mania. The "high" periods in this group are hypomanic (i.e., usually nonpsychotic, short-lived, and not incapacitating); indeed they may be welcomed by the patients as the "good" feature of the illness. By contrast, the defining characteristic of the Bipolar I group is the occurrence of at least one episode of an incapacitating or socially disruptive manic episode, usually psychotic and requiring hospitalization; depressive episodes commonly occur in Bipolar I disorder, although their presence is not necessary for including a patient in this category.

As shown in Table 2, slightly over a third of the 46 cyclothymic patients we studied progressed to spontaneous affective episodes that met the full duration and syndromal criteria for clinical depression ($N=11$), hypomania ($N=7$), and mania ($N=3$).[44] These episodes were "spontaneous"; that is they occurred over a 1- to 2-year drug-free follow-up. Thus 6% of the original cyclothymic group could be reclassifed as Bipolar I, and 38% as Bipolar II. This 34% progression from a cyclothymic affective personality to a clinical affective episode is significantly higher than the 5% risk in a nonaffective personality disorder group studied over an analogous drug-free period.

The tendency to switch to hypomania was further augmented by the administration of tricyclic antidepressants in 11 of the 25 cyclothymics who required this class of drugs for control of depressive symptoms. This 44% rate of pharmacologically occasioned hypomania was not significantly different from the 35% rate seen in Bipolar I controls, but was very significantly different from nonaffective personality controls where no patient exhibited pharmacologically induced hypomania.

Table 2 Affective Episodes in Cyclothymic and "Pseudocyclothymic" Groups Over a 1- to 2-Year Follow-Up[14]

Affective Episodes	Cyclothymic Group (N=46)		Pseudocyclothymic Group (N=50)	
	N	%	N	%
Drug-free course				
Depression	11	24	2	4
Hypomania or mania	10	22	0	0
Total [a]	16	35	2	4
Course on tricyclics [b]				
Hypomania	11[b]	44[b]	0	0

[a] The total number of patients is less than the number of episodes shown in the first row of both columns because several patients suffered both depressive and hypomanic episodes. The overall difference in the risk to develop clinical affective episodes for the cyclothymic and nonaffective personality groups was significant by the chi-square test ($p < .001$).
[b] Tricyclics were used, when clinically warranted, on 25 of 46 cyclothymic patients; 11 (44%) developed hypomania. This was very similar to the rate seen in bipolar controls (35%) and both were significantly different from the nonaffective personalities by chi-square analysis ($p < .001$).

Family History

In our study, cyclothymic and Bipolar I manic-depressive patients had similar patterns of familial affective illness (Table 3): 30% of the cyclothymics and 26% of the manic-depressives had first degree biological kin with manic-depressive illness, and the respective proportions of family history for suicide in the two groups were 22% and 18%. Very few of the nonaffective personalities had such histories.[44]

The pedigree of a cyclothymic proband is shown in Figure 1. This pedigree is loaded with affective and related disorders, that is, depressive illness, manic-depressive psychosis, suicide, alcoholism, and drug dependence. Furthermore, the transmission of the illness from generation III to generation I is accomplished through the intermediary of the cyclothymic prepositus in generation II, suggesting that cyclothymia itself is a phenotypical variant of the full-blown bipolar affective psychosis.

"Familial" is of course not synonymous with "hereditary." But the overall evidence, including that derived from adoption studies, converges in attributing the major variance of the familial distribution in affective disorders—particularly in the bipolar forms—to genetic factors.[51,52]

Conclusion

Two independent studies conducted in different populations, have provided strong evidence that cyclothymia is a subaffective disorder.[44,45] This evidence rests on (1) shared phenomenology with biphasic course; (2) familial distribution of affective illness similar to that found in classical manic-depressive illness; (3) high risk for hypomanic, manic, and depressive episodes during drug-free follow-up; and (4) high rates of tricyclic-induced hypomanic switches. A fifth line of evidence, response to lithium carbonate treatment, awaits studies with sufficient methodological rigor to address the question of measuring subtle diminution of moods in patients who tend to be highly mercurial in mood and noncompliant in treatment.*

The Question of Dysthymic Disorder

Clinical Identification

Describing dysthymia as subaffective expression of primary affective disorders is a more difficult task than identifying cyclothymia. The *DSM III*

---

* As previously noted, the modest prophylactic effect of lithium against depression in cyclothymia in the Peselow et al. study is conceivably caused by patient noncompliance. In our study, which had the limitation of being an open trial, significant *behavioral* improvement over several key clinical parameters (e.g., sleep, substance abuse, anger outbursts) could nevertheless be demonstrated during a 1-year period of lithium treatment. [20]

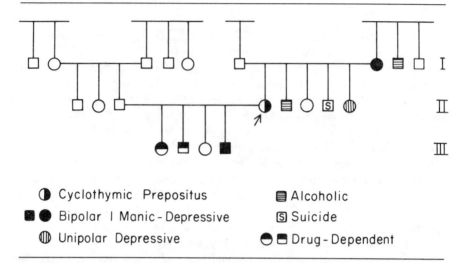

Figure 1 Pedigree of a cyclothymic proband
Source: From Akiskal et al. Cyclothymic temperamental disorders. *Psychiatr Clin North Am* 2(3):543, 1979.

(1980) criteria for dysthymia refer to a large and heterogeneous universe of chronically and intermittently depressed individuals. To select a *subaffective* group, we screened 137 chronic depressive probands who met the *DSM III* criteria for "dysthymic disorder." [53] Excluded were 1) adult onset chronic depressions that were the sequelae of unipolar depressive episodes; and 2) protracted, low-grade depressions in the setting of, or secondary to, validated nonaffective psychiatric diagnoses, as well as those secondary to longstanding and disabling medical disorders.[47] The 50 remaining subjects with early onset subsyndromal depressions and irregularly intermittent course were chosen for study. Such patients are often termed "characterologic depressives" because of their early onset prominent characterologic disturbances and dysphoric manifestations that are not easily separable from characterologic pathology.[54] We used a "crude" pharmacologic probe, response to thymoleptic agents such as tricyclic antidepressants and lithium carbonate, as a tentative attempt of subclassifying these subjects into "depressive" and "characterologic" groups. We viewed significant clinical response to these agents as compatible with primary affective disorder and, therefore, designated the 20 responders as "subaffective dysthymics." The chronic, intermittent, low-grade dysthymic illness in this group was hypothesized to represent a "true" subaffective disorder. By contrast, the fluctuating low-grade dysphoria of the 30 nonresponders was considered symptomatic of a predominately heterogeneous group of characterologic disorders, and this group was termed "character-spectrum disorder." We resorted to this pharmacologic "cleavage" of the charactero-

Table 3 History of Affective Illness in Biological Relatives of Cyclothymic, Bipolar I, and "Pseudocyclothymic" Groups

Affective Illness in Relative	Cyclothymic Group (N=46)		Bipolar I Group (N=50)		"Pseudocyclothymic" Group (N=50)		Significance
	N	%	N	%	N	%	
Depression	7	15	11	22	5	10	n.s.
Bipolar Illness	14	30	13	26	1	2	$p < .01$
Suicide	10	22	9	18	2	4	$p < .03$
Total[a]	30	65	28	56	7	14	$p < .001$

Note: The cyclothymic patients and the Bipolar I patients were very similar in these comparisons. The p values represent the cyclothymic and bipolar groups individually compared with the pseudocyclothymic group. In all cases the p values were the same for both comparisons.

[a] The total number of patients with a positive family history of affective illness is less than the sum of the first three rows in each column because some cases of suicide were from the ranks of either unipolar or bipolar patients.

logic sample because we could not decide on a reliable clinical or objective behavioral marker to accomplish this aim as we had done in cyclothymia. In brief, we hoped that this rough pharmacologic division could be validated by other findings.

Differentiating Characteristics of Subaffective Dysthymic and Character-Spectrum Disorders

In two reports we have provided evidence for the differentiation of true dysthymia from character-disorder-based dysphorias.[54,55] The strongest evidence comes from rapid eye movement (REM) latency findings. As shown in Figure 2, dysthymia proper (responder group) has short REM latency, similar to that of primary unipolar controls, and both groups differ significantly from nonaffective controls and the characterological group (or the nonresponder group). Other major supportive evidence for differences between the two groups is summarized in Table 4 and presented below.

In the **character-spectrum** group, women predominate, irritable dysphoria is seldom complicated by discrete major depressive episodes, REM latency is normal, substance abuse and familial alcoholism and sociopathy are common, and response to somatic therapies is rare (although a very small subgroup may respond to amphetamine-type drugs or tranylcypromine). We have suggested, based on phenomenology, course, family history, and sleep laboratory findings, that this group has a closer affinity to alcoholism, sociopathy, and somatization disorder than to primary affective illness. Unstable developmental histories, including multiple childhood losses, may partly explain the clinging and manipulative behavior of these subjects. What Klein and associates have described as "hysteroid dysphoria," with extreme rejection sensitivity in romantic relationships, may be a variant of the character-spectrum pattern.[56]

Sub-affective dysthymia has the clinical profile of a "true" subaffective disorder with intermittent subsyndromal depressions lasting days to weeks, often complicated by superimposed full-length syndromal depressive episodes. Sex ratio is almost even, REM latency is shortened to values observed in primary depressions, family history is positive for primary affective disorder, and response to secondary amine tricyclics is favorable. Many of these patients have hypersomnic-retarded phenomenology and familial bipolar illness, develop pharmacologic hypomania upon tricyclic challenge, and are lithium-responsive. Note that the 35% rate of pharmacologic hypomania in the dysthymic group is similar to that of cyclothymia and Bipolar I disorders described earlier, and significantly higher than the negligible rate in characterologic and unipolar controls (0%–5%). These findings suggest that a subgroup of subaffective dysthymic probands is related to cyclothymic disorders.

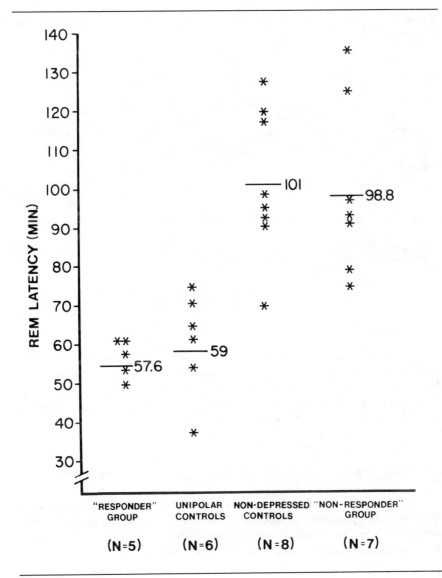

Figure 2 REM latency distribution in four groups of depressives
Note: Scheffé, $p < .05$.

Table 4 Comparison of Subaffective Dysthymic and Character Spectrum Disorders[a][54,55]

Variable	Subaffective Dysthymia[a] (N=20)		Character Spectrum[a] (N=30)		Significance[b]
	N	%	N	%	
Male sex[c]	9	45	5	17	$p < .05$
Family history					
Depression	6	30	1	3	$p < .01$
Bipolar disorder	7	35	1	3	$p < .01$
Alcoholism	2	10	16	53	$p < .01$
Assortative mating	2	10	14	47	$p < .05$
Developmental					
object loss	5	25	18	60	$p < .05$
Pharmacologic					
hypomania	7	35	0	0	$p < .001$

[a] Defined by response (subaffective) *versus* nonresponse (character spectrum) to thymoleptic drugs.
[b] By chi-square or Fisher exact tests.
[c] Subaffective dysthymics were similar to bipolar and different from unipolar controls.

Proposed Operational Criteria for Dysthymic Disorder

Based on the data summarized above, we have proposed operational criteria for identifying dysthymia conceived as a subaffective disorder. As described in Table 5, the salient features are insidious early onset; fluctuating, intermittent, and predominantly subsyndromal depressive course; subtle signs indicative of melancholia; and "stable" depressive personality attributes as defined by Schneider. [57]

External Validating Criteria for Dysthymia

Studies are in progress to test the validity of these operational criteria in a clinical population distinct from that which gave rise to them. Carroll's dexamethasone suppression test and Kupfer's REM latency technique are being used as biological markers.[58,59]

Cyclothymia and Dysthymia in the Offspring and Younger Sibs of Bipolar Probands

To ascertain the exact age and manner of onset of subaffective disorders, it is necessary to study a high-risk group for bipolar illness around the time of expected onset (i.e., adolescence and early adulthood). We recently completed a study (unpublished) of the offspring and younger sibs (< 25 years) of bipolar probands. Onset of psychopathology ranged from early to late teens; sex ratio was about even. As can be seen in Table 6, 54% of the sample had "typical" onset with "major episodes" (e.g., depression, often of psychotic proportions, mixed state, or manic psychosis). The remaining 46% had insidious onsets, and half of this group developed major episodes during a prospective course of 2–4 years. One subgroup within the insidious onset group was characterized by polydrug abuse—including ethanol—and temperamental deviations. However, even in this group, frank affective psychoses eventually made their appearance.

These data demonstrate that the onset of bipolar illness is often insidious, with subaffective manifestations, and frequent "masking" by substance use disorders. Dysthymic and cyclothymic manifestations were equally common in this insidious onset group. These data are consistent with the suggestion that the prepsychotic "personality" disturbances of bipolar patients represent early or subaffective manifestations of the illness.[20,44,50,66]

Table 5 Proposed Descriptive Criteria for Dysthymia as a Subaffective Disorder

1. Indeterminate onset, cardinal manifestations usually obvious before 21 years.
2. Fluctuating course over many years, but typically not free of depressive manifestations for more than a few weeks at a time.
3. Habitually subsyndromal in symptom profile, although the full range of depressive symptoms (which may even crystallize into superimposed syndromal episodes) occurs at various times.
4. At least two of the following melancholic manifestations:
   a. Psychomotor inertia
   b. Hypersomnia
   c. Anhedonia
   d. Diurnal variation (worse in a.m.).
5. Habitual introversion, with brief periods of extroversion sometimes seen in relatively "well" periods.
6. Presence of at least 5 of the 7 Schneiderian depressive personality traits:
   a. Quiet, passive, and indecisive
   b. Gloomy, pessimistic, and incapable of fun
   c. Self-critical, self-reproaching, and self-derogatory
   d. Conscientious and self-disciplining
   e. Brooding and given to worry
   f. Preoccupied with inadequacy, failure, and negative events to the point of morbid enjoyment of one's failures.
   g. Skeptical, hypercritical and complaining.
7. Absence of a diagnosable nonaffective disorder from the Washington University list of validated psychiatric disorders. Exception is made for sedativism (alcohol and drug abuse), which may serve to mask affective manifestations in the early course of the disorder.

Table 6 Manner of Onset of Affective "Spectrum" Disorders in the Children and Younger Sibs of Bipolar Patients (*N*=65)

Onset	Percentage
Episodic (N=35)	
Depression	37
Mania	12
Mixed State	5
Total	54
Insidious (N=30)	
Substance use disorders	
(polydrug ± ethanol)	17
Cyclothymia	15
Dysthymia	14
Total	46

A Proposed Dysthymic-Cyclothymic Continuum

The evidence reviewed in this chapter strongly suggests that dysthymic disorder (as defined by us) should be considered as a variant of cyclothymic disorder. Kretschmer had made a similar proposal when he stated that the depressive temperament

> is a soft temperament, which can swing to great extremes. The path over which it swings is a wide one, namely between cheerfulness and unhappiness. It does also swing towards the cheerful side, but not so often and not so far; on the other hand it lingers over in the unhappy direction.[4]

The evidence for this position based on our work can be summarized as follows: [54,55]

1. Although dysthymia pursues a "unipolar" course, pharmacologic challenge with tricyclic antidepressants mobilizes brief hypomanic responses—a feature characteristic of bipolar illness.[61]
2. About two-thirds of dysthymics suffer from hypersomnic-retarded-type depressions characteristic of bipolar illness.[62]
3. Like bipolar illness, onset is early, and the intermittent course can be considered a succession of "mini-episodes." Thus, dysthymia shares the high-frequency episode characteristic of the bipolar spectrum.[63,64]
4. The sex ratio is close to 1, a demographic characteristic of bipolar illness.[65]
5. Family history is often positive for bipolar illness.
6. Lithium carbonate response in our open trial, while in need of replication in a double-blind study, is also supportive of the concept of a subthreshold bipolar illness.

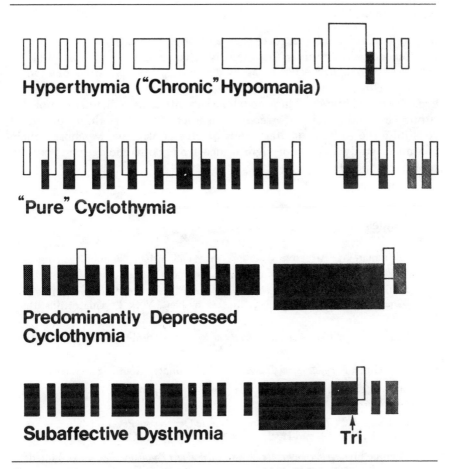

Figure 3 The spectrum of affective temperamental disorders

Source: Reproduced from Akiskal H, The Bipolar Spectrum in *Psychiatry Update: The American Psychiatric Association Annual Review, Vol. II.* Edited by Grinspoon L: Washington: American Psychiatric Press, Inc., 1983.

Figure 3 depicts the four types of overlapping subaffective disorders: predominantly hyperthymic disorder, where depressive swings rarely occur; "pure" cyclothymia, with an equal proportion of depressive and hypomanic swings; predominantly depressed cyclothymia, where syndromal depressive episodes are common and therefore designated as Bipolar II disorder; and subaffective dysthymia, where the "natural" (drug-free) course is that of subsyndromal depression, often complicated by syndromal depressions, but brief hypomanic switches on tricyclic challenge occasionally occur.

Summary

In this chapter I have argued that cyclothymia and dysthymia can be phenomenologically and operationally characterized and validated as subaffective disorders; that is, as milder and early expressions of bipolar illness. A clinical-familial continuum is postulated between dysthymic and cyclothymic subtypes. This model is submitted as a heuristic tool for future study in the subaffective disorders. Because these disorders constitute the earliest manifestations of bipolar affective psychoses, their continued study has major significance from both etiologic and public health standpoints.

References

1. Weissman M. Affective disorders in a U.S. urban community. *Arch Gen Psychiatry* 35:1304–11, 1978.

2. Spitzer RL and Endicott J. *Schedule for Affective Disorders and Schizophrenia: Life-Time Version.* New York: Biometrics Research, New York Psychiatric Institute, 1977.

3. Kraepelin E. *Manic-Depressive Insanity and Paranoia* Edinburgh: E&S Livingston, 1921.

4. Kretschmer E. *Physique and Character*, 2nd ed. London: Routledge, 1936.

5. Slater E. The inheritance of manic-depressive insanity. *Proc R Soc Med* 29:981–90, 1936.

6. Kallmann F. "Genetic Principles in Manic Depressive Psychosis" In *Depression.* edited by Zubin J. and Hoch P, pp. 1–24. New York: Grune & Stratton, 1954.

7. Campbell JD. *Manic-Depressive Disease: Clinical and Psychiatric Significance.* Philadelphia: Lippincott, 1953.

8. Kraines SH. *Mental Depressions and Their Treatment.* New York: MacMillan, 1957.

9. Winokur G, Clayton P, and Reich T. *Manic-Depressive Illness.* St. Louis: CV Mosby, 1969.

10. Von Zerssen D. "Premorbid Personality and Affective Psychosis." In *Handbook of Studies on Depression*, edited by Burrows GD, Amsterdam: Excerpta Medica, 1977. pp. 79–103.

11. Baldessarini R. Frequency of diagnoses of schizophrenia versus affective disorders from 1944 to 1968. *Amer J Psychiatry* 127: 759–63, 1970.

12. Lehmann H. "The Impact of the Therapeutic Revolution on Nosology." In *Problématique de psychose*, edited by Doucet P and Laurin C. New York: Excerpta Medica Foundation, 1969.

13. Pope H and Lipinski. Diagnosis in schizophrenia and manic-depressive illness. *Arch Gen Psychiatry* 35:811–28, 1978.

14. Akiskal HS and Puzantian VR. Psychotic forms of depression and mania. *Psychiat Clin North Am* 2:419–39, 1979.

15. Akiskal HS et al. The nosological status of neurotic depression: A prospective three-to-four year examination in light of the primary-secondary and unipolar-bipolar dichotomies. *Arch Gen Psychiatry* 35:756–66, 1978.

16. Rounsaville BJ, Sholomskas D, and Prusoff B. Chronic mood disorders in depressed outpatients: Diagnosis and response to pharmacotherapy. *J Aff Disorders* 2:73–88, 1979.

17. Klerman G. The spectrum of mania. *Compr Psychiatry* 22:11–20, 1981.

18. Akiskal HS et al. "The Joint Use of Clinical and Biological Criteria for Psychiatric Diagnosis: II. Their Application in Identifying Subaffective Forms of Manic-Depressive Illness." In *Psychiatric Diagnosis: Exploration of Biological Predictors.* edited by Akiskal HS and Webb WL. New York: Spectrum, 1978. pp. 219–29.

19. Akiskal HS. Subaffective disorders: dysthymic, cyclothymic and bipolar II disorders in the "borderline" realm. *Psychiatr Clin North Am* 4:25–46, 1981.

20. Akiskal HS, Khani M, and Scott-Strauss A. Cyclothymic temperamental disorders *Psychiatr Clin North Am* 2:527–54, 1979.

21. Leonard J, Korff J, and Schulz H. Die temperamente in deu familien der monopolaren und bipolarien pyasischen psychosen:*Psychiat Neurol* (Basel) 143:416–34, 1967.

22. Perris C. A study of bipolar (manic-depressive) and unipolar recurrent depressive psychoses. *Acta Psychiatr Scand* Supplement 194, 1966.

23. Wetzel RD et al. Personality as a subclinical expression of the affective disorders. *Compr Psychiatry* 21:197–205, 1980.

24. Gershon ES et al. Transmitted factors in the morbid risk of affective disorders: A controlled study. *J Psychiatr Res* 12:283–99, 1975.

25. Angst J et al. Bipolar manic-depressive psychoses: Results of a genetic investigation. *Hum Genet* 55:237–54, 1980.

26. Gershon E. "The Search for Genetic Markers in Affective Disorders." In *Psychopharmacology: A Generation of Progress,* edited by Lipton MA, DiMascio A, and Killam KF. New York: Raven Press, 1978. pp. 1197–1212.

27. Murphy DL and Weiss R. Reduced monoamine oxidase activity in blood platelets from bipolar depressed patients. *Am J Psychiatry* 128:1351–57, 1977.

28. Schooler C et al. Psychological correlates of monoamine oxidase activity in normals. *J Nerv Ment Dis* 166:177–86, 1978.

29. Buchsbaum MS, Murphy DL, and Coursay RD. The biochemical high risk paradigm: Behavioral and familial correlates of low platelet monoanime oxidase activity. *Science* 194:339–41, 1976.

30. Klein DF. "Drug Therapy as a Means of Syndrome Identification and Nosological Revision." In *Psychopathology and Psychopharmacology,* edited by Cole J. Baltimore: Johns Hopkins University Press, 1972. pp. 143–60.

31. Akiskal HS. "The Joint Use of Clinical and Biological Criteria for Psychiatric

Diagnosis: I. A Historical & Methodological Review," In *Psychiatric Diagnosis: Exploration of Biological Predictors,* edited by Akiskal HS and Webb WL. New York: Spectrum, 1978. pp. 103–32.

32. Murphy DL. Psychoactive Drug Responder Subgroups: Possible Contributions to Psychiatric Classification." In *Psychopharmacology: A Generation of Progress,* edited by Lipton MA, DiMascio A, and Killam KF. New York: Raven Press. pp. 807–20.

33. Jefferson JW and Greist JH. *Primer of Lithium Therapy.* Baltimore: Williams & Wilkins, 1977.

34. Klein DF, Honigfeld G, and Feldman S. Prediction of drug effect in personality disorders. *J Nerv Ment Dis* 156:184–98, 1973.

35. Peselow ED et al. Prophylactic effect of lithium against depression in cyclothymic patients: A life-table analysis. *Compr Psychiatry* 22:256–64, 1981.

36. Wold PN and Dwight R. Subtypes of depression identified by the KDS-3A: A pilot study. *Am J Psychiatry* 136:1415–19, 1979.

37. Tupin J. Lithium use in nonmanic depressive conditions. *Compr Psychiatry* 13:209–14.

38. Sheard MH and Marini JL. Treatment of human aggressive behavior: Four case studies of the effect of lithium. *Compr Psychiatry* 19:37–45, 1978.

39. Dyson W and Barcai A. Treatment of children of lithium-responding parents. *Curr Ther Res* 12:286–90

40. Van Putten T and Alban J. Lithium carbonate in personality disorders: A case of hysteria. *J Nerv Ment Dis* 164:218-222, 1977.

41. Van Putten T and Sanders DG: Lithium in treatment failures. *J Nerv Ment Dis* 161:255–64, 1975.

42. Flemenbaum A. Affective disorders & "chemical dependence": Lithium for alcohol and drug addiction? A Clinical note. *Dis Nerv Stst* 35:281–85, 1974.

43. Altamura AC. Therapeutic attempts with lithium in young drug addicts. *Acta Psychiat Scand* 52:312–19, 1975.

44. Akiskal HS et al. Cyclothymic disorder: Validating criteria for inclusion in the bipolar affective group. *Am J Psychiatry* 134:1227–33, 1977.

45. Depue RA et al. A behavioral paradigm for identifying persons at risk for bipolar depressive disorders: A conceptual framework and five validation studies. *J Abnor Psychology* 90 (Suppl): 381–438, 1981.

46. Spitzer R, Endicott J and Robins E. *Research Diagnostic Criteria (RDC) for a Selected Group of Functional Disorders.* 2nd ed. New York: New York Psychiatric Institute Biometrics Research Division, 1975.

47. Feighner JP et al. Diagnostic criteria for use in psychiatric research. *Arch Gen Psychiatry* 26:57–63, 1972.

48. Fieve RR and Dunner DL. "Unipolar and Bipolar Affective States." In *The Nature and Treatment of Depression,* edited by Flach FF and Draghi SC. New York: John Wiley & Sons, 1975. pp. 145–60.

49. Rifkin A et al. Emotionally unstable character disorder—A follow-up study. I. Depression of patients and outcome. *Biol Psychiatry* 4:65–79, 1981.

50. Waters BGH. Early symptoms of bipolar affective psychosis. *Can Psychiatr Assoc J* 24:55–60, 1979.

51. Mendlewicz J and Rainer JD. Adoption study supporting genetic transmission in manic depressive illness. *Lancet* 268:327–29, 1977.

52. Gershon ES, Dunner D, and Goodwin F: Toward a biology of affective disorders: Genetic contributions. *Arch Gen Psychiatry* 25:1–15, 1971.

53. Akiskal HS et al. Chronic depressions: Part 1. Clinical and familial characteristics in 137 probands. *J Affective Disorders* 3:297–315, 1981.

54. Akiskal HS et al. Characterological depressions: Clinical and sleep EEG findings separating "subaffective dysthymics" from "character-spectrum disorders." *Arch Gen Psychiatry* 37:777–83, 1980.

55. Rosenthal TL et al. Familial and developmental factors in characterological depressions. *J Affective Disorders* 3:183–92, 1981.

56. Leibowitz MR and Klein DF. Hysteroid dysphoria. *Psychiatr Clin North Am* 555–75, 1979.

57. Schneider K. *Clinical Psychopathology*. New York: Grune & Stratton, 1959.

58. Carroll BJ et al. A specific laboratory test for the diagnosis of melancholia. *Arch Gen Psychiatry* 38:15–27, 1981.

59. Kupfer DJ. REM latency: A psychobiological marker for primary depressive disease. *Biol Psychiatry* 11:159–74, 1976.

60. Waters BGW and Marchenko-Bouer I. Psychiatric illness in the adult offspring of bipolar manic-depressives. *J Aff Disorders* 2:119–26.

61. Akiskal HS et al. Differentiation of primary affective illness from situational, symptomatic and secondary depressions. *Arch Gen Psychiatry* 36:635–43, 1979.

62. Detre T et al. Hypersomnia and manic-depressive disease. *Amer J Psychiatry* 128:1303–5, 1972.

63. Akiskal HS and McKinney WT Jr. Overview of recent research in depression: Integration of ten conceptual models into a comprehensive clinical frame. *Arch Gen Psychiatry* 32:285–305, 1975.

64. Depue RA and Monroe SM. The unipolar-bipolar distinction in the depressive disorders. *Psychol Bull* 85:1001–29, 1978.

65. Weissman MM and Klerman GL. Sex differences and the epidemiology of depression. *Arch Gen Psychiatry* 34:98–111, 1977.

16

The Long-Term Effects of Depression

Giovanni B. Cassano, M.D. and Carlo Maggini, Ph.D.

Introduction

Between the extremes of full recovery and chronicity, depression shows variations of outcome that have not received the attention they deserve. When observations are extended to cover the intervals between depressive episodes, residual symptoms, signs of maladjustment, changes in personality, and other infraclinical disturbances emerge to complete the picture of the illness.

The boundaries between depressive phases and the intervening periods are blurred, and the continuity of the process underlying depression comes out clearly. Only in a limited number of cases can one discover intervals which are free from residual symptoms.[1]

A previous review identified and described the following long-term effects of depression: (1) residual symptoms, (2) social maladjustment, (3) personality changes, and (4) evolution toward chronicity.[2]

This chapter will consider the long-term effects of depression according to the above mentioned distinctions. Not discussed are the well-known forms of evolution and complications, such as acute confusional states, suicide, somatic and psychosomatic disorders, alcoholism, and drug addiction.

Residual Symptoms

As early as 1908 Weigandt noted a state of weakened psychic resistance and of permanent invalidity in some "cured depressives"; prolonged asthenia, incapacity to recover physical strength, and intellectual vigor were observed as well by Kraepelin and Benon.[3-5]

Various types of "residual phenomena" have been described, such as an excessive sensitivity to depression, a constant predisposition to anxiety and preoccupation;[6,7] dysphoric dissatisfaction and dry, authoritarian pessimism;[8] states of mild sadness and of inhibition (with diurnal variations);[9] persistent signs of vegetative irregularity;[7,10] sudden changes in mood;[11-14] prolonged cycles of dysphoria;[12] prolonged hyperthymic states; and states of anxiety involving agoraphobia. A growing number of subjects feel a depressive aftermath of a "watered down, faded" kind, which is the immediate sequel to depressive episode.

The expressions "depressive defect," "residual syndromes," and "interval symptomatology" have been used to refer to characteristic features such as a fall in levels of vital energy, a sensitiveness and dysphoria, and a striking vulnerability to events, which may follow the typical depressive symptoms of the central phase.[1,15,16] What is found is not exactly "mild chronicity," but a "non-specific residual syndrome immanent in the disorder."[17,18]

As a rule, the residual symptoms are the forms taken by a personality readjustment, and they gradually vanish during convalescence. If, however, environmental, psychological, or iatrogenic factors impede this delicate recovery phase, a subliminal residue—a real "depressive defect"—may take shape.

According to Weitbrecht, the fading away of depression and of its major symptoms leave behind a persistent weakness of mood and a fall in levels of vital energy;[8] reference may be made here to the concept of "dynamic emptying," and of "basic stadiums" or life stages.[17,19] Thus, there is a strong likelihood of fresh episodes or of evolution toward chronicity.

These residual states, which may be described as amorphous and featureless, may form part of the natural evolution of depression, especially in its unipolar forms, and may be strengthened by the subject's difficulty in recovering his or her role and by the fear of "jumping out of depression."[20]

It has also been hypothesized that some psychopharmacological treatments promote the maintenance of a residual syndrome by eliminating some symptoms at an early stage.[1,17,18,21-23]

Social Adjustment

Since 1954, the parameter of social adaptation allowed Kinkelin to distinguish between three forms of chronic depression: permanent social maladjustment with short, "free intervals;" a fair degree of social recovery, along with persistent residual states; and permanent social and medical disability.[24] A deterioration of the social role may be apparent at an early stage even before the typical symptoms become apparent. After clinical recovery, 4–12 months must pass before the subject can reach a satisfactory level of adaptation to his or her environment.[25] After a depressive phase a patient may be less enterprising than previously and find it hard to maintain his or her usual level of efficiency, although managing to carry out routine tasks.[26] Even when there is little real depressive content, a state of chronic invalidism may be maintained.[27] As much as 10 years after their latest depressive episode, about a quarter of Stensted's patients were unemployed.[28] The studies of Paykel et al. and Weissman et al. have shown that for a few months after their latest episode, clinically cured subjects showed an incomplete resumption of their roles, leaving them incapable of freely communicating or expressing their aggressiveness.[29-31] Social adaptation improves much more slowly than clinical symptomatology.[32] Even if they are slight and intermittent, residual depressive symptoms can endanger a patient's integration with his or her working environment, whereas conjugal roles and interpersonal relations are generally less strongly affected.[33,34] After a period of depression, reintegration into the family and the working environment is not always complete and, in any case, it only occurs after clinical remission.[25] This is the phase in which the patient can gain most from appropriate psychotherapeutic and sociotherapeutic treatment. The failure to assess the social integration achieved by depressives eliminates an essential parameter from the evaluation of treatment outcome.

Features of the Postdepressive Personality

The widespread concept that the personality can be fully recovered may derive from observing depressives who appear to have readjusted to the environment after an episode. As depressive symptomatology fades away, most personality changes appear in the form of a heightening or a flattening of previous individual traits, or else of a structural upheaval. The postdepressive personality often reproduces the premorbid profile of the candidate with certain traits exacerbated. Bipolar depressives, though often leaning toward a slightly hypomanic state, display a greater probability of returning to "normality." A unipolar depressive phase may be followed by emotional symptoms such as irritability, anxiety, phobias, a fall in vitality, and introversion, as well as by a personality profile indistinguishable from that of chronically anxious subjects.[35]

An unswerving acceptance of a rigidly self-imposed moral code and a dedication to their work that leaves no room for pleasure and interpersonal relations characterizes another type of postdepressive personality. Though socially integrated, such a compulsive personality conceals affective

235

coldness, an unstable form of adaptation, and little capacity for coping with changes. The self-esteem of such subjects is artificially buttressed by their dynamism, and their equilibrium is founded on an inflexible situation of dependence. Their "orderliness" is actually a weakened, vulnerable structure to compensate for their loss of postdepressive protection.

In another personality change, passive attitudes are prevalent, with a tendency to give up or to be lazily self-satisfied. Such subjects may display a negative cognitive set toward themselves, the world, and their own future.[36] In these subjects the learned helplessness and the fall off in aggressiveness may lead to withdrawal, a change in their life-style, or both as their ideology becomes melancholy.[37]

In others, egocentric and histrionic traits of personality become heightened. These subjects utilize their experience of depression to be demanding and manipulative. They are dysphoric, with an irritable affect sometimes giving rise to hostility and sociopathic behavior.

Last, pharmacological therapy has been recognized to have a favorable effect on readjusting personality development as well as on establishing an "anti-depressive personality" characterized by anedonia and flattening of affect, a clinical state which seems to correspond to a chronic depressive state.[38]

Chronic Depression

A diagnosis of chronic depression, recorded for fifteen percent of all depressives,[39,40] must be given in the case of persistent illness which, even if torpid and mild, maintains a clinically recognizable entity. According to Regis, chronic depression loses its painful hyperthymia and takes on a stable, mild form.[41] Depression and sadness appear dull and stereotyped as with plaintiveness and fixed ideas. Against this featureless, gloomy background, paroxysms of anxiety with suicidal tendencies may occur.[42] In the clinical picture described by Medow, the thymic component slowly fades, giving way to a striking rigidity of thought and behavior.[43] Feelings become crystallized around an "irreducible depressive" nucleus, and there are very few vital changes, as if everything were lost forever and irreparably burnt out. Within this emotional aridity, broken by outbursts of sad and painful feelings, patients live without positive feelings and are incapable of establishing emotional links with their ego or with the environment.

Other evolutional forms of depression are rarer nowadays; the postmelancholic delusions,[42] the continuous "folie circulaire" and the chronic mixed state.

Chronic depression may take on a variety of symptomatological features. In some cases, melancholy phenomena are prevalent, in others neurotic symptoms of anxiety, hysteria, or hypochondria prevail, and in still others, somatic or behavioral disorders are in the forefront. Depressive phenomena become persistent, or are separated by short, free intervals during which the patient's mood is normal, lasting at most 2 months.[44] In any case, the episodic course is lost.

Chronic depression often follows a melancholic episode; the fading away of depressive anguish is not accompanied by the recovery of the previous equilibrium. More rarely, the emergence of chronic depression passes unnoticed; in this case the deviation of mood toward sadness takes place slowly and insidiously, affecting every layer of the personality. This condition is often wrongly identified with the so-called depressive personality. The damage done to social and working relationships may only be slight; the slow emergence of a slight, mild symptomatology may permit a certain degree of adaptation.

The patient's persistent somatic disturbances induce them to apply frequently for laboratory analyses; they are regular users of medical services and considered to be neurotics, "crocks," hypochondriacs, hysterics, or neuroasthenics. Even in a psychiatric environment, chronic depressives are likely to be incorrectly diagnosed as neurotics or subjects with depressive personalities.[40] Ey used the term "chronic melancholia" to refer to the various kinds of personality structures deriving from an originally depressive pathology.[45] Neurotic mechanisms elaborate depression and anguish, and integrate them into the personality as a form of existence and a blueprint for living. Thus, in chronic cases, an evolutionary movement links melancholia with neurotic structure. In some subjects, chronicity is attributable to a special sensitivity to events and to the persistence of insurmountable problems.

Depressions other than those which depend on a nucleus of conflict for continuation are those characterized by a peculiar biochemical typology that cannot be corrected by current therapeutic means, and those arising from an organic pathology that deprives the ego of its normal adaptability in dealing with changing environmental conditions. And last, the fact that a depression becomes chronic is sometimes attributed to the use of inadequate, unduly short treatments.[40]

Conclusions

Nowadays the suffering and the degrees of disability of many depressives can be greatly alleviated. Pharmacotherapy makes it possible to reduce the duration and intensity of depressive episodes; to delay relapses; and to make them rarer, shorter, and less severe. In some cases, however, treatment must be prolonged; in others, depression loses its intermittent and self-limiting nature. When observation of the depressive disease is extended to include the period of remission, a more reliable picture of the affective pathology is obtained, which seems to evolve continuously and uninterruptedly throughout the patient's lifetime. Therefore, the attention of psychiatrists should be shifted from the acute phase of the illness to later periods, emphasizing long-term evolution, results, and treatments. Thus, any approach to rehabilitation and prevention of relapses calls for a thorough analysis of the types of recovery, with a careful inquiry into residual symptoms, kinds of readaptation to the environment, role resumption, and effects on personality.

This chapter attempted to provide a survey of the data available in the literature and to draw a distinction, if somewhat simplified, between chronic depression and residual symptoms and between personality changes and postdepressive maladjustment. Any treatment adopted after a depressive episode must be based on a careful examination of the "free intervals," which supposedly, by definition, present no psychopathological phenomena. Usually, however, these periods display recognizable residual symptoms and personality traits that are often a cause of suffering and disability, personally, within the family, and at work. If these features are ignored, therapeutic and preventive action is in danger of relying on nothing more systematic than the practitioner's personal empiricism.

References

1. Berner P et al. Zur frage des intervalls bein manisch depressiven krakheitge-schehen. *Ueivernatz.* 28:265, 1970.

2. Cassano GB and Maggini C. "Evoluzione ed Esiti della Depressione." In *La Condizione Depressiva*, edited by Cassano GB. Milano: Masson Italia Editeur, 1980.

3. Weygandt G. *Atlante e Manuale di Psichiatria.* Milano: Società Editrice Libraria, 1908.

4. Kraepelin E. *Psychiatrie,* 8th ed., Leipzig: Ed. Bart., 1913.

5. Benon R. *La Mélancolie.* Paris: G. Doin, 1925.

6. Gruhle (1950). cit. da WEITBRECHT (1969).

7. Vella G and Bollea E. Prime osservazioni sulle condizioni dei depressi nei periodi interfasici. *Riv. Psychiat.* 8:481, 1973.

8. Weitbrecht HJ. "Psicosi Endogene Depressive e Maniacali." In *Psichiatria del presente,* edited by Gruhle HW et al. Vadenz-Liechtenstein: Luxusangsdscu Rackford, 1969. p. 1.

9. Berner P, Krispin-Exner K, and Poeldinger W. Therapy possibilities for therapy-resistant depression. *Int. Pharmakopsychiat.* 7:189, 1974.

10. Kielholz P. *Diagnose und Therapie der Depressionen den Praktiken.* Munich: Lehmans, 1965.

11. Baastrup PC. Practical clinical viewpoints regarding treatment with Lithium. *Acta Psychiat. Scand.* (Suppl.) 207:12, 1969.

12. Freyhan FA. Treatment resistant or untreatable? *Compr. Psychiatry* 19:97, 1978.

13. Perris C. A study of bipolar (manic-depressive) and unipolar recurrent depressive psychoses. *Acta Psychiat. Scand.* (Suppl.) 42:194, 1966.

14. Weissman MM and Kasl SU. Help-seeking in depressed out-patient following maintenance therapy. *Br. J. Psychiat.* 129:252, 1976.

15. Helmchen H. Symptomatology of therapy-resistant depression. *Pharmakopsychiat.* 7:145, 1974.

16. Glatzel J. *Endogene Depressionen.* Stuttgart: Thiene, 1973.

17. Huber E. Reine defektsyndrome und baisstadien endogener psychosen. *Fortchr. Neurol. Pyschiat.* 34:409, 1966.

18. Greger J et al. Untersuchungen intervall phasicher psychosen. *Psychiat. Neurol. Med. Psychol.* (Lf2) 24, 12, p. 733, 1972.

19. Janzarik W. *Dynamische Grundkonstelationem in Endogenen Psychosen.* Berlin: Springer, 1959.

20. Klages W. "Zur Struktur der Chronischen Endogenen Depressionen." In *Problematik, Therapie und Rehabilitation der Chronischen Endogenen Psykhosen,* edited by Fr. Pause Enke, Stuttgart, 1967.

21. Huber G, Glatzel J, and Lungershausen E. Residual syndrome bei zyklothymien. *Fortrschr. Med.* 88:281, 1970.

22. Arnold OH and Krispin-Exner V. Zur frage der beeinflussung des verlanges des manischdepressiven krankriestgeschehens durch antidepressive. *Clin. Med. Wehr.* 115:929, 1965.

23. Peters UH and Gluck A. Die personlikeit am ende der depressiven phase. Bedsachtugen nach auskilingen endogen depressive phasen. *Nervenarta,* 44, 1, p. 14, 1973.

24. Kinkelin, M. Verlauf und prognose des manisch-depressiven irreseins. *Schweiz. Arch. Neurol. Psychiatr.* 73:101, 1954.

25. Weissman MM and Bothwell S. Assessment of social adjustment by patient self-report. *Arch. Gen. Psychiat.* 33:111, 1976.

26. Price JS. Chronic depressive illness. *Br. Med. J.* 1:1200, 1978.

27. Rennie TAC. Prognosis in manic-depressive psychoses. *Amer. J. Psychiat.* 98:801, 1942.

28. Stendstedt A. A study in manic-depressive psychosis. Clinical, social and genetic investigations. *Acta Psychiatr., Neurol. Scand.* (Suppl.) 79:1–111, 1952.

29. Paykel ES et al. Dimensions of social adjustment in depressed women. *J. Nerv. Ment. Dis.* 152, 1972.

30. Paykel ES et al. Maintenance therapy of depression. *Pharmakopsychiat.* 9:127, 1976.

31. Weissman MM et al. The efficacy of drugs and psychotherapy in the treatment of acute depressive episodes. *Am. J. Psychiatry* 136:555, 1979.

32. Paykel ES and Weissman MM. Social adjustment and depression: A controlled study. A longitudinal study. *Arch. Gen. Psychiat.* 28:659, 1973.

33. Murphy GE et al. Variability of the clinical course of primary affective disorder. *Arch. Gen. Psychiatry* 30:757, 1978.

34. Paykel ES, Klerman GL, and Prusoff BA. Prognosis of depression and the endogenous-neurotic distinction. *Psychological Medicine* 4:57, 1974.

35. Murray LG and Blackburn IM. Personality differences in patients with depressive illness and anxiety neurosis. *Acta Psychiat. Scand.* 50:183, 1974.

36. Beck AI. *Depression.* New York: Harper and Row, 1967.

37. Seligman M and Maier S. Failure to escape traumatic shock. *J. Exp. Psychol.* 74:1, 1967.

38. Mayer DY. Psychotropic drugs and the "anti-depressed" personality. *Br. J. Med. Psychol.* 43:349, 1975.

39. Robins E and Guze S. "Classification of Affective Disorders: The Primary-Secondary, the Endogenous, and the Neurotic-Psychotic Concepts." In *Recent Advances in the Psychobiology of the Depressive Illness.* Department of Health, Education and Welfare. Publication (HSM) 1969. pp. 70–9053,

40. Weissman MM and Klerman GL. The chronic depressive in the community: Unrecognized and poorly treated. *Comprehen. Psychiatry* 18:523, 1977.

41. Reges, E. *Precis Psychiatrie,* 1923.

42. Digo R. *Mélancholie. Étude Clinique. Encyclopédie Médico-chirurgicale,* Paris, 2, p. 37210 A10, 1955.

43. Medow, I. Zur eiblichkeitsfrage in der psychiatric. *J. Neurol.* 1:26, 1914.

44. American Psychiatric Association. *Diagnostic and Statistical Manual of Mental Disorders, DSM III.* Washington, D.C., 1980.

45. Ey H. *Études Psychiatriques,* Vol. III. Paris: Desclées de Brouwer et Cie. Edit., 1954.

PART TWO

Clinical Management and Psychopharmacology

How Do Antidepressants Work?

Ross J. Baldessarini, M.D.

Drug Actions and Drug Development

Antidepressants currently available in the United States are remarkably similar in their pharmacology, toxicology, and spectrum of clinical utility.[1] To a large extent, as with antipsychotic agents,[2] this outcome reflects the limitations of pharmacologic theory and pharmaceutical strategies in drug development. Monoamine neurotransmitter-based theories have continued to dominate current partial understanding of the actions of antidepressants, as well as oversimplified hypotheses concerning the pathophysiology of depression.[1,3,4] While intriguing new leads to common pharmacodynamic features of old and some unusual new "heterocyclic antidepressants" (HCAs), especially biochemical features, are highlighted below, the prediction of antidepressant activity has remained closely tied to screening for evidence of catecholamine enchancement in laboratory animals or uptake blockade in vitro (such as ability to reverse behavioral effects of reserpine or other amine-depleting agents, or to block the uptake of norepinephrine [NE] or related amines into brain tissue or isolated nerve endings). More recently, increased attention has also been given to drugs that selectively block the uptake (inactivation) of serotonin (5-hydroxy-tryptamine [5HT]), and those with low antimuscarinic (anti-acetylcholine [ACh]) activity. Of more than 75 currently available or experimental antidepressants, about half are structural analogs of imipramine or are

Supported in part by USPHS (NIMH) Career Award MH-47370 and Grant MH-21154. The manuscript was prepared by Mrs. Mila Cason; some of the material in this chapter was previously published.[1]

known to be inhibitors of NE uptake. Many of these represent minor alterations of older compounds, including three agents recently introduced in U.S. medical practice (trimipramine, amoxapine, and maprotiline). The close interdependence of theories of drug action and methods for their development may thus have contributed to the proliferation of many "me-too" drugs and to a still narrowly focused, circularly reasoned, and incomplete understanding of the mechanisms by which antidepressant effects occur.

Traditional Actions of Heterocyclic Antidepressants vs. Amine Uptake

Axelrod and his colleagues reported in the early 1960s that imipramine and other HCAs block the reuptake inactivation of NE at adrenergic nerve terminals in the peripheral sympathetic and central nervous systems (CNS).[5] Many studies have added to the evaluation of this phenomenon and extended it to measurements of the transport of other monoamine neurotransmitters of the CNS, particularly catecholamines and 5HT. Potency (IC_{50}) values for individual drugs have varied considerably among laboratories, and comparisons of large numbers of newer and older agents under the same conditions have been rare. Nevertheless, representative data of this kind are summarized in Table 1.[6-10] They indicate that most HCAs have very weak effects against the uptake of dopamine (DA) and variable effects against NE and 5HT. One fairly consistent finding is that desmethylated HCAs (*nor*-derivatives or secondary amines, many of which form spontaneously in vivo from tertiary amine precursors) such as protriptyline, desipramine, nomifensin, maprotiline, and amoxapine are highly potent against NE uptake, but relatively weak against 5HT uptake, and often less sedating than comparable tertiary amine compounds. In addition, N-desmethylation of some antipsychotic drugs reduces their sedative-neuroleptic activity and may result in mood-elevating products. A notable example is the new antidepressant amoxapine, which is a selective blocker of NE uptake.[7,11] Of the available antidepressants, trimipramine and doxepin are among the least potent against NE uptake (Table 1), and should interfere least with the hypotensive actions of postganglionic sympathetic blockers such as guanethidine; in vivo desmethylation of these antidepressants may alter this suggestion, as reported gradual effects of high doses of doxepin against guanethidine seem to illustrate.[12] In addition to in vitro evidence of NE-uptake blockade by many HCAs (Table 1), there is good evidence for similarly potent in vivo effects as evaluated by reduced accumulation of radiolabeled NE, or by diminished depletion of NE by the adrenergic neurotoxin, 6-hydroxydopamine (6-OHDA), which is taken up by NE nerve terminals—all as summarized in Table 2.[10,13] Although correlations between in vitro and in vivo potencies of HCAs

Table 1 In Vitro Inhibition of Uptake of Labeled Amines by Brain Tissue

Drug	Typical Clinical Dose (mg/d)	IC$_{50}$ (nM)			Potency Ratio (NE:5HT)
		NE	5HT	DA	
Protriptyline	30	2	1,600	5,200	800
Desipramine	100	2	2,000	15,000	1,000
Nomifensin	125	7	11,300	60	1,600
Nisoxetine	?	8	200	2,900	25
Maprotiline	150	20	24,000	9,300	1,200
Amoxapine[a]	250	23	566	—	25
Nortriptyline	100	30	1,400	5,300	6.7
Imipramine	150	60	490	15,600	7.3
Amitriptyline	150	130	300	6,200	3.5
Clomipramine	125	160	30	5,000	0.2
Doxepin	150	320	3,400	7,700	10.6
Mianserin	65	810	37,500	19,000	46.3
Viloxazine	225	1,400	64,000	56,000	45.7
Butriptyline	200	1,700	10,000	5,200	5.9
Iprindole	112	3,500	44,000	11,000	12.6
Trimipramine	100	4,400	5,400	6,700	1.2
Trazodone	300	(weak)	760	(weak)	—
Fluoxetine	60	740	270	12,000	0.4
d-Amphetamine	30	78	21,000	280	270
1-Amphetamine	30	150	77,000	1,300	500
Cocaine	?	126	850	400	6.7
Methylphenidate	50	200	81,000	700	400
Benztropine	4	450	14,000	425	30
Chlorpromazine	300	150	10,000	12,000	66.7
Thioridazine	300	4,000	5,500	3,500	1.4

Source of data: Randrup and Braestrup, 1977; Coupet et al., 1979; Möller-Nielsen, 1980; Sulser and Mobley, 1980; and Fuller 1981, (for synaptosomes of rat forebrain [NE, DA, 5HT] and mouse heart tissue [metaraminol as a model of NE]).[6-10]
[a] 7-OH and 8-OH amoxapine had similar activity against NE and 5-HT uptake.

against NE uptake are high ($r_s = .89$), the relationship between in vivo potency (*not* efficacy) in clinical use and potency against NE uptake in vivo and in vitro is weak ($r_s = .10$ to $.35$) (Table 3).

In general, in vivo evidence concerning 5HT-uptake blockade indicates limited potency of most HCAs, with the exception of clomipramine and newer experimental agents such as fluoxetine (Table 2). Whereas several such putatively selective anti-5HT-uptake agents are undergoing clinical trials and may have useful antidepressant or antineurotic effects,[1] it is *not proven* that their effects are due to facilitation of central 5HT neurotransmission. Clomipramine and fluoxetine, for example, have some activity against NE-uptake (Table 1). Moreover, paradoxically, at least two agents claimed to have antidepressant effects in European studies (methys-

Table 2 In vivo Inhibition of Amine Uptake

Drug	ED_{50} (mg/kg)			Potency Ratios
	^3H-NE (NE)	6-OH-DA (NE)	pCl-Amphetamine (5HT)	
Selective vs. NE				*NE:5HT*
Tandamine	—	.06	> 100	1,700
Protriptyline	.4	.12	~ 32	120
Desipramine	1.0	.25	> 100	160
Chlorodesipramine	—	1.6	> 32	20
Nisoxetine	—	.9	> 100	110
Nortriptyline	—	1.2	> 100	83
Imipramine	2.5	3.4	> 100	40
Nomifensin	3.0	1.9	—	—
Maprotiline	—	3.9	> 100	26
Amitriptyline	4.5	5.3	> 100	20
Viloxazine	8.0	5.3	> 100	15
Clomipramine	5.5	6.0	10	1.7
Doxepin	14	4.7	> 100	11
Selective vs. 5HT				*5HT:NE*
Fluoxetine	—	> 100	.4	250
Paroxetine	—	28	.9	31
Norfluoxetine	—	> 100	1.6	62
Zimelidine	—	> 32	2.8	11
Fluvoxamine	—	> 32	15	2.1
Weak vs. amine uptake				
Mianserin	22	> 48	> 100	—
Trazodone	> 100	> 32	> 100	—
Iprindole	> 100	> 100	> 100	—

Source of data: Clements-Jewery et al., 1980; and Fuller, 1981.[10,13]
Note: Tests include blockade of uptake of ^3H-NE by heart, depletion of cardiac NE after 6-OH-DA, and loss of brain 5HT after p-Cl-amphetamine—all in mouse.

ergide and cyproheptadine)[8] are believed to have 5HT-receptor *blocking* actions.[14] While facilitation of 5HT in the brain might be expected to produce sedation or anxiolytic effects, production of true antidepressant activity by 5HT-facilitating agents, especially in severe melancholia, requires further critical appraisal.

Of the many experimental antidepressants, most are pharmacologically similar to older HCAs. A few, such as iprindole, mianserin, trazodone, alprazolam and S-adenosylmethionine are intriguing as their action mechanisms are obscure.[1,15] These atypical antidepressants are not blockers of uptake of NE 5HT, or DA, nor are they monoamine oxidase (MAO) inhibitors (virtually all new HCAs are not). The first two have recently been suggested to have subtle NE-release modifying actions[10] and trazodone may have some 5HT-uptake blocking action (Table 1). These agents raise serious doubts as to the generality of the monoamine-uptake blockade hypothesis of the action of HCAs, assuming that encouraging support for the clinical efficacy of newer atypical agents is sustained.[1,15] Although several exceptions to the rule that NE-uptake blockers are usually antidepressant can be cited (amphetamines, cocaine, methylphenidate, mazindol), these do have short-lasting stimulant actions in man. On the other hand, chlorpromazine is also an effective blocker of NE uptake (similar in potency to amitriptyline, clomipramine, or even cocaine [Table 1]). Yet chlorpromazine, a potent DA-receptor antagonist, has antiagitation effects and is antipsychotic, although its status in nonpsy-

Table 3 Correlations Among Clinical Potency and Actions of Antidepressants

Factors (potencies)	r	N	P
Adrenergic			
1. *In vitro* vs. *in vivo* NE-uptake	+.89	14	<.001
2. Clinical vs. *in vitro* NE-uptake			
a. all available agents	+.31	19	NS
b. imipramine analogs only (r_s)	+.81	7	<.05
c. imipramine analogs only (r_{xy})	+.63	7	~.05
3. Clinical vs. *in vivo* NE-uptake	+.10	16	NS
4. Clinical vs. NE:5HT anti-uptake ratio	−.06	19	NS
5. NE-uptake vs. α_1 receptor blockade	+.32	10	NS
6. Clinical vs. anti-α_1 receptor	−.73	10	<.02
7. Clinical vs. anti-NE uptake: anti-α_1 ratio	+.65	10	<.04
8. Clinical vs. anti-DA receptor	−.20	10	NS
Serotonergic			
9. Clinical vs. 5HT-uptake *in vitro*	+.15	19	NS
10. Anti-5HT$_1$ vs. 5HT$_2$ receptors	+.88	7	<.02
11. Clinical vs. anti-5HT$_1$	−.10	8	NS
12. Clinical vs. anti-5HT$_2$	−.31	6	NS
Histaminergic and Muscarinic			
13. Anti-H$_1$ vs. H$_2$ receptors	+.49	9	NS
14. Clinical vs. H$_1$	−.41	8	NS
15. Clinical vs. H$_2$	−.51	9	NS
16. Clinical vs. ACh (muscarinic)	−.10	11	NS

Source of data: From Tables 1, 2 and 4; clinical potency (*not* efficacy) data are from Paykel and Baldessarini.[1,46]

Note: Correlations are by non-parametric rank method (Spearman, r_s) for N agents; an evaluation of linear regression (r_{xy}) of clinical potency vs. anti-NE uptake for imipramine analogs (item 2c) reveals a suggestive correlation ($r_{xy} = +.63$ of low power, as slope = .24). Anti-β activity (*in vitro*) is too weak to justify analysis.

The general impressions given by the above are as follows: (a) lower potency correlates with more anti-ACh, anti-H$_1$ and anti-α_1 effect (and possibly greater risk of toxicity, sedation, and hypotension); (b) among similar agents greater potency tends to correlate with greater anti-NE uptake effect (but this may be an artifact of drug development procedures) and less anti-α_1 effect; (c) most agents are weak β-blockers (may *permit* β-down-regulation); (d) there is little effect on DA uptake or receptors; and (e) none of these effects, alone, seems to account for antidepressant effects.

chotic depressions is obscure.[2] The psychomotor stimulant and agitation-inducing effects of stimulants (or of other DA-agonists such as L-dopa and bromocriptine), believed to be mediated by their DA-enhancing actions, limit their usefulness in depression. A sustained vs. quick time-course of action may also help to differentiate stimulants from true antidepressants. Although at least two new antidepressants have some effect against the uptake of DA (nomifensin and bupropion), nomifensin is also an extremely potent blocker of NE uptake (Table 1) and the clinical status and actions of buproprion are still highly tentative.[1,15] Nomifensin may also have stimulant properties in patients.

Interactions of Antidepressants with Neurotransmitter Receptors

Recent advances in the technology of evaluating the abundance and affinity of binding sites for drugs and neurotransmitters in brain tissue have led to many evaluations of older antidepressants and some experimental antidepressants. These evaluations have been complemented by other biochemical and physiological methods, such as stimulation of the formation of cyclic-AMP or cyclic-GMP, changes in transmitter turnover or firing rates of aminergic neurons, responses to microapplication of amines to neurons in the CNS, and behavioral responses to amine agonists. Receptors or binding sites evaluated thus far (Table 4) include traditional α_1 (postsynaptic) and α_2 (presynaptic) noradrenergic receptors, β-adrenergic receptors, dopamine (DA) receptors, histamine (H) receptors (types 1 and 2), muscarinic acetylcholine (ACh) receptors, and serotonin receptors (labeled by 5HT, type 1; by spiroperidol in some brain areas, type 2; or by LSD, a mixed and complex interaction).[8,10,16-18] Most of the available reports are incomplete or difficult to compare and summarize, but several patterns seem to be emerging.

There are few consistent relationships between the in vitro potency of interaction with the above receptors or binding sites and clinical potency (Table 3), even among agents that are similar chemically or in some independent pharmacologic characteristic (such as ability to inhibit uptake of NE; see Table 1). One of the few correlations with limited success in predicting clinical side-effects is the apparent anticholinergic activity of antidepressants, as assayed by competition with a potent muscarinic antagonist such as ^{3}H-QNB (quinuclidinyl benzylate), or by the stimulation of cyclic-GMP synthesis by neural tissues.[16-19] These studies reveal that among traditional antidepressants, amitriptyline is most potent, followed closely by protriptyline, doxepin, and imipramine; whereas the desmethylated products, desipramine and nortriptyline, are much less potent in vitro, and somewhat less anticholinergic in man (although less strikingly so than is sometimes supposed). Moreover, some new agents,

Table 4 Antidepressants vs. Amine Receptors: In Vitro Inhibition Constants (nM)

Drug	Typical Clinical Dose (mg/d)	Adrenergic			DA	ACh_{mus}	Serotonin		Histamine		Antidepressant
		α_1	α_2	β			$5HT_1$	$5HT_2$	H_1	H_2	
Protriptyline	30	265	>1,000	3,100	360	115	—	640	48	420	—
Fluoxetine	60	8,000	—	>10,000	6,600	>10,000	10,000	1,300	—	—	—
Mianserin	65	86	35	4,400	2,200	3,900	500	41	3.3	67	—
Nortriptyline	100	71	1,700	15,000	800	950	920	41.	17	417	100
Desipramine	100	140	>1,000	4,200	980	2,200	9,500	540	250	317	125
Iprindole	112	9,600	>1,000	21,000	6,300	>10,000	>10,000	1,900	105	200	40,000
Clomipramine	125	55	—	—	—	500	—	—	—	50	8
Amitriptyline	150	24	620	6,800	290	50	1,480	13	0.13	54	20
Imipramine	150	56	1,000	38,000	610	280	5,000	245	16	153	10
Doxepin	150	23	890	7,100	380	200	720	246	0.4	160	300
Trimipramine	150	45	1,430	—	—	125	42	—	0.1	—	—
Trazodone	300	103	1,500	>10,000	3,000	>50,000	1,700	111	460	50,000	—
Chlorpromazine	300	4.3	—	>10,000	25	5,700	3,500	15	28	41	300
(³H-Ligand, or Test Used):		(WB-4101)	(Clonidine)	(Dihydroxy-alprenolol)	(Spiroperidol, striatum)	(ligand)ᵃ + (ileum)	(5HT)	(Spiroperidol, cortex)	Mepyramine or cGMP	cAMP	Imipramine

Note: Data are summarized and averaged from Richelson and Divinitz-Romero, 1977; Peroutka and Synder, 1980, 1981; Fuller, 1981; Möller-Nielsen, 1980; and Richelson, 1981.[8, 10, 16, 19] *Note:* Rank-correlations with clinical potency are poor (even excluding neuroleptics).
ᵃ ACh data are averages of data using guinea pig ileum, or ³H-quinuclidinyl benzilate (QNB) or other anticholinergic agents as ligands in brain as results were very similar.

such as iprindole, fluoxetine, trazodone, alprazolam, and mianserin are virtually without anticholinergic activity (Table 4). Because the correlation between anti-ACh activity and *clinical* potency generally is rather weak (Table 3), an antimuscarinic hypothesis of HCA antidepressant action is not supported. Nevertheless, since there is a rough correspondence between these anti-ACh actions and ability to induce atropinelike poisoning in patients, and to some degree cardiac toxicity, screening of new agents in this way may lead to less toxic medications.

Other short-term receptor interactions have been much less helpful in suggesting an hypothesis of drug action or a generally useful principle to guide drug development. There is some tendency for strong anti-α_1 interactions to correlate roughly with hypotensive or sedative actions: notably, of doxepin and amitriptyline (as well as chlorpromazine), which are the most potent (Table 4). Interactions with α_2 receptors are generally very weak, with the notable exception of mianserin, leading to the hypothesis that this agent may facilitate the release of NE from nerve terminals by blocking presynaptic α_2 receptors believed to throttle the release of NE.[10] If potentiation of action of NE is an important effect of many HCAs, that effect is especially likely to be mediated by postsynaptic α_1 receptors. This hypothesis is suggested by the correlational analyses summarized in Table 3. Thus, although the potency vs. NE uptake (in vitro or in vivo) correlates only weakly with clinical potency of HCAs, there is a significant *inverse* correlation of the latter ($r_s = -.73$) with α_1-blocking potency. Moreover, clinical potency correlates significantly with the ratio of potencies of blocking NE uptake: NE α_1 receptors ($r_s = +.65$), although the effects on uptake and α_1 sites themselves are not significantly intercorrelated ($r_s = +.32$). These relationships thus suggest that increased availability of NE (by potent uptake blockade) along with *weak* α_1 blockade may be desirable characteristics in an antidepressant. The β-receptor *desensitizing* action of repeated HCA treatment (discussed below) provides further support for this hypothesis. Although this approach of correlating in vivo potencies with antidepressant potencies in test systems (Table 3) is of much more limited power and generality than, say, the correlation of neuroleptic potency with antagonism of ^{3}H-butyrophenone binding,[20,21] it does yield some interesting relationships.

Interactions of HCAs with DA receptors are generally weak and, again, the relatively sedative agents doxepin and amitriptyline, as well as the 7-OH metabolite of amoxapine (rare in man), but (paradoxically) also the non–sedating agent protriptyline, have moderate potency in one or both of two test systems (binding of ^{3}H-spiroperidol or formation of cyclic-AMP in tissue of basal ganglia)[7,16] (Table 4). Similarly, several of these agents are relatively potent histamine (especially H_1) receptor antagonists--particularly doxepin, which is one of the most potent antihistamines known; but there is only weak potency-order correspondence with either H_1 or H_2 interactions and clinical potency, at least for the rather small number of agents so tested (Tables 3 and 4).

Long-Term Effects of HCAs

Later changes in the characteristics of amine receptors following 1–3 weeks of antidepressant treatment, in contrast to immediate interactions, are more promising in providing clues to actions of HCAs that may underlie clinical effects. Notably, there is growing support for the impression that presynaptic (α_2) noradrenergic receptors may become less sensitive (or abundant) after repeated treatment with an antidepressant. This change may lead to increased release of NE per nerve impulse in cardiac or brain tissue, as well as to decreased responsiveness to exogenous α_2 but not α_1 (postsynaptic) agonists.[22] This change appears to be correlated with a rise of NE turnover and of the firing rates of NE neurons in the locus coeruleus of the brainstem.[10,22] These effects are best evaluated with desipramine. Amitriptyline recently also has been reported to lead to increased binding of α_1 and muscarinic agents to receptors in brain tissue,[23] although others do not agree (Table 5).[24] The duration, functional significance, and generality of these effects among chemically dissimilar antidepressants require further study.

Note that for several years, repeated administration of antidepressants of dissimilar chemical types (including MAO inhibitors and some atypical newer agents such as iprindole, which lacks acute effects on NE metabolism or actions), as well as electroconvulsive therapy (ECT)—but not treatment with other classes of neuropharmaceuticals—led to *diminished* sensitivity of β-adrenergic responses in brain tissue. This change has been well evaluated with NE- or isoproterenol- sensitive formation of cyclic-AMP as well as with binding methods (notably, with ^{3}H-β-antagonists such as dihydroalprenolol).[9,16,24–27] Although such a "down-regulation" of sensitivity to NE (typically by 20-30%) seems counterintuitive in view of traditional hypotheses concerning NE insufficiency in depression, the *physiological* significance of such a change is uncertain. Some evidence exists, however, that NE microiontophoretically applied to β-sensitive CNS neurons may be less effective.[28,29] Such changes are likely to represent one of several mechanisms that attempt to restore homeostasis of central neurotransmission, the postsynaptic effects of which are complex and poorly understood neurophysiologically.[30] It is likely that β-blockade, per se, is *not* an adequate explanation for antidepressant effects; indeed, the beta-antagonist propranolol is even suspected of inducing depression in some patients.[31] Moreover, chlorpromazine and amphetamine can exert

Table 5 Diminution of Receptor Binding in Cerebral Cortex After Anti-depressant Treatment

Treatment	Norepinephrine		Serotonin			Dopamine	
	Beta-adrenergic		Binding		Iontophoretic Actions	Postsynaptic Binding	Presynaptic Stimulation
	Cyclase	Binding	$5HT_1$	$5HT_2$			
ECT	+	+	?	?	+	0	+
imitriptyline	+	+	0	+	+	0	+
Amipramine	+	+	+	+	+	0	+
Clomipramine	+	+	?	?	+	?	?
Doxepin	?	+	?	?	?	?	?
Nortriptyline	?	+	?	?	?	?	?
Desipramine	+	+	+/0	+	+	0	?
Nisoxetine	+	0	?	?	?	?	?
Iprindole	+	+/0	0	+	+	0	+
Trazodone	?	+/0	?	+	?	?	?
Bupropion	?	+	?	+	?	?	?
Mianserin	+/0	+/0	?	+	?	?	+
Methysergide	?	0	?	0	?	?	?
Fluoxetine	+	0	0	0	?	?	?
Zimelidine	+	?	?	?	0	?	?

Phenelzine	?	?	?	?	?
Nialamine	+	+	+	?	?
Pargyline	+	+/0	+/0	0	?
Tranylcypromine	+	+	?	?	?
Clorgyline	?	+	+	?	?
Deprenyl	?	0	0	?	?
d-Amphetamine	+	+	?	?	+
Cocaine	?	0	?	?	?
Chlorpromazine	+	0	?	?	?
Haloperidol	0	0	?	?	?
Diazepam	0	?	?	?	?
Lithium	?	+	+	0	?

Source: Based on data in Serra et al., 1979; Peroutka and Snyder, 1980, 1981; Savage et al., 1980; Sellinger-Barnette et al., 1980; Sulser et al., 1978, 1980; Charney et al., 1981; Chiodo and Antelman, 1980; and Wielosz, 1981.[9,16,17,25,26,32,33,39,40,42]

Note: Binding sites ([3H]-labeling agent) *without* consistent changes include: $5HT_1$ (unless inhibitors of MAO-A were given, α_1 (WB-4101) with few agents tested, H_1 (mepyramine), DA (spiro-peridol in striatum), muscarinic-ACh (QNB). $5HT_2$ is defined by spiroperidol in cortex; LSD binding ($5HT_{1+2}$) also decreases; α_2 may also diminish, based on indirect evidence (mostly, desipramine). The effect on β-receptors disappears within a week after stopping desipramine. There are no effects after single doses. Rats were typically treated for 2-3 weeks with large doses of drugs with tissue taken one day after the end of treatment. Experimental conditions included: stimulation of cAMP formation in cerebral cortex slices by NE or isoproterenol; binding with [3H]-dihydroalprenolol (β), [3H]-5HT ($5HT_1$), [3H]-spiroperidol ($5HT_2$ in cortex; DA in striatum); or behavioral or neurophysiologic evidence of decreased responsiveness of DA cells to low "presynaptic" doses of the direct DA agonist, apomorphine. Symbols represent: (+) effect reported, (0) effect not found, (?) effect not evaluated.

effects like those of imipramine on β-receptors (Table 5). Irrespective of the functional significance of such a short-lived and reversible change in beta adrenergic sensitivity, the generality of the effect across many classes of agents is striking and might lead to new methods for predicting antidepressant activity of new substances.[32] A summary of findings based on receptor binding, or cyclic-AMP synthesis-stimulating assays is provided in Table 5.

Although there are few reports of consistent long-term changes in the binding of labeled ligands to α_1, ACh, histamine, or DA receptors,[16,23,24] some interesting findings with serotonin and dopamine systems are emerging. For the binding of ^{3}H-serotonin itself (5HT$_1$ receptors), there have been reports of variable and somewhat inconsistent decreases in binding site density after treatments that produce sustained increases in the levels of 5HT in the brain, notably with inhibitors of MAO-type A,[33] but less consistently with HCAs.[24,34] (See Table 5.) More intriguing, however, are data indicating a *fall* of 20–40% in binding of ^{3}H-spiroperidol, which is believed to bind to a class of 5HT receptors in the cerebral cortex called type-2 (in contrast to selective labeling of DA sites in the basal ganglia with this ligand).[16] (See Table 5.) Curiously, these chemical observations seem to contradict results of behavioral and neurophysiological studies, which consistently indicate an *increased* sensitivity to 5HT in several brain regions after repeated treatment (weeks) with typical and even some atypical antidepressants, such as iprindole.[35-38] In the DA system, there is still no evidence of altered receptor binding sites or of postsynaptic changes in sensitivity to this catecholamine.[24] Nevertheless, there have been intriguing recent reports of behavioral and neurophysiological changes consistent with a *decrease* in sensitivity of putative *pre*synaptic DA receptors that are believed to throttle the production and release of DA.[39-41] In addition, ECT may alter presynaptic as well as postsynaptic receptors so as to enhance DA neurotransmission, perhaps especially in the mesolimbic DA system.[41-42] These effects may thus *increase* the functional availability to, or effects of, DA at *post*-synaptic DA receptors, and may contribute to the mood- and behavior-activating effects of antidepressant treatments.[39-42]

Despite these interesting leads, current knowledge of the physiological relations between membrane binding changes and regulation of neurotransmitter function is too incomplete to permit a coherent interpretation of these complex and sometimes seemingly paradoxical findings. Yet, their fair consistency across classes of antidepressant treatments (including some atypical agents and ECT) is quite compelling,[32,39-41] and this approach deserves further attention as a contribution to understanding the actions of antidepressant treatments or to the development of more powerful predictive tests to aid in the development of new treatments.

The application of tritium-labeled antidepressants themselves in search of unique tissue binding sites or receptors has not led to important insights to date, although they may permit development of radioreceptor assays for antidepressant drugs. A major problem has been that potencies of interaction of drugs in such binding assays correlate poorly with clinical potency to the extent that they have been studied (Table 3). This result may reflect the complex interactions of such labeled compounds with tissue—including cholinergic, serotonergic, and histaminergic receptors—and, especially likely, to serotonin transport sites or other sites on 5HT cells.[17,43,44]

How Do Antidepressants Work?

The short answer to this difficult question is that no one knows how antidepressants work. Because so little is known about the biological basis of depression itself, it may not yet be possible to know.[1,3,4] The pharmacological work previously summarized is almost certainly biased by the rediscovery of more and more NE-uptake blocking and some 5HT-uptake blocking agents, and by the still uncertain *clinical* status of the more provocatively atypical new agents that do not block amine uptake sites or receptors. Although sustained NE-potentiating effects caused by uptake blockade may contribute to the actions of many antidepressants, this is not a universal feature of all antidepressants, especially not the newer, atypical putative ones. (See Tables 1 & 2.) Because it may be possible to obtain useful antidepressant effects by more than one mechanism and because there are almost certainly several biologically dissimilar varieties of depression,[3,4] it may not be reasonable to seek common actions for *all* antidepressants. Nevertheless, some promising leads have come from evaluations of β-NE and 5HT$_2$ receptors which appear to have a remarkably broad range of positive findings across many classes of agents (Tables 3 & 5). In addition, findings already discussed concerning gradual increases of physiological sensitivity to 5HT or diminishing sensitivity of presynaptic α_2-NE receptors, possibly increasing NE release in brain, are very provocative. Suggested effects at DA presynaptic receptors are also intriguing. While it is difficult to conclude that temporary and reversible loss of sensitivity of β-NE receptors itself is "therapeutic" it also remains uncertain how such receptors relate to modified function of the CNS or how they contribute to homeostatic responses to foreign chemical agents. A summary of reported effects of antidepressants is provided in Table 6.

Conclusions

Clearly, this is a most exciting time in the development and evaluation of antidepressants since the introduction of modern antidepressants in the 1950s and 1960s, and the work leading to amine hypotheses of their

Table 6 Summary of Actions of Heterocyclic Antidepressants

Acute (hours)

- Block uptake of NE $\geq$ 5HT (except iprindole and few other atypical agents) but not DA.
- Reduce synthesis/turnover of NE or 5HT.
- Reduce firing rates of NE or 5HT neurons.
- Block 5HT, ACh (muscarinic), NE (α_1), and histamine ($H_1 > H_2$) receptors (inversely with potency).

Later (weeks)

- Block of amine uptake continues.
- Return of turnover and firing rates, possibly increased.
- Decrease NE (β) and (α_2, presynaptic) receptor sensitivity.
- Increase NE release (α_2 effect?).
- Probably no change or some increase in NE (α_1) receptor sensitivity.
- Uncertain effects of 5HT receptors (increased physiological responses, but decreased binding to $5HT_2$ and perhaps to $5HT_1$ sites).
- No change or some increase in ACh_m receptors.
- No change in DA receptor binding, but possible increase in presynaptic DA receptor function to increase DA release.

actions in the 1960s.[3] There is now an unprecedented array of new agents[45–51] and of new techniques and ideas concerning drug actions.[1,9,10,15,17,19,24,32,39,40] Yet there are limitations and remaining problems, both theoretical and practical[1] (Table 7). Apparently, we are still faced with an irreducible residue of 20 to 30 percent of patients who respond poorly or not at all to any of the available or experimental treatments for depression.[1,2,52,53] Newer agents, the clinical efficacy of which remains uncertain in most cases of severe depression, at least promise alternatives and additional safety for some patients.[15,45,49,54,55] A more coherent theory to predict antidepressant activity, thereby aiding the development or discovery of more nearly ideal antidepressants, is needed. Needed, too, are more consistently effective agents for use in severe as well as mild depression; agents that are less toxic in therapeutic doses, especially in the elderly, not

Table 7 Problems in the Pharmacology of Antidepressants

1. *Efficacy:* 20–30% of cases respond poorly.
2. *Toxicity:* Newer agents seem less toxic to heart and CNS, but efficacy not always well supported.
3. *Pharmacokinetics:* Generalizations about "therapeutic levels" are uncertain.
4. *Pharmacodynamics:* Lack of coherent theory or method to predict new agents (short of clinical trials) vs. more "me too" drugs.

lethal in suicidal or accidental overdoses, and less likely to interact unfavorably with other medicinal agents.

The present overview suggests several tentative conclusions. It is almost certain that no single biochemical or neurophysiological hypothesis accounts for the clinical actions of all antidepressants. Although many have a NE-uptake blocking action, this may reflect some circularity of reasoning and of the process of pharmaceutical development. In fact, correlations between anti-uptake potency and clinical potency are rather weak (Table 4), although the range of clinical potencies is limited. Receptor binding analyses suggest that antihistamine effects (especially at H_1 receptors) are most striking in some agents of low clinical potency that are also relatively sedative. Anticholinergic effects (muscarinic receptors) may help to predict some toxic in vivo actions. The hypothesis is suggested that the combination of high anti-NE uptake potency, low anti-α_1 blocking potency, and a tendency to down-regulate β-NE-receptors may be especially characteristic of antidepressants with relatively low sedative and hypotensive actions. Increased *function* via postsynaptic α_1, $5HT_1$, and DA receptors may occur. A major theoretical limitation to addressing the question of how antidepressants work is our limited understanding of the pathophysiology of depressive illnesses and the growing impression that they are biologically heterogeneous.[1]

References

1. Baldessarini, RJ. *Biomedical Aspects of Depression and its Treatment*. Washington, D.C.: American Psychiatric Press, 1983.

2. Baldessarini, RJ. "Drugs and the Treatment of Psychiatric Disorders." In: *The Pharmacologic Basis of Therapeutics*, edited by Gilman AG, Goodman LS and Gilman A. VI Edition, New York: MacMillan Co., 1980. pp. 391–447.

3. Baldessarini RJ. The basis for amine hypotheses in affective disorders. A critical evaluation. *Arch Gen Psychiatry* 32:1087–93, 1975.

4. Baldessarini RJ. Biomedical aspects of mood disorders. *McLean Hospital J.* 6:1–34, 1981.

5. Axelrod J, Whitby LG, and Hertting G. Effect of psychotropic drugs on the uptake of H^3-norepinephrine by tissues. *Science* 133:383–84, 1961.

6. Randrup A and Braestrup C. Uptake inhibition of biogenic amines by newer antidepressant drugs: relevance to the dopamine hypothesis of depression. *Psychopharmacology* 53:309–14, 1977.

7. Coupet J et al. Amoxapine, an antidepressant with antipsychotic properties— a possible role for 7-hydroxyamoxapine. *Biochem. Pharmacol.* 28:2514–15, 1979.

8. Möller-Nielsen I. "Tricyclic Antidepressants: General pharmacology." In *Psychotropic Agents: Antipsychotics and Antidepressants, Handbook of Experimental*

Pharmacology, edited by Hoffmeister F and Stille G. Vol. 55, Part I. Berlin: Springer-Verlag, 1980. pp. 399–410.

9. Sulser F and Mobley PL. "Biochemical Effects of Antidepressants in Animals." In *Psychotropic Agents: Antipsychotics and Antidepressants, Handbook of Experimental Pharmacology*, edited by Hoffmeister F and Stille G. Vol. 55, Part I. Berlin: Springer-Verlag, 1980. pp. 471–410.

10. Fuller RW. "Enhancement of Monoaminergic Neurotransmission by Antidepressant Drugs." In *Antidepressants: Neurochemical, Behavioral and Clinical Perspectives*, edited by Enna SJ, Malic JB, and Richelson E. New York: Raven Press, 1981. pp. 1–12.

11. Ban TA. Amoxapine and viloxazine: review of literature with special reference to clinical studies. *Psychopharmacology Bull*. 15:22–25, 1979.

12. Oates JA, Fann WE, and Cavanaugh JH. Effect of doxepin on the norepinephrine pump. A preliminary report. *Psychosomatics* 10, (No. 3, Section 2):12–13, 1969.

13. Clements-Jewery S, Robson PA, and Chidley LJ. Biochemical investigations into the mode of action of trazodone. *Neuropharmacology* 19:1165–73, 1980.

14. Stewart RM et al. Receptor mechanisms in increased sensitivity to serotonin agonists after dihydroxytryptamine shown by electronic monitoring of muscle twitches in the rat. *Psychopharmacology* 60:281–89, 1979.

15. Baldessarini RJ. Overview of recent advances in antidepressant pharmacology. *McLean Hospital J*. 7:1–27, 1982.

16. Peroutka SJ and Snyder SH. Long-term antidepressant treatment decreases spiroperidol-labeled serotonin receptor binding. *Science* 210:88–90, 1980.

17. Peroutka SJ and Snyder SH. "Interactions of Antidepressants with Neurotransmitter Receptor Sites." In *Antidepressants: Neurochemical, Behavioral and Clinical Perspectives*, edited by Enna SJ, Malick JB, and Richelson E. New York: Raven Press, 1981. pp. 75–90.

18. Richelson E and Divenetz-Romeros. Blockade by psychotropic drugs of the muscarinic acetylcholine receptor in cultured nerve cells. *Biol. Psychiatry* 12:771–85, 1977.

19. Richelson E. "Tricyclic Antidepressants: Interactions with Histamine and Muscarinic Acetylocholine Receptors." In *Antidepressants: Neurochemical, Behavioral and Clinical Perspectives*, edited by Enna SJ, Malick JB, and Richelson E. New York: Raven Press, 1981. pp. 53–73.

20. Baldessarini RJ. Schizophrenia. *New Engl. J. Med*. 297:988–95, 1977.

21. Creese I, Burt DR, and Snyder SH. "Biochemical Actions of Neuroleptic Drugs: Focus on the Dopamine Receptor." In *Handbook of Psychopharmacology*, Vol. 10. Edited by Iversen LL, Iversen SD, and Snyder SH. New York: Plenum Press, 1978. pp. 37–89.

22. McMillen BA et al. Effects of chronic desipramine treatment on rat brain noradrenergic responses to β-adrenergic drugs. *Eur. J. Pharmacol*. 61:239–46, 1980.

23. Rehavi M et al. Amitryptyline: long-term treatment elevates α-adrenergic and muscarinic receptor binding in mouse brain. *Brain Res*. 194:443–53, 1980.

24. Enna SJ et al. "Effect of Chronic Antidepressant Administration on Brain Neurotransmitter Receptor Binding." In *Antidepressants: Neurochemical, Behavioral and Clinical Perspectives*, edited by Enna SJ, Malick JB, and Richelson E. New York: Raven Press, 1981. pp. 91–105.

25. Sulser F, Vetulani J, and Mobley PI. Mode of action of antidepressant drugs. *Biochem. Pharmacol.* 27:257–61, 1978.

26. Sellinger-Barnette MM, Mendels J, and Frazer A. The effect of psychoactive drugs on beta-adrenergic receptor binding sites in rat brain. *Neuropharmacology* 19:447–54, 1980.

27. Crews FT, Paul SM, and Goodwin FK. Acceleration of β-receptor desensitization in combined administration of antidepressants and phenoxybenzamine. *Nature* 290:787–89, 1981.

28. Siggins GR and Schultz JE. Chronic treatment with lithium or desipramine alters discharge frequency and norepinephrine responsiveness of cerebellar Purkinje cells. *Proc. Natl. Acad. Sci. U.S.A.* 76:5987–91, 1979.

29. Olphe HR and Schellenberg A. Reduced sensitivity of neurons to noradrenaline after chronic treatment with antidepressant drugs. *Eur. J. Pharmacol.* 63:7–13, 1980.

30. Szabadi E. Review: Adrenoceptors on central neurons: Microiontophoretic studies. *Neuropharmacology* 18:831–43, 1979.

31. Waal HJ. Propranolol-induced depression. *Br. Med. J.* 2:50, 1967.

32. Charney DS, Menkes DB, and Henninger GR. Receptor sensitivity and the mechanism of action of antidepressant treatment. *Arch. Gen. Psychiatry* 38:1160–80, 1981.

33. Savage DD, Mendels J, and Frazer A. Monoamine oxidase inhibitors and serotonin uptake inhibitors: Differential effects on [3 H]serotonin binding sites in rat brain. *J. Pharmacol. Exp. Ther.* 212:259–63, 1980.

34. Maggi A, U'Prichard DC, and Enna SJ. Differential effects of antidepressant treatment on brain monoaminergic receptors. *Eur. J. Pharmacol.* 61:91–98, 1980.

35. Friedman E and Dallob A. Enhanced serotonin receptor activity after chronic treatment with imipramine or amitriptyline. *Commun. Psychopharmacol.* 3:89–92, 1979.

36. Mogilnicka E and Klimek V. Mianserin, danitracen and amitryptyline withdrawal increases the behavioral responses of rats to L-5HTP. *J. Pharm. Pharmacol.* 31:704–05, 1979.

37. Gallagher DW and Bunney WE, Jr. Failure of chronic lithium treatment to block tricyclic antidepressant-induced 5HT supersensitivity. *Naunyn-Schmiedeberg's Arch. Pharmacol.* 307:129–33, 1979.

38. Menkes DB, Aghajanian GK, and McCall RB. Chronic antidepressant treatment enchances α-adrenergic and serotonergic responses in the facial nucleus. *Life Sciences* 27:45–55, 1980.

39. Serra G et al. Chronic treatment with antidepressants prevents the inhibitory effect of small doses of apomorphine on dopamine synthesis and motor activity. *Life Sciences* 25: 415–24, 1979.

259

40. Chiodo L and Antelman SM. Repeated tricyclics induce a progressive dopamine autoreceptor subsensitivity independent of daily drug treatment. *Nature* 287:451–54, 1980.

41. Chiodo L and Antelman SM. Electroconvulsive shock: progressive dopamine autoreceptor subsensitivity independent of repeated treatment. *Science* 210:799–801, 1980.

42. Wielosz M. Increased sensitivity to dopaminergic agonists after repeated electroconvulsive shock (ECS) in rats. *Neuropharmacology* 20:941–45, 1981.

43. Kinnier WJ et al. Characteristics and regulation of high-affinity [^{3} H] imipramine binding to rat hippocampal membranes. *Neuropharmacology* 20:411–19, 1981.

44. Sette M et al. Localization of tricyclic antidepressant binding sites on serotonin nerve terminals. *J. Neurochem.* 37:40–42, 1981.

45. Pinder RM et al. Maprotiline: A review of its pharmacologic properties and therapeutic efficacy in mental depressive states. *Drugs* 13:321–52, 1977.

46. Paykel ES. "Management of Acute Depression." In *Psychopharmacology of Affective Disorders*, edited by Paykel ES and Coppen A. New York: Oxford University Press, 1979. pp. 235–47.

47. Zis AP and Goodwin FK. Novel antidepressants and the biogenic amine hypothesis of depression. *Arch. Gen. Psychiatry* 36:1087–1107, 1979.

48. Feigner JP. Pharmacology: new antidepressants. *Psychiat. Ann.* 10:388–95, 1980.

49. Montgomery SA. Review of antidepressant efficacy in inpatients. *Neuropharmacology* 19:1185–90, 1980.

50. Settle EC, Jr. and Ayd FJ, Jr. Trimipramine: twenty years' worldwide clinical experience. *J. Clin. Psychiatry* 41:255–74, 1980.

51. Shopsin B. Second generation antidepressants. *J. Clin. Psychiatry* 41: (No. 12, Section 2):45–6, 1980.

52. Morris JB and Bect AT. The efficacy of antidepressant drugs. *Arch. Gen. Psychiatry* 30:667–74, 1974.

53. Kupfer DJ and Detre TP. "Tricyclic and Monoamine-Oxidase-Inhibitor Antidepressants: Clinical Use." In *Handbook of Psychopharmacology*, Vol. 14, edited by Iversen LL, Iversen SD, Snyder SH. New York: Plenum Press, 1978. pp. 199–232.

54. Burgess CD and Turner P. Cardiotoxicity of antidepressant drugs. *Neuropharmacology* 19:1195–99, 1980.

55. Smith RC et al. Cardiovascular effects of therapeutic doses of tricyclic antidepressants: importance of blood level monitoring. *J. Clin. Psychiatry* 41:(No. 12, Section 2):57–63, 1980.

18

Antidepressant Treatments: Regulation and Adaptation of Functional Receptor Systems

Fridolin Sulser, M.D.

Past hypotheses on the mode of action of antidepressant treatments, both pharmacotherapy and electroconvulsive shock treatment (ECT), have been mainly based on acute pharmacological effects elicited by a number of clinically effective antidepressant drugs at presynaptic neuronal sites. Neurohormonal substances such as norepinephrine (NE) and serotonin (5HT) convey their chemical signals through specific membrane surface receptors to the inside of the cell. It is surprising therefore, that so little emphasis has been placed on postsynaptic receptor mediated events and on the pharmacology of antidepressant drugs following their chronic administration on a clinically relevant time basis. At the International Catecholamine Symposium in Strasbourg, Lipton made the following comments: "Significant gaps in information remain. One of these is in the area of understanding the receptors and their alterations. Another is in the almost certain interaction of the various aminergic systems with each other."[1] Since 1973, some of these gaps slowly have been filled with pertinent information.

Two discoveries made in the second half of the 1970s have shifted the research emphasis from acute presynaptic neuronal actions of drugs to postsynaptic receptor mediated events. First, in 1975, our laboratory reported that the chronic but not acute administration of antidepressant drugs and ECT induce subsensitivity of central noradrenergic receptor systems.[2] The second important discovery was the demonstration that this

The original studies from this laboratory have been supported by USPHS grant MH-29228 and by the Tennessee Department of Mental Health and Mental Retardation.

noradrenergic subsensitivity in brain was linked to a decrease in the density of beta adrenergic receptors.[3] Our understanding of what receptors are, how they work, and how antidepressant drugs elicit alterations in their sensitivity and number has increased spectacularly in the past 6 years. This chapter discusses the current status of the regulation of central noradrenergic receptor function and its relevance to the therapy of depression.

Down-Regulation of the NE Receptor Coupled Adenylate Cyclase System by Clinically Effective Antidepressant Treatments

The NE receptor coupled adenylate cyclase system in brain, with its subpopulation of beta adrenergic receptors, has been characterized as a functional receptor system that displays the two essential properties of receptors: recognition function (stereospecificity for agonists and antagonists) and action function, that is, a biological response upon activation by agonists (formation of the second messenger cyclic AMP). Receptors, whose excitation is closely coupled to a measurable biochemical response, are attractive for studying function, but have to be distinguished from "acceptors," which may solely represent membrane surface binding sites for particular ligands without a known biological function. In brain, the NE receptor coupled adenylate cyclase system shows stereospecificity for agonists and antagonists,[4,5] and develops supersensitivity following chemical or surgical denervation.[6-13] The beta adrenergic receptors represent a subpopulation of NE receptors that are coupled to adenylate cyclase.[4,14]

Although our knowledge of the molecular mechanism of receptor excitation by agonists is still scanty, a fascinating picture has emerged of the molecular mechanisms involved in the coupling of beta adrenergic receptors to the catalytic unit of adenylate cyclase. Concerning beta adrenergic receptor coupled adenylate cyclase systems, the flow of information across the phospholipid membrane proceeds from the receptor via the nucleotide regulatory protein (G-protein) to the catalytic unit of the enzyme. Our current understanding of the role of GTP binding protein(s) as macromolecular messenger(s) in the receptor-cyclase coupling has recently been authoritatively reviewed by Limbird.[15]

Although drugs such as reserpine (which can precipitate depressive reactions in man) up-regulate this functional NE receptor system with its beta adrenergic receptor subpopulation, a number of antidepressant treatments have been shown to induce subsensitivity of the NE receptor coupled adenylate cyclase system that is generally, but not invariably, linked to a reduction in the density of beta adrenergic receptors.[16] Antidepressant treatments that have been reported to down-regulate the NE receptor coupled adenylate cyclase system in brain are listed in Table 1.

Table 1 Antidepressant Treatments Which Elicit Subsensitivity of the NE-Receptor Coupled Adenylate Cyclase System in Brain.

	Subsensitivity to NE and/or Isoproterenol	*Reduction in the Density of β-adrenergic Receptors*
Antidepressant drugs which block uptake of 5HT and/or NE		
Chlorimipramine	yes	yes
Imipramine	yes	yes
Amitriptyline	yes	yes
Zimelidine	yes	yes,no
Antidepressant drugs which block predominantly uptake of NE		
Desipramine	yes	yes
Nisoxetine	yes	no
Oxaprotiline	yes	yes
Drugs which block selectively uptake of 5HT		
Fluoxetine	no	no
Alaproclate	no	ND
Antidepressant drugs which do not block uptake of NE and/or 5HT		
Iprindole	yes	yes
Mianserin	yes	yes,no
Trazodone	ND	yes
Bupropione	ND	yes
Andidepressant drugs which block MAO		
Pargyline	yes	yes
Nialamide	yes	yes
Tranylcypromine	yes	yes
Electroconvulsive treatment	yes	yes
Chlorpromazine	yes	yes
REM sleep deprivation	ND	yes

Source: The data have been observed in the author's laboratory or computed from the literature.
Note: ND is not determined.

Note that ECT, which is generally considered to have a faster onset of antidepressant action in man, also rapidly down-regulates the NE receptor system.[17] Moreover, the ECT induced reduction in the density of beta adrenergic receptors[17-19] occurs following clinically equivalent treatment schedules and is still present four days after the last of 12 ECTs when other biochemical changes disappear (Belmaker, personal communication). Because the specific 5HT uptake inhibitors fluoxetine and alaproclate did not alter noradrenergic receptor functon, we have concluded that the action of the more selective 5HT uptake inhibitors—chlorimipramine and amitriptyline—are the consequence of their in vivo conversion to their secondary amines, desmethylchlorimipramine and nortriptyline, respectively. These metabolites are known to inhibit the neuronal uptake of NE. It remains to be seen whether fluoxetine and alaproclate possess true antidepressant efficacy in man and thus would represent exceptions to the rule. Note also that the so-called atypical and/or second generation antidepressants such as oxaprotiline, zimelidine, iprindole, mianserin, trazodone, and bupropion reportedly reduce the sensitivity of the NE receptor coupled adenylate cyclase system or the density of beta adrenergic receptors, or both.[2,3,20-25] The finding that the antipsychotic drug chlorpromazine shares this down-regulating action with antidepressants is not surprising;[26] chlorpromazine also increases the availability of NE at postsynaptic receptor sites as a consequence of alpha$_2$ receptor blockade and the inhibition of neuronal reuptake of NE. Clinically, chlorpromazine has also exerted antidepressant activity. However, this therapeutic action may be marked by other pharmacological effects, such as blockade of dopamine receptors, that are elicited by this drug.

As far as the decrease in the number of beta adrenergic receptors is concerned, all published studies on antidepressant treatments—with the exception of REM sleep deprivation[27]—have shown that this reduction in the number of receptors is due to a decrease in the ^{B} max value without changes in K_d values.[3,17-21,23-25,28,29] It is pertinent that the decrease in the density of beta adrenergic receptors following chronic treatment with psychotropic drugs appears to be quite specific for clinically effective antidepressants; whereas as other central nervous system-active drugs—such as cocaine, barbiturates, anticonvulsants, benzodiazepines, and antihistaminics—are inactive in this regard.[30]

In considering the multicomponent system of the NE receptor coupled adenylate cyclase system, subsensitivity and/or supersensitivity of the system are functional definitions, and sensitivity changes need not necessarily be reflected in corresponding changes in the number of beta adrenergic receptors. For example, subsensitivity following the antidepressant drugs nisoxetine, mianserine, and zimelidine is not consistantly linked to a decrease in the density of beta adrenergic receptors.[21,31] However, these dissociations are probably reflecting different stages of the same process of down-regulation, that is, an alteration in coupling (uncoupling) that may proceed the actual loss of receptor sites. Finally, a drug might cause subsensitivity by specifically inhibiting the catalytic unit of adenylate cyclase without major changes in either receptor number or coupling. Indeed, Ebstein et al., have provided evidence that therapeutic concentrations of lithium inhibit the beta adrenergic receptor coupled adenylate cyclase at a site distal to the receptor recognition site.[32] This raises the possibility that the antidepressant effect of lithium is also related to its ability to cause subsensitivity of the NE receptor coupled adenylate cyclase system.[33] By and large, both the subsensitivity of the noradrenergic receptor system in brain and/or the decrease in the number of beta adrenergic receptors, recover or return to normal values, respectively, within one to two weeks following discontinuation of drug treatment.

Noradrenergic subsensitivity following chronic treatment with antidepressant drugs has been verified electrophysiologically. Thus, subsensitivity to iontophoretically applied NE has been demonstrated in both cerebellar Purkinje cells and in cortical pyramidal cells following the chronic but not the acute administration of tricyclic antidepressants and monoamine oxidase inhibitors (MAOI).[34,35] The time course of recovery from subsensitivity evidenced electrophysiologically, parallels that of the return of sensitivity of the NE receptor coupled adenylate cyclase system to control value.

The Use of Antidepressant Drugs to Study Molecular Mechanisms of the Plasticity of Functional Noradrenergic Receptor Systems in Brain

The process of activation of receptors resulting in either the formation of second messengers or a change in passage of specific ions appears to be regulated in part by the specific agonist that binds to the recognition site of its receptor. Work with antidepressant drugs has indicated that an increased availability of the agonist NE and, thus, a persistent occupancy of the receptor by the agonist, is but one of the prerequisites for down-regulation of the NE receptor coupled adenylate cyclase system with its subpopulation of beta adrenergic receptors. Some of this evidence is listed in Table 2. Thus, tricyclic antidepressants cannot down-regulate the NE receptor system if NE receptors are blocked by propranolol or if the presynaptic nerve endings have been destroyed by 6-hydroxydopamine.[23,36] A number of experiments conducted in our laboratories support such a view. Thus, while amphetamine per se is a weak down-regulator of the NE receptor coupled adenylate cyclase system in brain of rats, a marked noradrenergic subsensitivity linked to a decreased density of beta-adrenergic receptors occurs following inhibition of the aromatic hydroxylation of the drug.[37] Such a procedure prolongs the half-life of amphetamine about

Table 2   NE-Receptor Interaction as a Prerequisite for Down-Regulation

1. No down-regulation by DMI if NE receptor is blocked by propranolol.
2. No down-regulation by DMI or iprindole following 6-OHDA or electrolytic lesions of the locus coeruleus.
3. Down-regulation by nisoxetine (short half-life) following multiple doses and by amphetamine following inhibition of its aromatic hydroxylation (prolongation of half-life and no accumulation of the partial antagonist p-hydroxy-norephedrine).
4. Down-regulating property of oxaprotiline resides in its (+)-enantiomer, a potent inhibitor of neuronal uptake of NE.
5. α_2-blockade plus DMI and/or MAO inhibitor shortens onset of down-regulation.

five fold and reduces the accumulation of parahydroxynorephedrine,[38] which has been shown to be a partial NE antagonist.[39] The consequence of such metabolic interactions is a more persistent NE receptor occupancy following the administration of amphetamine. More recently, Mishra et al., have shown that the marked down-regulation of the NE receptor coupled adenylate cyclase system by the new tetracyclic antidepressant drug oxaprotiline is due to the action of its (+)-enantiomer, a potent inhibitor of the neuronal reuptake of NE.[20] Subsensitivity is not induced by (−)-oxaprotiline, which does not inhibit the neuronal uptake of NE. Finally, the combination of an alpha₂ blocker with either tricyclic antidepressants or MAO inhibitors accelerates and intensifies the reduction in the density of beta-adrenergic receptors.[40-42] Additional support for the view that NE signal input is essential for the regulation of sensitivity of the NE receptor coupled adenylate cyclase system comes from experiments conducted in animals with unilateral lesions of the locus coeruleus.[43] Thus, while DMI and iprindole reduced the sensitivity of the receptor system on the non lesioned side, both drugs failed to down- regulate the system in the cortex ipsilateral to the lesion of the locus coeruleus. The finding that the non-NE uptake inhibitor, iprindole, fails to down-regulate the NE receptor system in the absence of signal input rules out a direct effect of the drug at postsynaptic sites. These results and the finding that cocaine, a potent inhibitor of neuronal reuptake of NE, does not down-regulate the density of beta adrenergic receptors,[25,44] indicate that the NE signal input—though a prerequisite—is not sufficient per se to elicit down-regulation. Additional regulatory or coregulatory factors (perhaps involved in the processing of the NE signal at its receptor) are suggested to be essential in the regulation of receptor sensitivity and thus the neuronal signal transfer through the membrane. The suggestion that neuropeptides existing as cotransmitters in terminal axons could function as neuromodulators by changing properties and/or the sensitivity of receptors for primary transmitters is provocative and deserves further study.[45,46]

In view of the observed dissociation of noradrenergic subsensitivity from a reduction in the density of beta adrenergic receptors following treatment with some antidepressants, studies on the effect of drugs on the coupling mechanism of receptors to the enzyme and on guanine nucleotide regulatory proteins are indicated.[21,31] Dissociations between sensitivity and receptor number have been reported to occur in other cell systems and are compatible with the view that desensitization may proceed in two steps, one being the modification of the coupling process between the receptor and the catalytic unit of the cyclase and the other the actual loss of the receptors.[47-49] Recent results from Axelrod's laboratory at the National Institute of Mental Health have shown that the beta receptor mediated phospholipid methylation changes membrane fluidity and coupling of the beta adrenergic receptor with adenylate cyclase. This increase in coupling can be blocked by inhibiting phospholipid methylation with S-adenosyl-homocysteine.[50,51] These results draw attention to the importance of lipids in the microenvironment of the beta adrenergic receptor coupled adenylate cyclase system in membranes, and to the role of membrane lipids in receptor mechanisms in general.[52,53]

Considerable evidence exists for a role of steroid hormones (adrenal corticoids, estrogens) in the regulation of central noradrenergic sensitivity and the number of beta adrenergic receptors.[54-56] Cytoplasmic receptors have been demonstrated in brain for both adrenal corticoids and estrogens.[57-59] The steroids could act as endocrine regulators of central noradrenergic sensitivity independent of or in concert with antidepressant drugs.

Neurobiological Consequences of Down-Regulation of the NE Receptor Coupled Adenylate Cyclase System by Antidepressant Treatments

Changes in sensitivity of the NE receptor coupled adenylate cyclase system by antidepressant treatments and in membrane properties through beta receptor activation probably will not only alter the signal transfer of NE, but also the transfer of other receptor mediated neuronal signals such as 5HT and dopamine (DA). In this regard, it is noteworthy that ECT enhances 5HT and dopamine mediated behaviors and that this enhancement is abolished by bilateral lesions of the locus coeruleus.[60] Assuming that the noradrenergic input from the locus coeruleus is inhibitory at dopaminergic and/or serotonergic effector sites, down-regulation of the NE system by ECT would lead to disinhibition or facilitation of DA or 5HT mediated behaviors that would be prevented by lesions of the locus coeruleus. The following could be interpreted this way: (*a*) the increased behavioral responsiveness to the 5HT agonist 5-methoxy-N, N-dimethyl-tryptamine after chronic treatment with imipramine or amitriptyline;[61] (*b*) the potentiation of apomorphine induced aggressive behavior following chronic treatment with typical (amitriptyline, desipramine, chlorimipramine) and atypical (iprindole, mianserin) antidepressants;[62] and (c) perhaps, the enhanced sensitivity to iontophoretically applied 5HT in various brain areas following chronic treatment with tricyclic antidepressants.[63]

The changes in sensitivity of the NE receptor coupled adenylate cyclase system following chronic treatment with antidepressants represent an important step in the regulation and adaptation of a specific biological response. Though the changes in the cyclic AMP response to NE are relatively small and the number of NE fibers terminating in a given area is sparse, the NE receptor coupled adenylate cyclase system functions as a highly efficient kinetic amplification system.[64] Consequently, small changes in the membrane transfer of the NE input signal and the formation of the second messenger cyclic AMP will be profoundly amplified or deamplified. Although implications for the etiology of affective disorders are premature at this time, the delayed down-regulation of central adrenergic receptor systems by clinically effective antidepressant treatments (pharmacotherapy and ECT) with the resulting deamplification of the NE signal may represent a therapeutically relevant biochemical action.

References

1. Lipton MA. In *Frontiers in Catecholamine Research*, edited by Usdin E and Snyder SH. New York: Pergamon Press, 1973. pp. 1181–85.

2. Vetulani J and Sulser F. Action of various antidepressant treatments reduces reactivity of noradrenergic cyclic AMP generating system in limbic forebrain. *Nature* 257:495–96, 1975.

3. Banerjee SP et al. Development of β-adrenergic receptor subsensitivity by antidepressants. *Nature* 268:455–56, 1977.

4. Robinson SE et al. Structural and steric requirements of β-phenethylamines as agonists of the noradrenergic cyclic AMP generating system in the rat limbic forebrain. *Naunyn-Schmiedeberg's Arch. Pharmacol.* 303:175–80, 1978.

5. Robinson SE and Sulser F. The noradrenergic cyclic AMP generating system of the rat limbic forebrain and its stereospecificity for (+) butaclamol. *J. Pharm. Pharmacol.* 28:645–46, 1976.

6. Palmer GC. Increased cyclic AMP response in norepinephrine in the rat brain following 6-hydroxydopamine. *Neuropharmacology* 11:145–48, 1972.

7. Weiss B and Strada S. Neuroendocrine control of the cyclic AMP system of brain and pineal gland. *Adv. Cyclic. Nucl. Res.* 1:357–74, 1972.

8. Huang M, Ho AKS, and Daly JW. Accumulation of adenosine 3', 5' monophosphate in rat cerebral cortical slices. *Mol. Pharmacol.* 9:711–17, 1973.

9. Kalisker A, Rutledge CHO, and Perkins JP. Effect of nerve degeneration by 6-hydroxydopamine on catecholamine-stimulated adenosine 3', 5' monophosphate formation in rat cerebral cortex. *Mol. Pharmacol* 9:619–29, 1973.

10. Dismukes RJ and Daly JW. Norepinephrine sensitive systems generating adenosine 3', 5' monophosphate: Increased responses in cerebral cortical slices from reserpine-treated rats. *Mol. Pharmacol.* 10:933–40, 1974.

11. Blumberg JB et al. The noradrenergic cyclic AMP generating system in the limbic forebrain: Pharmacological characterization and possible role in the mode of action of antipsychotics. *Europ. J. Pharmacol.* 37:357–66, 1976.

12. Vetulani J et al. A possible common mechanism of action of antidepressant treatments: Reduction in the sensitivity of the noradrenergic cyclic AMP generating system in the rat limbic forebrain. *Naunyn Schmiedeberg's Arch. Pharmcol.* 293:109–14, 1976.

13. Mishra R et al. The noradrenaline receptor coupled adenylate cyclase system in brain: Lack of modification by changes in the availability of serotonin. *Naunyn-Schmiedeberg's Arch. Pharmacol.* 316:218–24, 1981.

14. Mobley PL and Sulser F. Norepinephrine stimulated cyclic AMP accumulation in rat limbic forebrain slices: Partial mediation by a subpopulation of receptor with neither α- or β characteristics. *Europ. J. Pharmacol.* 60:221–27, 1979.

15. Limbird LE. Activation and attenuation of adenylate cyclase. The role of GTP binding proteins as macromolecular messengers. *Biochem. J.* 195:1–13, 1981.

16. Sulser F. New perspectives on the mode of action of antidepressant drugs. *Trends Pharmacol. Sci.* 1:92–94, 1979.

17. Gillespie DD, Manier DH, and Sulser F. Electroconvulsive treatment: rapid subsensitivity of the norepinephrine receptor coupled adenylate cyclase system in brain linked to down-regulation of β-adrenergic receptors. *Comm. Psychopharmacol.* 3:191–95, 1979.

18. Bergstrom DA and Kellar KJ. Effect of electroconvulsive shock on monoaminergic receptor binding sites in rat brain. *Nature* 278:464–66, 1979.

19. Pandey GN et al. Beta-adrenergic receptor function in affective illness. *Am. J. Psychiat.* 136:675–78, 1979.

20. Mishra R et al. Oxaprotiline: Induction of central noradrenergic subsensitivity by its (+)-enantiomer. *Life Sci.* 30:1747–55, 1982.

21. Mishra R, Janowsky A, and Sulser F. Action of mianserin and zimelidine on the norepinephrine receptor coupled adenylate cyclase system in brain: Subsensitivity without reduction in β-adrenergic receptor binding. *Neuropharmacol.* 19:983–87, 1981.

22. Ross SB et al. Effects of zimelidine on serotonergic and noradrenergic neurons after repeated administration in the rat. *Psychopharmacol.* 72:219–25, 1981.

23. Wolfe BB et al. Presynaptic modulation of beta adrenergic receptors in rat cerebral cortex, after treatment with antidepressants. *J. Pharmacol. Exp. Ther.* 207:446–57, 1978.

24. Clements-Jewery S. The development of cortical β-adrenoceptors subsensi-

tivity in the rat by chronic treatment with trazodone, doxepin and mianserin. *Neuropharmacology* 17:779–81, 1978.

25. Pandey GN and Davis JM. In *Neuroreceptors, Basic and Clinical Aspects*, edited by Usin E, Bunney WE, and Davis JM. New York: John Wiley and Sons, 1981. pp. 99–120.

26. Schultz J. Psychoactive drug effects on a system which generates cyclic AMP in brain. *Nature* 261:417–18, 1976.

27. Molginicka E et al. Rapid eye movement sleep deprivation decreases the density of ^{3}H-imipramine binding sites in the rat cerebral cortex. *Europ. J. Pharmacol.* 65:289–92, 1980.

28. Sarai K et al. Desmethylimipramine induced decrease in β-adrenergic receptor binding in rat cerebral cortex. *Biochem. Pharmacol.* 27:2179–81, 1978.

29. Bergstrom DA and Keller KJ. Adrenergic and serotonergic receptor binding in rat brain after chronic desmethylimipramine treatment. *J. Pharmacol. Exp. Ther.* 209:256–61, 1979.

30. Sellinger MD, Mendels J, and Frazer A. The effect of psychoactive drugs on β-adrenergic receptor binding sites in rat brain. *Neuropharmacology* 19:447–54, 1980.

31. Mishra R, Janowsky A, and Sulser F. Subsensitivity of the NE receptor coupled adenylate cyclase system in brain. Effects on nisoxetine or fluoxetine. *Europ. J. Pharmacol.* 60:379–82, 1979.

32. Ebstein RP, Hermon M, and Belmaker RH. The effect of lithium on noradrenaline induced cyclic AMP accumulation in rat brain: Inhibition after chronic treatment and absence of supersensitivity. *J. Pharmacol. Exp. Ther.* 213:161–67, 1980.

33. Belmaker RH et al. "The adrenergic receptor as the Locus of Antidepressant Therapy in Humans." In *Neurotransmitters and their Receptors*, edited by Littauer UZ, Dudai Y, Silman I, Teichberg VT, and Vogel Z, New York: John Wiley & Sons, 1980. pp. 139–47.

34. Siggins GR and Schultz JE. Chronic treatment with lithium or desipramine alters discharge frequency and norepinephrine responsiveness of cerebellar Purkinje cells. *Proc. Natl. Acad. Sci.* USA 76:5987–91, 1979.

35. Olpe HR and Schellenberg A. Reduced sensitivity of neurones to noradrenaline after chronic treatment with antidepressant drugs. *Europ. J. Pharmacol.* 63:7–13, 1980.

36. Schweitzer JW, Schwartz R, and Friedhoff AJ. Intact presynaptic terminals required for beta-adrenergic receptor regulation by desipramine. *J. Neurochem.* 33:377–79, 1979.

37. Manier DH, Gillespie DD, and Sulser F. Development of and recovery from subsensitivity of the noradrenergic cyclic AMP generating system in brain: Effect of amphetamine following inhibition of its aromatic hydroxylation by iprindole. *Naunyn-Schmiedeberg's Arch. Pharmacol.* 313:113–18, 1980.

38. Freeman JJ and Sulser F. Iprindole-amphetamine interactions: The role of aromatic hydroxylation of amphetamine in its mode of action. *J. Pharmacol. Exp. Ther.* 183:307–15, 1972.

39. Mobley PL et al. Modification of the noradrenergic cyclic AMP generating system in the rat limbic forebrain by amphetamine: Role of its hydroxylated metabolites. *Naunyn-Schmiedeberg's Arch. Pharmacol.* 306:267–73, 1979.

40. Johnson RW et al. Effect of desipramine and yohimbine on α_2 and β-adrenoreceptor sensitivity. *Europ. J. Pharmacol.* 67:123–27, 1980.

41. Wiech NL and Ursillo RC. Acceleration of desipramine induced decrease of rat corticocerebral β-adrenergic receptors by Yohimbine. *Comm. Psychopharmacol.* 4:95–100, 1980.

42. Crews FT, Paul SM, and Goodwin FK. Acceleration of β-receptor desensitization in combined administration of antidepressants and phenosybenzamine. *Nature* 290:787–89, 1981.

43. Janowsky AJ et al. Role of neuronal signal input in the down-regulation of central noradrenergic receptor function by antidepressant drugs. *J. Neurochem.* 39:290–92, 1982.

44. Sethy VH and Harris DW. Effect of norepinephrine uptake blockers on β-adrenergic receptors of the rat cerebral cortex. *Europ. J. Pharmacol.* 75:53–56, 1981.

45. Hökfelt T et al. "Coexistence of Peptides and Putative Transmitters in Neurons." In *Neuralpeptides and Neuronal Communication,* edited by Costa E, and Trabuech M. New York: Raven Press, 1980. pp. 1–12.

46. Costa E. "The modulation of Postsynaptic Receptors by Neuropeptide Cotransmitters: A Possible Site of Action for a New Generation of Psychotropic Drugs." In *Neuroreceptors, Basic and Clinical Aspects,* edited by Udsin E, Bunney WE, Jr., and Davis JM. New York: John Wiley & Sons, 1981. pp. 15–25.

47. Harden TK, Su YF, and Perkins JP. Catecholamine induced desensitization involves and uncoupling of β-adrenergic receptors and adenylate cyclase. *J. Cyclic Nucl. Res.* 5:99–106, 1979.

48. Su VF, Harden TK, and Perkins JP. Isoproterenel induced desensitization of adenylate cyclase in human astrocytoma cells. Relation of loss of hormonal responsiveness and decrement in β-adrenergic receptors. *J. Biol Chem.* 254:38–41, 1979.

49. Homburger V et al. Further evidence that desensitization of β-adrenergic sensitive adenylate cyclase proceeds in two steps. *J. Biol. Chem.* 255:10436–444, 1980.

50. Hirata F and Axelrod J. Enzymatic methylation of phosphatidylethanolamine increases erythrocyte membrane fluidity. *Nature* 275:219–20, 1978.

51. Hirata F, Strittmatter WJ, and Axelrod J. β-adrenergic receptor agonists increase phospholipid methylation, membrane fluidity and β-adrenergic receptor adenylate cyclase coupling. *Proc. Natl. Acad. Sci.* 76:368–72, 1979.

52. Hirata F and Axelrod J. Phospholipid methylation and the transmission of biological signals through membranes. *Science* 209:1082–90, 1980.

53. Loh HH and Law PY. The role of membrane lipids in receptor mechanisms. *Ann. Rev. Pharmacol. Toxicol.* 20:201–33, 1980.

271

54. Wagner HR, Crutcher KA, and Davies JN. Chronic estrogen treatment decreases β-adrenergic responses in rat cerebral cortex. *Brain Res.* 171:147–51, 1979.

55. Mobley PL and Sulser F. Adrenal corticoids regulate sensitivity of noradrenaline receptor coupled adenylate cyclase in brain. *Nature* 286:608–09, 1980.

56. Wagner DA and Davies JN. Decreased β-adrenergic responses in the female rat brain are eliminated by ovariectomy: correlation of (^{3}H)-dihydroalprenolol binding and catecholamine stimulated cyclic AMP levels. *Brain Res.* 201:235–39, 1980.

57. McEwen BS. "Steroid Hormone Interactions with the Brain: Cellular and Molecular Aspects." In *Reviews of Neuroscience*, edited by Schneider DM, Vol. 4. New York: Raven Press, 1979. pp. 1–30.

58. Heritage AS et al. Brain stem catecholamine neurons are target sites for sex steroid hormones. *Science* 207:1377–79, 1980.

59. Sar M and Stumpf WE. Central noradrenergic neurons concentrate ^{3}H-oestradiol. *Nature* 289:501–02, 1981.

60. Green AR and Deakin JFW. Brain noradrenaline depletion prevents ECS-induced enhancement of serotonin and dopamine mediated behavior. *Nature* 285:232–33, 1980.

61. Friedman E and Dallob A. Enhanced serotonin receptor activity after chronic treatment with imipramine or amitriptyline. *Commun. Psychopharmacol.* 3:89–92, 1979.

62. Maj J, Mogilnicka E, and Kordeka A. Chronic treatment with antidepressant drugs: potentiation of apomorphine-induced aggressive behavior in rats. *Neurosci. Lett.* 13:337–41, 1979.

63. de Montigny C and Aghajanian GK. Tricyclic antidepressants: Longterm treatment increases responsitivity of rat forebrain neurons to serotonin. *Science.* 202:1303–06, 1978.

64. Walsh DA and Ashby CS. Protein kinase: Aspects of their regulation and diversity. *Recent Prog. Horm. Res.* 29:329–59, 1973.

19

Beta-Adrenergic Stimulants and Depressive States

Pierre Simon, Ph.D., Yves Lecrubier M.D., Alain Puech, M.D. and Daniel Widlöcher, M.D.

The antagonism of different effects of apomorphine by neuroleptics is well known. With the discovery of different dopaminergic pathways and of different types of dopaminergic receptors, this antagonism was extensively studied in order to show differences between neuroleptics. We previously showed that apomorphine-induced hypothermia especially fits this aim.[1] Some neuroleptics, such as chlorpromazine, antagonize the other effects of apomorphine, but not the hypothermia; others, such as haloperidol, antagonize all the effects of apomorphine in the same range of doses.

Apomorphine-induced hypothermia is also antagonized by imipramine-like drugs.[2] It was a surprise to find that the higher the dose of apomorphine, the more pronounced the antagonism induced by the same dose of imipramine.[3] On the contrary, the higher the dose of apomorphine, the less pronounced the antagonism induced by the same dose of neuroleptics.

Using pharmacological reagents, we were able to confirm that hypothermia induced by low doses of apomorphine is clearly related to a dopaminergic medication. On the contrary, the hypothermia induced by very high doses of apomorphine is related to a decrease in the activity of the noradrenergic system. All the drugs activating this system, and especially the stimulants of the beta-adrenergic receptors (isoproterenol, salbutamol), are efficient on this model.

Because imipramine-like drugs and beta-adrenergic stimulants have in common this specific antagonism of high doses of apomorphine-induced hypothermia, we decided to systematically study the central nervous system (CNS) effects of beta stimulants in mice. These effects can be summarized as follows:[4]

- Decrease of motor activity.
- Lack of stereotyped behavior, even at very high doses.
- Antagonism of reserpine-induced hypothermia without modification of ptosis and akinesia.
- Antagonism of oxotremorine-induced hypothermia without modification of tremor and peripheral symptoms.
- Potentiation of yohimbine toxicity.
- Lack of modification of barbiturate-induced anesthesia.
- Lack of effect on the "behavioral despair" test.

Table 1 shows a comparison with the psychopharmacological profiles of imipramine and d-amphetamine.

To determine if the effects of salbutamol are related to a central or a peripheral effect, we compared the intraperitoneal and intraventricular

Table 1 Comparative Profile of Activity of Imipramine, Dexamphetamine, Isoprenaline, and Salbutamol

	Imipramine	Dexamphetamine	Isoprenaline	Salbutamol
Reserpine				
Ptosis	+	+	0	0
Akinesia	0	+	0	0
Hypothermia	+	+	+	+
Oxotremorine				
Tremor	+	0	0	0
Peripheral	+	0	0	0
Hypothermia	+	+	+	+
Yohimbine				
Toxicity	+	+	+	+
Apomorphine				
($16 \ mg/kg^{-1}$)				
Climbing	0	0	0	0
Stereotypes	0	0	0	0
Hypothermia	+	+	+	+
Motor Activity	0	↗	↘	↘
Stereotyped Behavior	0	+	0	0
Toxicity (aggregated mice)	0	+	+	0

routes of administration. The antagonism of oxotremorine-induced hypo-thermia was obtained with lower doses by the intraventricular route. This can be considered as an indirect proof for a central mechanism of action, but the other effects seem to be, at least partly, of a peripheral origin.[5]

We also showed that the effects of salbutamol are antagonized by propranolol (Table 2).[6] It is interesting that imipramine effects are also antagonized by propranolol.[7] This fact and the similarity between imipra-mine and salbutamol profiles led us to look for an antidepressant effect of salbutamol in patients.

Some biochemical data were also in favor of this research. After chronic administration of most of the drugs considered as antidepressants, the number of beta-adrenergic receptors decreased. Such a decrease was observed after imipramine-like drugs, MAO inhibitors, mianserin, and also after electroshock.[8–11]

Salbutamol was chosen because toxicity, side effects, and contraindi-cations were known, because of previous clinical utilization in asthmatic patients, and to prevent premature uterine contractions. Knowing the low bioavailability of oral administrations, we decided to use intravenous route using 6 mg/day, the dose used in pregnant women.

For the first open-label clinical study, we selected a limited number of depressed patients, whose disorders for the most part contraindicated imipramine-like drugs. This preliminary study suggested antidepressant properties with a rapid onset of action.[12]

A first controlled study comparing salbutamol (6 mg/day) to clomi-pramine (150 mg/day), both given by intravenous infusion, was performed on depressed inpatients (10 per group).[13] The symptomatology was evaluated by two blind observers at days 0, 5, and 15, using the Hamilton Rating Scale (hrs). Both treatments were effective on the overall sympto-matology, but the onset of action of salbutamol was more rapid (Table 3). These results were confirmed by others.[14–17]

A second controlled study (not yet published) was undertaken in a larger number of newly admitted depressed inpatients ($n = 126$) to confirm previous findings. During the first 10 days one of the two treatments (either salbutamol 6 mg/day or clomipramine 150 mg/day, both i.v.) was randomly allocated. Then all patients received clomipramine 150 mg orally between days 10 and 28. As in the previous study, we used blind observers because the very distinct side effects of the two treatments made a double-blind study unrealistic.

The main results at day 8 can be summarized as follows: Dropout rates were identical owing to side effects (salbutamol—2 and clomipramine—1), or because of interfering concomitant therapy (1 in each group). Improve-ment was not significantly greater in the salbutamol group (Table 4). However, the histogram of improvements in the two groups is very

Table 2 Antagonism by Propranolol of Some Pharmacological Effects of Imipramine, D-amphetamine, Isoprenaline and Salbutamol

	Reserpine Hypoth.	Ptosis	Oxotremorine Hypoth.	Tremor	Apomorphine 16 mg/kg Hypoth.	S.B.	Yohimbine Toxicity	Stereotyped Behavior
Isoprenaline								
saline	+	+	+	0	+	0	+	0
propra.	−	±	−		−		−	
Salbutamol								
saline	+	0	+	0	+	0	+	0
propra.	−		−		−		−	
Imipramine								
saline	+	+	+	+	+	0	+	0
propra.	−	+	−	+	−		−	
D-Amphetamine								
saline	+	+	+	+	+	0	+	+
propra.	−	+	−	−	−		−	+

Note: propra = propranolol; hypoth = hypothermia; S.B. = stereotyped behavior.

Table 3 Changes in Hamilton Score

	Day 0—5	Day 0—15
Clomipramine	− 4.35	− 5.30
N = 10	± 1.34	± 1.72
Salbutamol	− 9.9[a]	− 12.9[a]
N = 10	± 1.94	± 2.8

Note: Student *t* Test. $p < .05$.
[a] Difference between treatment groups.

different, especially if we take into consideration only the 74 patients with primary affective disorders (Figure 1). Most of the patients of the clomipramine group showed a moderate and partial improvement. In the salbutamol group, more patients had no improvement yet more patients had a significant improvement. If we consider recovery to be a significant improvement—Hamilton Rating Scale Global Score at day 8 of less than 10, and improvement of HRS of 10 points or more—there is a significant difference in endogenous patients in favor of the salbutamol (Table 5). However, this analysis was not planned in the original design and this difference can only be considered as a trend that would have to be proven by future experiments. Table 6 shows the results according to the diagnosis. The superiority of salbutamol for bipolar patients is very clear.

At day 28, the results have less meaning. The population is smaller because more patients dropped out of the study for various reasons. Also, both treatments were about equally effective after the 10th day (Table 7). One point should be noted: the mean length of hospitalization was slightly shorter for patients of the salbutamol group, especially for endogenous patients.

Regarding the side effects, those of salbutamol are well known. Tremor (especially during the infusion) and tachycardia, for which a tolerance appears within 3 to 6 days, were constant. Anxiety caused by tachycardia was expected; it was only noticed by some patients on the first day.

Table 4 Hamilton Rating Scale at Day 0 and Day 8

	Day 0	Day 8	Δ %
Salbutamol	23.5	11.8	51.3
N = 59	± 7.2	± 8.8	± 33
Clomipramine	22.9	12.3	43.8
N = 62	± 6.7	± 6	± 29

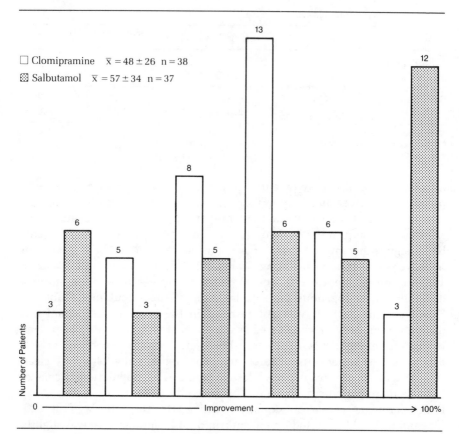

Figure 1 Improvement at day 8: Hamilton Rating Scale, patients with primary affective disorder[a]

[a] Bipolar, unipolar or single episode.

Table 5 Number of Complete Recovery at Day 8

	Salbutamol	*Clomipramine*
All Patients	25 /59	16/62
Endogenous	16*/25	7/25
Other Patients	9 /34	9/37

HRS Global Score ≤ 10
HRS Improvement ≥ 10

Table 6 Improvement at Day 8: Hamilton Rating Scale Scores

	Salbutamol			Clomipramine		
	Day 0	Day 8	% of Success[a]	Day 0	Day 8	% of Success[a]
All Patients	23.49 ± 7.25	11.78 ± 8.84	42	22.89 ± 6.67	12.32 ± 6.06	26
Bipolar (I)	20.89 ± 7.42	4.44 ± 4.39	78	22.70 ± 6.60	12.70 ± 5.25	20
Unipolar (II)	23.69 ± 6.83	11.19 ± 8.93	56	24.73 ± 5.90	11.87 ± 6.49	33
Single episode (IV)	20.67 ± 6.10	12.00 ± 9.47	33	22.77 ± 7.88	10.92 ± 5.54	38
Neurotic (V)	20.92 ± 4.94	11.83 ± 7.23	33	19.79 ± 5.71	12.05 ± 6.29	16
Delusional (III)	32.00 ± 5.44	19.01 ± 8.22	10	29.80 ± 2.59	17.60 ± 6.19	20

[a] The criteria for "success" were D0-D8 (Hrs) ≥ 10 and D8 (Hrs) ≤ 10.

Table 7

	Salbutamol N = 57		Clomipramine N = 60	
	D28	%	D28	%
HRS Scores	5.5	75	6	71.5
	± 6	± 30	± 5	± 25
Retardation Scale	7.7	64	8.3	67
	± 8	± 48	± 9	± 33
Mean Length Hospitalization (Days)	All M = 29 Endogenous : M = 26		All M = 33 Endogenous : M = 34	

We think that these results confirm the existence of the antidepressant properties of salbutamol. The onset of action is rapid, especially in endogenous patients. The occurrence of a complete, early response in some patients and of no response in others may be due to the specificity of the mechanism of action of salbutamol, the direct stimulation of beta-adrenergic receptors. This may be an important tool for biological classification of depressive states.

One other point should be discussed: Are the central beta-adrenergic receptors involved in the mechanism of action of antidepressants of the β_1 or of the β_2 type? Preliminary unpublished experiments seem to show that the sensitivity of central beta-adrenergic receptors to β_1 or β_2 stimulants or blockers is different from β_1 receptors and from β_2 receptors. Moreover, it is possible that the interaction of salbutamol with the serotonergic system explains some of its central effects.[18]

Because salbutamol cannot be used orally and because it poorly crosses the blood/brain barrier, we decided to study clenbuterol, which presents a good bioavailability by oral route, crosses the blood/brain barrier, and is a very specific β_2 stimulant (more than β_1). Preliminary results from an open-label study seem to confirm our hopes.

References

1. Puech AJ, Simon P, and Boissier JR. Benzamides and classical neuroleptics: Comparison of their actions using 6 apomorphine-induced effects. *Eur J Pharmacol* 50:291–300, 1978.

2. Lapin IP and Samsonova ML. Apomorphine-induced hypothermia in mice

and the effect on it of adrenergic and serotoninergic agents (in Russian). *Farmakol Toksikol* 31:563–70, 1968.

3. Puech AJ, Frances H, and Simon P. Imipramine antagonism of apomorphine-induced hypothermia: A non dopaminergic interaction. *Eur J Pharmacol* 47:125–27, 1978.

4. Frances H and Simon P. Isoproterenol and psychopharmacological tests: Antagonism by beta-adrenergic antagonists. *Pharmacol Res Comm* 10:211–17, 1978.

5. Frances H et al. Are psychopharmacological effects of beta-adrenergic stimulants central of peripheral? *Pharmacol Res Comm* 2:273–78, 1979.

6. Frances H, Puech AJ, and Simon P. Profil psychopharmacologique de l'isoprenaline et de salbutamol. *J Pharmacol* (Paris) 9:25–34, 1978.

7. Souto M et al. Antagonism by d,l-propranolol of imipramine effects in mice. *Eur J Pharmacol* 60:105–8, 1979.

8. Banerjee SP et al. Development of beta-adrenergic receptor subsensitivity by antidepressants. *Nature* 268:455–56, 1977.

9. Vetulani J et al. A possible common mechanism of action of antidepressant treatments. *Arch Pharmacol* 293:109–14, 1976.

10. Clements-Jewery S. The development of cortical beta-adrenoceptor subsensitivity in the rat by chronic treatment with trazodone, doxepin and mianserin. *Neuropharmacol* 17:779–81, 1978.

11. Bergstrom DA and Kellar KT. Effects of electroconvulsive shock on monoaminergic receptor binding sites in rat brain. *Nature* 273:464–66, 1979.

12. Lecrubier Y et al. Effet antidepresseur d'un stimulant beta-adrenergique. *Nouv Press Med* 6:2786, 1977.

13. Lecrubier Y et al. A beta-adrenergic stimulant (salbutamol) versus clomipramine in depression: A controlled study. *Br J Psychiatry* 136:354–58, 1980.

14. Bille J et al. Note preliminaire sur les effets antidepresseurs d'un beta stimulant. *Ann Med Psychol* 137:9–12, 1979.

15. Goudemand M et al. Medication beta sympathomimetique et depression. *Lille Med* 25:522–25, 1980.

16. Lerer B, Ebstein RP, and Belmakerr RM. "Salbutamol treatment of depression induces subsensitivity of beta-adrenergic adenylate cyclase." 12th CINP Congress, Goteborg, June 1980.

17. Agnoli A et al. "Antidepressive action of selective beta stimulant drugs." Abstract III, World Congress of Biological Psychiatry, Stockholm, 1981.

18. Ortmann R et al. Interaction of beta-adrenoceptor agonists with the serotonergic system in rat brain. *Naunyn-Schmiedeberg's Arch Pharmacol* 316:225–30, 1981.

Cardiovascular Effects of Tricyclic Antidepressants

Alexander H. Glassman, M.D.

Tricyclic antidepressant drugs (TCAs) have been in widespread clinical use for more than 20 years. It has long been apparent that an overdose of these drugs has serious toxic effects on the heart,[1] and it was originally believed that these deleterious effects would exist in attenuated forms when the drugs are administered at usual therapeutic doses. Although this seems obvious, it has not proven to be the case. Only after 20 years have we gradually acquired an accurate understanding of the cardiovascular effects of TCAs. This chapter will review our current knowledge of the cardiovascular effects of the tricyclics with an emphasis on implications for both the clinician and researcher.

Case Report and Survey Studies

Early clinical testing of psychotropic drugs, often done in a population free of any preexisting cardiovascular disease, can miss real cardiovascular effects. Case reports are the general clinical sequence by which a drug is associated with a previously unsuspected cardiovascular effect. After sufficient case reports appear in the literature, large epidemiological surveys can be used in hopes of clarifying the situation.

Unfortunately, both of these methods have major limitations. The difference between cause and effect and coincidence is rarely established in a case report because of the clinician's understandable reluctance to reexpose a patient to a drug he now holds responsible for a serious side effect. However, among the myriad case reports are a few that carefully document cardiovascular complications from standard doses of TCAs, the most convincing of which implicate TCAs in the development of heart block.[2-4]

Two epidemiologic studies have attempted to assess the relationship between the tricyclic drugs and cardiovascular death rate. The Boston Collaborative Drug Surveillance Program reported no difference in the overall death rate or occurrence of sudden death between the TCA recipients and the controls.[5] Among 4,074 hospitalized patients with a diagnosis of cardiovascular disease 80 were taking TCAs. Regarding the frequency of arrhythmias, heart block, shock, syncope, hypotension, cardiac failure, or fatality rate during hospitalization, no difference existed between patients with diagnosed cardiovascular disease taking TCAs and the control group without cardiac disease. However, the conclusions that can be drawn are limited because of small mean dose (72 mg/day), the lack of matching for cardiovascular disease, the lack of analysis for individual tricyclic antidepressant drugs, and, most of all, the relatively small number of cardiac patients receiving tricyclics.

The Aberdeen General Hospitals Group also studied the adverse effects of TCAs using a hospital-based drug information system.[6-8] Of 864 patients who received amitriptyline, 119 had a diagnosis of cardiac disease. An identical number of nondepressed patients who matched the tricyclic antidepressant cases for age, sex, cardiac diagnosis, and length of hospital stay were selected as controls. The overall mortality rate in both the index cases and controls was high; 19% of the index cases and 12% of the controls died during hospitalization. Although this difference is not significant, 13 of 23 deaths in the amitriptyline-treated cases were sudden and unexpected as contrasted with 3 of 15 controls. This difference in sudden deaths was significant. However, although this Scottish study is apparently well matched for cardiovascular disease and carefully separated outcomes by drug, it does not specify dose and the observations concerning sudden death were retrospective and, therefore, less powerful than they might first appear. The question also arises whether or not the controls were appropriate. As Avery and Winokur have emphasized, it is possible that the high mortality rate associated with depressive illness rather than with the drugs, accounts for differences in mortality between cases and controls in the Scottish study.[9,10] Recently, Weeke and Tsuang presented data indicating an increased incidence of cardiovascular deaths in a depressed population.[11,12] But the Aberdeen group was reporting sudden death, not total deaths, and as a result, Avery and Winokur's criticism would not be germane.

In summary, the case report literature is generally unconvincing, with the notable exception of those authors reporting heart block. The two survey studies yielded contradictory findings; thus, it remained for prospective studies controlling for plasma level measurements to determine the cardiovascular effects of therapeutic doses of the TCAs.

In order to answer the question "What are the cardiovascular effects of the TCAs?" — the question itself must be subdivided into a number of discrete queries that more precisely address the different components of the cadiovascular system. Thus, it is more useful to ask, "What are the effects of TCA in cardiac rate, conduction, rhythm, left ventricular performance, and blood pressure?"

Effects of Therapeutic Doses of TCA on the ECG

In one of the first cardiovascular studies to incorporate blood level measurements, Vohra et al. examined the effect of nortriptyline and doxepin on the ECG.[13] The average age of the 32 depressed patients was 42; and 20 were treated with nortriptyline and 8 with doxepin. The data showed a significant drug-related increase in the PR interval in the group as a whole ($p < .05$) suggesting that the change in PR interval was more marked with nortriptyline than doxepin.

In a subsequent effort to clarify the possible differences between the cardiac effects of nortriptyline and doxepin, Burrows et al. did a crossover study using 150 mg/day doses for each drug.[14] He found that nortriptyline caused a significant increase in the QRS duration but doxepin did not. However, this result was produced by comparing levels of nortriptyline that were more than therapeutic for depression to levels of doxepin that were undoubtedly less than therapeutic. Despite this weakness, Burrow's study and the one by Vohra constitute an important part of the evidence for the frequently heard claim that doxepin has less cardiovascular effects than other TCA drugs. To meaningfully compare the cardiovascular effects of the different TCAs, the drugs—or for that matter any pharmacological effect of any drug—must be given at doses that produce comparable efficacy.

Unfortunately, defining therapeutic doses of the TCA drugs is a difficult task. This is because the large interindividual differences in the metabolism characteristic of these drugs necessitate plasma level measurements. Even when these measurements are available, however, only nortriptyline and imipramine, of the tricyclics marketed in this country, have well-established relationships between these plasma level measurements and antidepressant response.

Nortriptyline has a therapeutic window with a maximum clinical response, whereas imipramine has no such therapeutic window. [15,16] Increased plasma levels of imipramine produce increasing side effects, but the antidepressant effect seems to reach a plateau. With both drugs, 80–90% of endogenously depressed nondelusional patients will respond at therapeutic plasma levels.[17] However, the clinical response to nortriptyline occurs at about one-half the plasma concentration required for imipramine. In addition, because of nortriptyline's longer half-life and smaller volume of distribution, the equivalent therapeutic dose of nortriptyline is approximately one-third that of imipramine. Thus, to be most clinically meaningful, a study should compare the cardiovascular effects of a dose of imipramine three times that of nortriptyline. This dose ratio would usually produce approximately equal antidepressant therapeutic efficacy. Comparable therapeutic ratios between other tricyclics are less clear.

Further studies of the ECG effects of nortriptyline in patients within the therapeutic window were conducted by Freyschuss and Ziegler. [18,19] These studies are comparable in that they both included relatively young patients essentially free from cardiovascular disease. Among the total of 57 patients, only 2 developed modest ECG changes while on nortriptyline. Thus, the studies to date indicate that in middle aged, depressed patients, free from serious cardiovascular disease, therapeutic plasma levels of nortriptyline are unlikely to increase either the PR or QRS measurements. However, changes in these measurements do occur more often at plasma level concentrations only slightly higher than the upper limit of the therapeutic window.

Having established that nortriptyline can effect the conducting system as evidenced by PR prolongation, Vohra sought to more precisely identify where nortriptyline was exerting its major impact.[20] Because the PR interval is a rough measure of AV conduction, an increased PR interval could be the result of either AVnodal AH or intraventricular HV prolongation. Vohra's bundle electrocardiography is a technique by which the components of AV conduction can be isolated and evaluated separately. Vohra performed this study in 12 patients prior to and while taking nortriptyline. He found that the AH interval was unaffected, but a prolongation of the HV interval occurred in 1 of 8 patients with plasma concentrations less than 200 ng/ml and in all 4 patients with plasma levels above 200 ng/ml. This data further supports the notion that usual therapeutic concentrations of nortriptyline are unlikely to cause any change in PR interval in patients without preexisting conduction abnormality; but that delays in intraventricular conduction become likely at only slightly higher than therapeutic plasma concentrations. Perhaps more importantly this study demonstrated that nortriptyline, like quinidine, affected primarily the HV interval. This led Vohra to speculate on other quinidine-like characteristics for the tricyclic drugs.

In contrast to the effect reported for nortriptyline, we have studied the ECG effects of imipramine in 44 depressed patients and found that therapeutic plasma concentrations regularly produced increases in the PR, QRS and QT$_c$ measurements.[21] In one patient who developed 2:1 heart block, catheter studies showed that imipramine's effect was predominantly on the HV system.[3] The potency of imipramine's action on intraventricular conduction is also supported by the electrophysiological studies of Weld and Bigger and Rawling and Fozzard.[22,23] These studies support the observations of Vohra and emphasize the quinidine-like quality of the tricyclics.

We have now seen five cases of second-degree heart block develop among 21 TCA-treated patients who had preexisting PR or QRS abnormalities. In contrast, second- or third-degree block never developed in more than 200 TCA-treated patients who did not have preexisting conduction abnormalities. This clinical data is consistent with the expectation—based in part on experience with quinidine—that patients with conduction abnormalities are at increased risk during treatment with a TCA.

By far, the most widely used tricyclic in this country is amitriptyline. Despite its widespread use, however, very little data are available concerning its cardiovascular effects at therapeutic plasma concentrations. Whether a relationship exists between amitriptyline plasma levels and antidepressant response is in dispute, and only a few prospective studies of its cardiovascular effects are in existence.[24-29] The data that are available suggest that, like imipramine at therapeutic doses, amitriptyline prolongs cardiac conduction; in overdose it seems to be at least as toxic as the other tricyclic antidepressant drugs.[24,27,28,30] With the information currently available, it is not possible to make specific comparisons with other tricyclic antidepressant drugs.[30]

Summarizing the literature, we can say that TCA drugs at or just above therapeutic plasma levels frequently prolong PR and QRS intervals, and that these changes reflect an action in the specialized ventricular conducting system and ventricular muscle. Modest to moderate increases in either the PR or QRS are not by themselves dangerous. These changes are rarely, if ever, clinically significant with any available TCA at normal therapeutic antidepressant plasma concentrations in patients free of conduction disease. At therapeutic plasma concentrations, the only depressed patients in danger of AV or HV block are those with preexisting conduction defects, particularly those that involve the His Purkinje system. The major determinants of high degrees of block are probably the type and degree of preexisting disease. Although it seems likely that there are differences between the propensity of various TCAs to produce conduction delays, it is unclear that the safest TCA presently available would be safe if the underlying conduction disease were sufficiently severe.

During the past 10 years, the clinical significance of sinus node dysfunction has become widely recognized.[31] This so-called Sick Sinus Syndrome is now the most common indication for insertion of a permanent cardiac pacemaker. Although the TCA drugs do show a preferential effect on HV conduction, experience with quinidine suggests that tricyclics will occasionally aggravate sinus node disease when the underlying pathology is severe.[32] Unlike the tricyclics, lithium seems to have a predilection for the sinus node and little effect on HV conduction.[33,34]

Heart Rate

Tachycardia is a crucial issue in the treatment of patients with coronary artery disease. Increased heart rate increases oxygen consumption and the resulting increase in oxygen demand can only be met by increased coronary blood flow. If coronary flow cannot keep pace with the increased demand, the patient could experience angina pectoris, or even infarction.

Reporting on an assortment of TCAs, Vohra noted an average increase of 9 beats per minute (bpm) in the resting heart rate, and this increase tended to be greater if the pre-drug heart rate was slower.[13] Unfortunately, Vohra reported neither the number of measurements this average was based on, nor how long the patients were on medication. Freyschuss and Ziegler have studied a combined total of 57 patients with therapeutic plasma concentrations of nortriptyline.[18,19] They both report a drug-associated increase in pulse rate averaging 16 bpm, which, on medication, resulted in an average resting pulse of 96 bpm.

Two studies reported on the effect of amitriptyline on heart rate. Ziegler, who studied 15 patients averaging 32 years of age, found an average increase of 16 bpm with the larger increases associated with higher plasma levels of the drug.[27] Peet studied a similar group of patients and found an average increase of 10 bpm on amitriptyline.[28]

We have reported heart rate data on imipramine that was collected by a continuously recorded, computer-analyzed 24-hour Holter ECG recording.[21] This means that rate estimates are based on a sample of approximately 100,000 beats per day. We found that imipramine caused trivial increases in heart rate. The rise was maximal in the first week, averaging 7 bpm. The pulse returned toward baseline rates during the second and third weeks of treatment even though blood levels of the drug continued to rise. By the fourth week of treatment, pulse increase measured over 24 hours averaged less than 3 bpm. Like Vohra, we found larger increases more frequently in those patients with lower initial heart rates.

In summary, amitriptyline and nortriptyline may have more effect on heart rate than imipramine or desmethylimipramine, but the data for the former pair have been collected in a much less precise manner and from a significantly younger population than that for the latter. Finally, tricyclic-induced sinus tachycardia probably does occur, but it seems to be an uncommon event.

Therapeutic Plasma Levels and Cardiac Rhythm

Because TCAs can cause severe arrhythmias in overdose, it has been widely believed that their use is contraindicated in patients with arrhythmias. Although seemingly logical, it is not necessarily true that a drug will have the same cardiovascular effects at a therapeutic level as it does at a toxic level. A case in point is quinidine, which is a potent antiarrhythmic at a therapeutic level but actually causes arrhythmias when at a toxic level. This is particularly pertinent to our work because of the similar effects that quinidine and imipramine have on intraventricular conduction.

In 1977 we reported two cases in which plasma concentrations of imipramine that were therapeutic for depression, dramatically reduced ventricular arrhythmias.[35] We have now observed 11 additional depressed patients with an incidental finding of ventricular arrhythmia.[21] Of these 11 patients, 10 experienced more than 90% reduction in their arrhythmias while being treated with imipramine for their depression. This astounding degree of antiarrhythmic activity leaves no doubt that among its other pharmacological properties, imipramine has powerful antiarrhythmic action. A similar antiarrhythmic action for both imipramine and nortriptyline has now been demonstrated in cardiac patients free of depression.[36] This observation is also supported by animal studies which have demonstrated that imipramine has a major effect on the initial inward sodium current of the Purkinje fiber[22,23] that is characteristic of type I antiarrhythmic compounds such as quinidine, procainamide, and disopyramide.

The observation that imipramine is a powerful antiarrhythmic drug at normal plasma concentrations has the obvious implication that these drugs can be used safely in depressed patients with ventricular "extra beats." In fact, it is likely, although it has not been proven, that if a depressed patient receiving quinidine or procainamide for an arrhythmia were given imipramine, his usual antiarrhythmic drug could be reduced or discontinued.

Perhaps the most important implication of imipramine's antiarrhythmic activity is for the treatment of tricyclic antidepressant overdose. Increasingly, evidence indicates that the tricyclic antidepressant drugs have become the most common cause of deliberately ingested toxic overdose. In severe overdose, there is no question that ventricular arrhythmias do occur, and the emergency room physician might easily consider treating these arrhythmias with quinidine or other similar antiarrhythmic drugs. However, only if the physician realizes that the tricyclics themselves are type I antiarrhythmic drugs does the danger of this procedure become apparent. In fact, the arrhythmias seen in TCA overdose are similar to those seen in quinidine toxicity.[37] Although no systematic studies are yet available, it seems reasonable to treat TCA overdoses that develop arrhythmias as one would quinidine overdoses; that is, with sodium lactate and pacing.[38] This therapeutic rationale should significantly increase the percentage of patients surviving tricyclic antidepressant overdose.

Except for nortriptyline it is not clear to what extent other TCA drugs share imipramine's antiarrhythmic activity at therapeutic antidepressant concentrations. It is likely that many share this quality to some extent. Data from dog experiments support this contention;[39] however, no observations have been reported in human subjects with tricyclic antidepressants other than imipramine, maprotiline, and recently nortriptyline.[36,40]

Effects on Mechanical Functioning of the Heart

Only a few groups have attempted to study the effects of TCAs on the mechanical function of the heart in adults. Taylor and Braithwaite studied 8 depressed patients receiving nortriptyline; and Burckhardt and Muller examined a group of 66 depressed patients receiving an assortment of tricyclic and tetracyclic antidepressants.[41-43] In both of these studies, patients were examined after being on medication for a number of weeks. In a different approach, Burgess studied a group of normal volunteers given single doses of amitriptyline.[29] Using the systolic time interval (STI) as the method of evaluation, all three groups found evidence for deteriorating ventricular function on TCAs. However, the validity of the STI as an indicator of myocardial function in patients taking drugs that are known to prolong intraventricular conduction time has been questioned for technical reasons.[44]

Recently we studied 20 depressed patients in a double-blind, randomized, crossover study comparing the effects of imipramine and desmethylimipramine on the ECG and left ventricular function.[44] We evaluated ventricular performance by the STI and by echocardiogram, a noninvasive method of assessing the mechanical function of the ventricles that is not dependent on intraventricular conduction. Though the STI measurements indicated deteriorating ventricular performance on TCA, this was not corroborated by the echocardiograms. This further substantiates the contention that the STI may be misleading when used to evaluate the TCAs effect on ventricular performance.

Furthermore, in a study evaluating TCA effect on ventricular performance at toxic levels of drug, Thorstrand found no impairment of the heart's mechanical performance in 10 patients who attempted suicide with tricyclic drugs.[45] Even during coma, Thorstrand found evidence of high cardiac output. Thorstrand's data are most impressive because they were obtained directly by cardiac catheterization, a direct and reliable method. In a similar situation Langou recently replicated and extended these observations.[46]

At this point, it would seem unlikely that tricyclic antidepressant drugs have an adverse effect on the mechanical performance of the heart at therapeutic plasma concentration in spite of the impairment seen in the STI studies. Certainly, in patients without prior evidence of impaired left ventricular function, there is no evidence that these drugs would cause such a clinically significant impairment. The problem comes in treating depressed patients with overt heart failure, a history of failure, or an enlarged heart without clinical failure. We have recently undertaken a study of such patients using radionuclide techniques. The preliminary results suggest that even in patients with preexisting impaired left ventricular function, tricyclics do not adversely affect ventricular performance. However, the problem has been that this group of patients has had an extraordinarily high rate of severe orthostatic hypotension.[47]

Orthostatic Hypotension

One of the most frequent and potentially serious side effects of tricyclic antidepressant treatment is orthostatic hypotension. Fractures, lacerations, myocardial infarctions, and sudden deaths have all been reported.[48,49]

By far, the most studied drug in this context is imipramine. An early study by Muller et al., observed "moderate to severe" postural hypotension in 24% of 82 depressed patients treated with imipramine.[48] The patients were split into two groups; half with a mean age of 70, all of whom had some cardiovascular disease; and half with a mean age of 39, all free from cardiovascular disease. Most of the untoward reactions attributed to orthostatic hypotension, including two myocardial infarctions in patients with preexisting angina, occurred in the older age group.

We have examined the effects of imipramine on blood pressure in 148 patients in a retrospective study and 44 patients in a prospective study.[49] In the retrospective study, the average age was 59 and the dose of drug 225 mg. Almost 20% of the 148 patients had symptoms associated with orthostatic hypotension that were severe enough to interfere with their treatment (e.g., drug discontinued, dose reduced, or dose unable to be increased to desired level). Of these, 4% sustained significant physical injuries such as lacerations or fractures.

In the prospective study, 44 depressed patients with an average age of 59 were treated with therapeutic plasma levels of imipramine. One minute after standing, the average fall in systolic blood pressure was 26mmHg, which represented a statistically significant increase ($p < .001$) as compared to the pre-drug orthostatic drop. An important clinical characteristic of this on-drug orthostatic fall was that there was no tendency for patients to accommodate to the effect of the drug. The other surprising observation was that the orthostatic drop in pressure was maximal far below therapeutic blood levels of imipramine. In clinical terms, this means that a patient on any usual oral dose of imipramine (75 mg or more/day) can have that dose increased without the risk of concomitantly increasing the postural drop. Whatever drop that patient is experiencing is likely to remain the same. If it is safe to continue, it is safe to raise the dose. Conversely, moderately decreasing the dose of imipramine is not likely to alter orthostatic hypotension if it is a serious problem.

Recently we have had the opportunity to study a group of depressed patients treated with imipramine many of whom had severe cardiovascular disease. Among those patients with more severe heart disease the incidence of severe orthostatic hypotension increased dramatically.[47] This group was likely to have or have had congestive heart failure and to be on multiple cardiovascular medications. Whether the increase is due to the heart disease per se or to interaction with the cardiac drugs this group was taking is unclear. However, it was clear that there was a five- or sixfold increase in the number of patients falling from postural hypotension.

The data available on the orthostatic effect of other tricyclics are not as complete as that with imipramine, but the works of Hayes, Kopera, and others strongly imply that this orthostatic effect exists for amitriptyline and desmethylimipramine as well.[50–52] Interestingly, for more than a decade doxepin has been marketed as the safest tricyclic in patients with cardiovascular disease, even though almost nothing is known concerning doxepin's potential to cause orthostatic hypotension.

The only TCA presently marketed where there is a disagreement in the literature on its orthostatic effect is nortriptyline. Freyschuss et al. reported that orthostatic effect of nortriptyline in 40 healthy and relatively young (mean age 44) depressed patients was negligible.[18] In a study of 20 patients with a mean age of 42 and no cardiovascular illness, Vohra also reported that there were no postural systolic drops with nortriptyline.[13]

In contrast, Reed et al., found that nortriptyline caused a significant orthostatic drop: mean drop on-drug of 24 mmHg compared to pre-drug drop of 10 mmHg.[53] This study, however, included only 8 patients (3 with a mean age of 25 and 5 with a mean age of 68), and orthostatic averages were based on blood pressures taken only two or three times per week. No statistical analysis is presented, but the small number of both patients and blood pressure measurements makes drawing conclusions from this study difficult.

We recently completed a study of the orthostatic effects of nortriptyline in 15 patients with an average age of 59, and compared the results to orthostatic effects of imipramine in a comparable group of patients.[54] The average orthostatic drop on nortriptyline was 13 mmHg, which is significantly less than the 26 mmHg average orthostatic drop for the patients on imipramine. Furthermore, we treated 8 patients with both imipramine and nortriptyline, thereby allowing a comparison of the differential orthostatic effects of the two drugs, using the patient as his own control. In this group, which included a number of patients with very large orthostatic drops, nortriptyline caused significantly less orthostatic hypotension.[54] In fact, the patients who were forced to stop their imipramine because they repeatedly fell or passed out when standing, showed no clinical orthostatic hypotension at all when switched to nortriptyline.

The mechanism by which tricyclics induce orthostatic hypotension is unclear. It has been suggested that this effect is a result of alpha-1-adrenergic blockade. This, in our opinion, is not supported by the clinical evidence. U'Prichard et al., have shown that nortriptyline and imipramine have equivalent alpha-1-adrenergic blocking effects, whereas desmethylimipramine has significantly less.[55] If orthostatic hypotension were a direct function of alpha-1-blockade, it would suggest that nortriptyline and imipramine should cause the same degree of orthostatic hypotension and desmethylimipramine should induce substantially less. Evidently, this is not the case. Imipramine and desmethylimipramine appear to possess essentially equivalent orthostatic effects, and it is nortriptyline that causes less. Therefore, the clinical data make the direct alpha-1-adrenergic blockade theory untenable.

Recently, des Lauriers et al., reported that in 10 of 11 patients treated with chlorimipramine, the addition of 12 mg of yohimbine, an alpha-II-adrenergic agonist, substantially reduced the systolic orthostatic drop observed after standing 1 minute.[56] The observation that an alpha-II-agonist can reverse tricyclic-induced orthostatic hypotension, however, should not be taken to mean necessarily that orthostatic drop itself is caused by alpha II blockade. For instance, recent work by Talman et al. has shown that L-glutamate may be involved in the mechanism by which baro-receptor stimulation can trigger systemic hypotension.[57]

Clinical and Research Implications

A critical review of the cardiovascular effects of the TCA drugs shows that the risks associated with these drugs have been poorly understood for many years. For healthy adult patients with no cardiac disease these drugs given at therapeutic levels appear to be free of significant risk except for postural hypotension. Even in those patients with overt heart disease, tricyclic antidepressant drugs do not necessarily pose a threat. In fact, those depressed patients with ventricular arrhythmias are likely to experience improvement in their arrhythmias during antidepressant drug treatment. The one group at increased risk are those depressed patients with preexisting intraventricular conduction abnormalities. Fortunately, most of these patients can be identified from a routine pretreatment ECG. Certainly, a pretreatment ECG should be obtained in any depressed patient over 50 or any patient with a history of or reason to suspect cardiac disease. A prolonged PR or QRS interval or other evidence of ventricular conduction disease undoubtedly carries a markedly increased risk of inducing serious degrees of heart block.

Presently, the effects of TCA drugs on left ventricular function are still unclear. Several studies suggest that tricyclic antidepressants impair the heart's mechanical function. However, this conclusion is suspect because neither case reports nor direct intracardiac measurements in toxic overdose support it. Although tricyclics probably do not adversely affect left ventricular function, those depressed patients with preexisting left ventricular impairment are at much higher risk for orthostatic hypotension.

Undoubtedly, the most common serious cardiovascular complication of the tricyclic drugs at normal therapeutic levels is orthostatic hypotension. Postural drops in systolic pressure of more than 35 mm will occur in more than 20% of the population. Although major drops can occur at any age, the risk of serious sequelae increases dramatically with age and with either coronary or cerebral insufficiency. This problem is well documented with imipramine and there is little evidence to indicate that amitriptyline, doxepin, or desmethylimipramine are significantly different. The use of tricyclic antidepressants in patients with a history of myocardial infarction or symptoms of angina but free of conduction abnormalities is primarily limited by the degree and frequency to which these patients develop postural hypotension. The only presently marketed tricyclic antidepressant documented to carry a lower risk of orthostatic hypotension is nortriptyline.

The treatment of tricyclic overdose should reflect the recently recognized antiarrhythmic activity of the tricyclic antidepressant drugs. The failure to recognize this has been detrimental to the treatment of these patients. Survival from TCA overdose should be improved by treating the cardiovascular complications as if they resulted from an overdose of quinidine. In fact, the tricyclics can be understood as a quinidine-like compound. At usual therapeutic levels they moderately slow ventricular conduction and are markedly antiarrhythmic, whereas in overdose they can cause severe conduction block and occasional ventricular arrhythmia. Certainly, the cardiovascular effects of the tricyclic drugs at both therapeutic and toxic concentrations become much clearer when viewed from this perspective.

Finally, the antiarrhythmic properties of the tricyclics may tell us something about the effect of these drugs on the brain. It is far easier to examine isolated cardiac tissue than it is to examine isolated brain tissue. The work of Weld and Rawling on the effects of tricyclic antidepressants on isolated Purkinje tissues as well as on ventricular muscle, has shown that imipramine has striking effects on the fast sodium channels.[22,23] This startling observation on isolated cardiovascular tissue raises the question of whether imipramine also affects sodium channels in nerve fibers. Cases of death from imipramine overdose have long been known to show imipramine tightly bound to the heart.[58] Imipramine is also known to bind tightly to isolated Purkinje fibers, though it is not clear whether sodium channels are involved in this phenomenon. One might even wonder if there is any connection between this binding and the recently described high affinity site for imipramine on human platelets.[59] The relevance of these cardiovascular effects to the mode of action of imipramine on the brain remains to be seen; however, it is tempting to speculate that imipramine's effect on the fast sodium channel in some way relates to what we refer to as "reuptake blockage" in neuronal tissue. It is difficult to imagine that a pharmacological effect so dramatic as that seen in cardiac tissue does not exist in some form in neuronal tissue as well.

References

1. Williams RB, Jr. and Sherter C. Cardiac complications of tricyclic antidepressant therapy. *Ann Intern Med* 74:395–98, 1971.

2. Smith RB and Rusbatch BJ. Amitriptyline and heart block. *Br. Med. J.* 3:311, 1967.

3. Kantor SJ et al. Imipramine induced heart block: A longitudinal case study. *JAMA* 231:1364–66, 1975.

4. Kristjansen P and Poulsen H. Grenblok som bivirkning ved amitriptylinbehandling. *Ugeskr Laeg* 125:394–95, 1963.

5. Boston Collaborative Drug Surveillance Program. *Lancet* 1:529–31, 1972.

6. Coull DC et al. Amitriptyline and cardiac disease: Risk of sudden death identified by monitoring system. *Lancet* 2:590–91, 1970.

7. Moir DC et al. Cardiotoxicity of amitriptyline. *Lancet* 2:561–64, 1972.

8. Moir DC, Dingwall-Fordyce I, and Weir RD. Medicines evaluation and monitoring group—A follow up study of cardiac patients receiving amitriptyline. *Eur. J. Clin. Pharmacol.* 6:98–101, 1973.

9. Avery D and Winokur G. Mortality in depressed patients treated with electroconvulsive therapy and antidepressants. *Arch. Gen. Psychiatry* 33:1029–37, 1976.

10. Malzberg B. Mortality among patients with involutional melancholia. *Am J. Psychiatry* 93:1231–38, 1937.

11. Weeke A. Cause of death in manic-depressives. Workshop: Klinische Relevanz der Kardiodepressiven Wirkung von Psychopharmaka, Geneva, Switzerland, April 1981.

12. Tsuang MT, Woolson RF, Fleming JA. Premature deaths in schizophrenia and affective disorders. *Arch. Gen. Psychiatry* 37:979–83, 1980.

13. Vohra J, Burrows GD, and Sloman G. Assessment of cardiovascular side effects of therapeutic doses of tricyclic antidepressant drugs. *Austr. N.Z.J. Med.* 5:7–11, 1975.

14. Burrows GD et al. "TCA Drugs and Cardiac Conduction." In *Proceedings of the 10th Congress, Colleqium Internationale Neuropsychopharmacologicum.* London: Pergamon Press, 1977.

15. Asberg M et al. Relationship between plasma level and therapeutic effect of nortriptyline. *Br. Med. J.* 3:331–34, 1971.

16. Kragh-Sorensen P, Hansen CE, and Asberg M. Plasma levels of nortriptyline in the treatment of endogenous depression. *Acta. Psychiat. Scand.* 49:444–56, 1973.

17. Glassman AH et al. Clinical implications of imipramine plasma levels for depressive illness. *Arch. Gen. Psychiat.* 34:3, 197–204, 1977.

18. Freyschuss U et al. Circulatory effects in man of nortriptyline, a tricyclic antidepressant drug. *Pharmacol. Clin.* 2:68–71, 1970.

19. Ziegler VE, Co BT, and Biggs JT. Plasma nortriptyline levels and ECG findings. *Am. J. Psychiat.* 134:441–43, 1977.

20. Vohra J et al. The effect of toxic and therapeutic doses of tricyclic antidepressant drugs on intracardiac conduction. *Eur. J. Cardiol.* 3/3:219–27, 1975.

21. Giardina EGV et al. The electrocardiographic and antiarrhythmic effects of imipramine hydrochloride at therapeutic plasma concentrations. *Circulation* 60:5,1045–52, 1979.

22. Weld FM and Bigger JT, Jr. Electrophysiological effects of imipramine on ovine cardiac Purkinje and ventricular muscle fibers. *Circ. Res.* 46:167–75, 1980.

23. Rawling D and Fozzard HA. Electrophysiological effects of imipramine on cardiac Purkinje fibers. *Am. J. Cardiol.* 41:387, 1978.

24. Kupfer DJ et al. Amitriptyline plasma levels and clinical response in primary depression: II. *Commun. Psychopharmacol.* 2:441–50, 1978.

25. Robinson DS et al. Plasma tricyclic drug levels in amitriptyline-treated depressed patients. *Psychopharmacology* 63 (3):223–31, 1979.

26. Montgomery SA et al. Amitriptyline plasma concentration and clinical response. *Br. Med. J.* 1:230–31, 1979.

27. Ziegler VE, Co BT, and Biggs JT. Electrocardiographic findings in patients undergoing amitriptyline treatment. *Dis. Nerv. Syst.* 38 (9):697–99, 1977.

28. Peet M, Tienari P, and Jaskari MO. A comparison of the cardiac effects of mianserin and amitriptyline in man. *Pharmakopsychiatr. Neuropsychopharmakol.* 10:309–12, 1977.

29. Burgess CD, Turner P, and Wadsworth J. Cardiovascular responses to mianserin hydrochloride: A comparison with tricyclic antidepressant drugs. *Br. J. Clin. Pharmacol.* 5 (suppl. 1):21s–28s, 1978.

30. Petit JM et al. Tricyclic antidepressant plasma levels and adverse effects after overdose. *Clin. Pharmacol. Therap.* 21:47–51, 1977.

31. Bigger JT, Jr. and Reiffel JA. Sick sinus syndrome. *Ann. Rev. Med.* 30:91–118, 1979.

32. Short DS. The syndrome of alternating bradycardia and tachycardia. *Br. Heart. J.* 16:208–14, 1954.

33. Roose SP. et al. Cardiac sinus node dysfunction during lithium treatment. *Am. J. Psychiatry* 136:6, 804–06, 1979.

34. Wellens HJ, Cats VM, and Duren DR. Symptomatic sinus node abnormalities following lithium carbonate therapy. *Am. J. Med.* 59:285–87, 1975.

35. Bigger JT, Jr. et al. Cardiac antiarrhythmic effect of imipramine hydrochloride. *N. Eng. J. Med.* 296:206–08, 1977.

36. Giardina EGV, Bigger JT, Jr., and Johnson LL. The effect of imipramine and nortriptyline on ventricular premature depolarizations and left ventricular function. *Circulation* 64 (IV):316, 1981.

37. Hoffman BF, Bigger JT, Jr. "Antiarrhythmic drugs." In *Drill's Pharmacology of Medicine*, edited by DiPalma JR. New York: Raven Press, 1978. pp. 1033–46.

38. Kantor SJ et al. Imipramine-induced heart block: A longitudinal case study. *JAMA* 231:1364–66, 1975.

39. Wilkerson, RD. Antiarrhythmic effects of tricyclic antidepressant drugs in ouabain-induced arrhythmias in the dog. *J. Pharmacol. Exp. Ther.* 205:666–74, 1978.

40. Raeder EA, Zinsli M, and Burckhardt D. Effect of maprotiline on cardiac arrhythmias. *Br. Med. J.* 2:102, 1979.

41. Taylor DJ and Braithwaite RA. Cardiac effects of tricyclic antidepressant medication: A preliminary study of nortriptyline. *Br. Heart. J.* 40:1005–09, 1978.

42. Muller V and Burckhardt D. Die Wirkung tri- und tetrazyklischer Antidepressiva auf Herz und Kreislauf. *Schweiz. Med. Wschr.* 104:1911–13, 1974.

43. Burckhardt D et al. Cardiovascular effects of tricyclic and tetracyclic antidepressants. *JAMA* 239:3:213–16, 1978.

44. Giardina EGV et al. A comparison of desmethylimipramine and imipramine on electrocardiogram and left ventricular function. (Submitted for publication.)

45. Thorstrand C. Cardiovascular effects of poisoning with tricyclic antidepressants. *Acta. Med. Scand.* 195:505–14, 1974.

46. Langou RA et al. Cardiovascular manifestations of tricyclic antidepressant overdose. *American Heart J.* 100:458–64, 1980.

47. Glassman AH et al. Factors related to orthostatic hypotension associated with tricyclic antidepressants. *J. Clin. Psychiatry* 43:35–38, 1982.

48. Muller OF, Goodman N and Bellet S. The hypotensive effect of imipramine hydrochloride in patients with cardiovascular disease. *Clin. Pharmacol. Ther.* 2:300–07, 1961.

49. Glassman AH et al. Clinical characteristics of imipramine-induced orthostatic hypotension. *Lancet* 1:468–72, 1979.

50. Hayes JR, Born GF, and Rosenbaum AH. Incidence of orthostatic hypotension in patients with primary affective disorders treated with tricyclic antidepressants. *Mayo Clin Proc* 52:509–12, 1977.

51. Kopera H. Anticholinergic and blood pressure effects of mianserin, amitriptyline and placebo. *Br. J. Clin. Pharmacol.* 5, Suppl. 1:29s–34s, 1978.

52. Roose SP et al. Tricyclic-induced postural hypotension: Comparative studies. New Research. Presented at APA, San Francisco, May 1980.

53. Reed K et al. Cardiovascular effects of nortriptyline in geriatric patients. *Am. J. Psychiatry* 137:986–89, 1980.

54. Roose SP et al. Comparison of imipramine- and nortriptyline-induced orthostatic hypotension: A meaningful difference. *Psychopharmacol.* 1:316–19, 1981.

55. U'Prichard DC et al. Tricyclic antidepressants: therapeutic properties and affinity for alpha-noradrenergic receptor binding sites in the brain. *Science* 199:197–98, 1978.

56. des Lauriers A et al. Effet favorable de la Yohimbine sur l'hypotension orthostatique induite par la clomipramine. (unpublished.)

57. Talman WT, Perrone MH, and Reis DJ. Evidence for L-glutamate as the neurotransmitter of baroreceptor afferent nerve fibers. *Science* 209:813–14, 1980.

58. Moccetti T et al. Kardiotoxizitat der trizyklischen Antidepressiva. *Schweiz. Med. Wschr.* 101:1, 1971.

59. Briley MS et al. Tritiated imipramine binding sites are decreased in platelets of untreated depressed patients. *Science* 209:303–05, 1980.

21

Monoamine Neuronal Firing as a Tool to Predict Antidepressant Activity in Animals

Albert Dresse, M.D. and J. Scuvee-Moreau, Ph.D.

Introduction

Because it is difficult to assess a selective effect of antidepressants in the usual pharmacological tests, we decided some years ago to study the central action of these drugs by means of electrophysiological techniques. This approach had the advantage of allowing a fairly critical investigation of the action of antidepressants on the functional activity of central neurons containing a given neurotransmitter. Noradrenaline (NA) and/or 5-hydroxytryptamine (5HT) have been implicated in the mechanism of action of antidepressants both for clinical and experimental reasons.[1] Therefore, the effect of well-known or newly developed antidepressants on the spontaneous firing rate of rat brain noradrenergic and serotonergic neurons was recorded by means of extracellular microelectrodes. The experimental conditions have been described.[2,3]

Effect of Antidepressants on the Monoaminergic Neurons

The noradrenaline neuronal systems of the rat brain have been well documented by many authors since the first description by Dahlstrom and Fuxe.[4] To study the effect of antidepressants, one homogeneous group of

For generous gift of drugs we thank the companies Astra-Nobelpharma (zimelidine, alaproclate); Boehringer-Ingelheim (clonidine); Ciba-Geigy (desipramine, imipramine, clomipramine); Hoechst (nomifensine); Lilly (nortriptyline); Merck Sharp & Dohme (amitriptyline); Organon (mianserin); and Upjohn (alprazolam, 41-123).

noradrenaline cells, the A6 group or locus coeruleus, was chosen. The axons of these cells go to many cerebral structures, mainly the cerebral and cerebellar cortex.[5] In collaboration with Maeda, we have observed that in the newborn rat it is possible to follow these axons in the mesencephalon and the lateral hypothalamus.[6] It is important to notice that one locus coeruleus neuron may contact hundreds of cells in the cortex. This

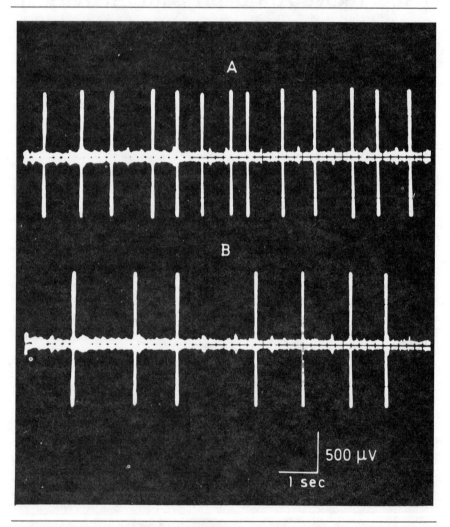

Figure 1 Electrical activity of a noradrenergic neuron of the locus coeruleus before (A) and after (B) an i.v. perfusion of desipramine
Note: Total dose: .3 mg/kg.

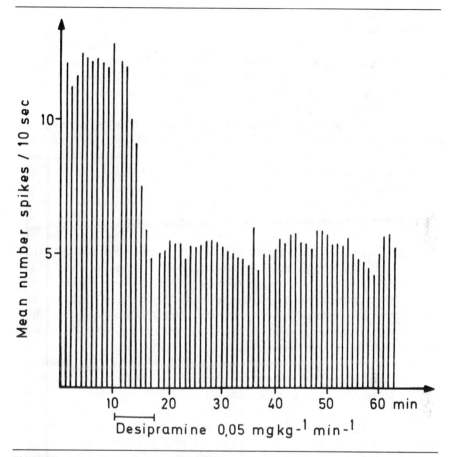

Figure 2 Progressive decrease of the frequency of discharge of a locus coeruleus neuron during the i.v. perfusion of desipramine
Note: The frequency of discharge in spikes/10 sec is expressed against time in minutes.

organization has important functional implications. By approaching one of these noradrenaline containing cells with a microelectrode, it is possible to record its spontaneous electrical activity, characterized by a frequency of discharge of .5 to 5 spikes/sec (Figure 1A).[7] The shape and amplitude of these spikes are reproducible. An antidepressant given parenterally to the animal decreased the spontaneous firing rate of the neuron. For example, by infusing desipramine at a dose as low as .05 mg/kg/min it is possible to obtain a progressive decrease in the firing rate of the NA cells. No modification in the amplitude nor in the shape of the spike is observed but only a reduction of the spontaneous rate of firing (Figures 1B and 2). It is possible to compute the total dose necessary to produce a 50% decrease of the spontaneous firing rate of these noradrenergic cells (ID_{50}). For desipramine, the ID_{50} is .3 mg/kg.

The spontaneous activity of the serotonergic neurons of the nucleus raphe dorsalis (B7 group) has been similarly recorded. Theses neurons are also characterized by a low frequency of discharge (.2 to 2 spikes/sec).[8] The i.v. perfusion of some antidepressants, for instance clomipramine (.05 mg/kg/min), decreases their spontaneous firing rate.

The rat brain contains dopaminergic cells forming the nigrostriatal, mesolimbic, mesocortical, and hypothalamo-hypophyseal systems.[9] We were interested in the mesolimbic system and have recorded the electrical activity of the dopamine (DA) containing cells of the A10 group. The spontaneous activity of these DA containing cells has another pattern from the NA and 5-HT neurons. The cells fire in bursts with spikes of progressively decreasing amplitude.[10] Besides dopamine, some of these cells also contain an intestinal peptide, cholecystokinin.[11] We have observed that some dopamine cells are activated by the intravenous administration of a neuroleptic, haloperidol, while other cells of the same area are not activated despite similar electrophysiological characteristics. Differences in reactivity are perhaps related to the presence or absence of a concomitant transmitter. We have not studied the effect of antidepressants on these dopaminergic cells except for nomifensine, which is known to have an inhibitory action on dopamine uptake.

Five classical tricyclic antidepressants, (TCAs) have been studied in this electrophysiological model: desipramine, imipramine, clomipramine, amitriptyline, and nortriptyline inhibitors of NA and/or 5HT uptake.[12,13] These TCAs are secondary or tertiary amines (Figure 3). The effect of new substances (Figure 4) has also been studied: mianserin, a weak inhibitor of amine uptake; nomifensine, a potent inhibitor of NA and DA uptake; and zimelidine, a potent inhibitor of 5HT uptake.[14-16] All of these drugs more or less potently decrease the firing rate of locus coeruleus or raphe dorsalis cells (Table 1). An infusion of .3 mg/kg of desipramine is sufficient to produce a 50% decrease of the firing rate of locus coeruleus cells ($N = 6$). A dose of up to 12 mg/kg of the same substance does not reduce the activity of the raphe dorsalis cells. Desipramine is thus a selective inhibitor of the activity of noradrenaline containing cells after an acute injection. The reverse is true for clomipramine, which is about 10 times more active on locus coeruleus and raphe dorsalis cells. Nortriptyline selectively acts on noradrenaline cells and amitriptyline is about equipotent on both types of cells. An examination of the results obtained with the other substances shows that nomifensine is a very potent inhibitor of the noradrenaline cells in this model. It is about 100 times more active on locus coeruleus than on raphe dorsalis cells. The reverse is true for zimelidine, which reduces the activity of raphe dorsalis cells (.9 mg/kg) without decreasing the activity of

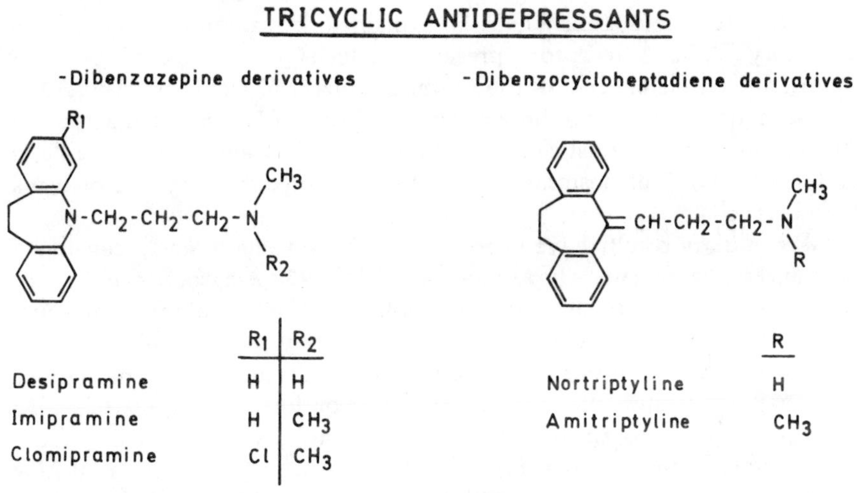
TRICYCLIC ANTIDEPRESSANTS
-Dibenzazepine derivatives
-Dibenzocycloheptadiene derivatives
R1
N-CH2-CH2-CH2-N
CH3
R2
CH-CH2-CH2-N
CH3
R
R1 R2
Desipramine H H
Imipramine H CH3
Clomipramine Cl CH3
R
Nortriptyline H
Amitriptyline CH3

Figure 3 Chemical structures of the tricyclic antidepressants tested

locus coeruleus cells. Note that zimelidine is the only antidepressant so far investigated that produces an increase of the spontaneous firing rate of the noradrenaline cells. Thus, this drug decreases the spontaneous firing of 5-HT cells and simultaneously increases the firing of noradrenaline cells.

Mianserin in this model does not modify the firing rate of the NA cells and is only a weak inhibitor of the spontaneous firing of 5HT cells. However, an effect of mianserin on the NA cells may be demonstrated indirectly by the use of clonidine, an alpha 2 agonist.[17] Perfusion of this

Table 1 Effect of the Antidepressant on NA and 5HT Containing Cells

	locus coeruleus DI_{50} (*mg/kg* ± *E.S.*)	*n*	*raphe dorsalis* DI_{50} (*mg/kg* ± *E.S.*)	*n*
Desipramine	.29 ± .02	6	> 12	5
Imipramine	1.30 ± .11	6	1.63 ± .33	6
Clomipramine	3.08 ± .3	6	.34 ± .02	6
Nortriptyline	.66 ± .06	6	9.16 ± 1.6	5
Amitriptyline	1.42 ± .24	6	1.78 ± 0.27	6
Nomifensine	.07 ± .004	7	> 8	6
Mianserin	> 15	5	9.03 ± 1.03	6
Zimelidine	> 13	5	.9 ± .11	9

Note: DI_{50}: mean total dose necessary to produce a 50% inhibition of the firing rate.
n = number of animals.

drug at a very low dose (2 mcg/kg) decreases the spontaneous firing rate of the locus coeruleus cells. This is explained by a stimulation of the inhibitory alpha 2 receptors present on locus coeruleus cell bodies.[18] Mianserin completely blocks the inhibitory effect of clonidine. Therefore, mianserin has no effect on the spontaneous firing of NA cells but acts as an alpha 2 antagonist against clonidine. In our model, mianserin is also able to inhibit the action of desipramine on the spontaneous firing rate of locus coeruleus cells.

Preliminary results have been obtained with some recently developed substances: alaproclate, alprazolam, and U41,123. Alaproclate is a very specific inhibitor of the 5HT neuronal uptake in the animal (Svär, personal communication). It is metabolized to a completely inactive substance. As little as .05 mg/kg/min of this drug produces a diminution of the activity of the raphe dorsalis cells without any effect on locus coeruleus (ID_{50} : .35 mg/kg). Contrary to zimelidine, alaproclate produces no increase of the spontaneous firing of the noradrenaline cells. Alprazolam is a new benzodiazepine which is reported to produce antidepressant activity in patients.[19] No effect is observed on the noradrenaline cells. On the contrary, alprazolam was surprisingly able to decrease the spontaneous firing of the 5HT neurons. The ID_{50} was about 3 mg/kg. Similar results have been obtained with another substance, U41,123, which is a derivative of alprazolam. With this substance an effect is also observed on the 5HT containing cells without any effect on the noradrenaline containing neurons. The ID_{50} is about 5 mg/kg.

Experiments have been performed after chronic administration of antidepressants, but they will not be described in detail here. Desipramine, nomifensine, clomipramine, and zimelidine have been injected daily intraperitoneally during 14 days. After repetitive administration, the

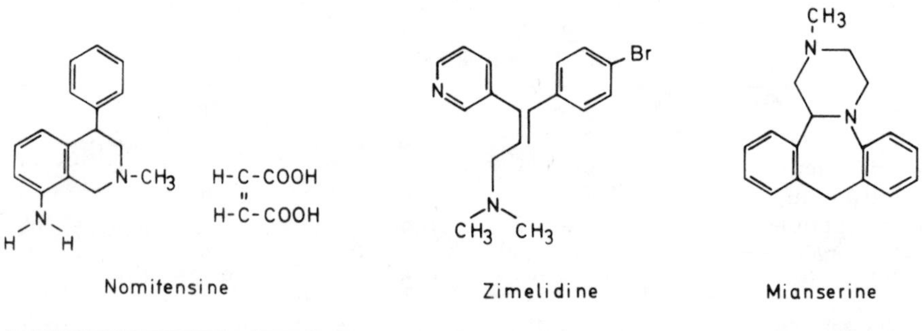

Figure 4 Chemical structures of the new antidepressant drugs: nomifensine, zimelidine and mianserin

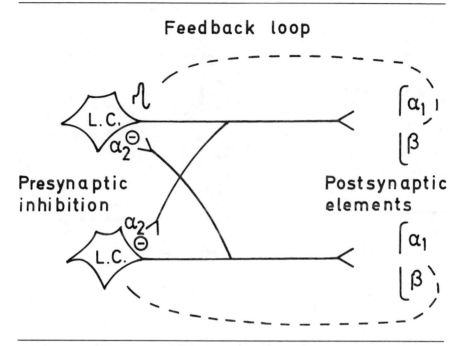

Figure 5 Schematic representation of two interlinked locus coeruleus neurons

results differ greatly from those obtained after acute experiments. For desipramine, after 14 days of repetitive administration of 5 mg/kg/day, an attenuation of the inhibitory effect on locus coeruleus cells is observed. That is partly caused by hyposensitivity of alpha 2 receptors (see Discussion section). The situation is not the same as concerns the serotonergic neurons. No modification of the inhibitory effect of clomipramine is observed after repetitive administration of clomipramine.[20]

Discussion

How is it possible to interpret all these data? A possible explanation is given in Figure 5. The transmitter synthesized in the perinuclear region or at the level of the terminal is released in the synaptic cleft to act on various types of receptors situated on the postsynaptic elements. To interpret the effect of antidepressants, the presence of somatodendritic and presynaptic receptors (the so-called alpha 2 receptors) must be considered.[18,21] These receptors are located both on the perikaryon and on the presynaptic terminals. The role of these alpha 2 receptors is not the same at these two locations. At the cellular body level, the alpha 2 receptor regulates the

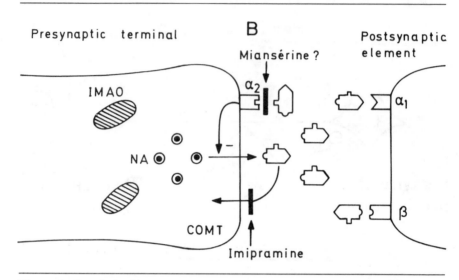

Figure 6 Detailed schematic representation of a noradrenergic synapse

firing rate of the cell; at the terminal level, the presynaptic alpha 2 receptor regulates the release of the transmitter. In spite of their pharmacological similarity, their physiological actions are different. It has also been demonstrated histochemically and electrophysiologically that the locus coeruleus cells are interlinked by axonal collaterals going from one cell to another.[22] The noradrenaline released from these collaterals reduces the firing rate by stimulation of the alpha 2 perikaryon receptors. An inhibition by antidepressants of the uptake mechanism at the terminal level increases the quantity of noradrenaline available at the alpha 2 perikaryon receptors. This may explain the observed inhibitory action of desipramine, nomifensine, or other drugs on the spontaneous firing of the locus coeruleus cells. The possible effect of a multineuronal feedback loop is also considered. The same regulatory mechanisms seem to appear at the level of the 5HT cells of the raphe dorsalis.

Another view of our interpretation is given in Figure 6, which represents a terminal with the presynaptic and postsynaptic sites. The noradrenaline molecules are released in the synaptic cleft. Desipramine and the other substances inhibit the uptake mechanism. Therefore, the presence of noradrenaline in the synaptic cleft is prolonged. In our experiments it seems that mianserin inhibits the effect of noradrenaline on the alpha 2 receptors. This confirms the observations of Bauman and Maitre.[14]

If it is possible to further establish that some depressive states are related to a deficiency in the noradrenaline or serotonin neurons, the experimental demonstration of selective antidepressant drugs may be useful for a more selective treatment of these patients.

Summary

Various antidepressants studied in this electrophysiological model have a specific action on the noradrenaline neurons. That is the case for desipramine, nortriptyline, and nomifensine. A small dose of nomifensine is sufficient to produce a diminution of the spontaneous firing rate of noradrenaline cells; a very high dose is necessary to obtain a diminution of the firing rate of the serotonergic cells. The reverse is true for substances like clomipramine, zimelidine, and alaproclate. They have a potent inhibitory action on 5HT containing cells and at best, a very weak effect on the noradrenaline containing cell. This selectivity of action of antidepressants on NA or 5HT containing cells may have important therapeutic consequences.

References

1. Carlsson A. The contribution of drug research to investigating the nature of endogenous depression. *Pharmakopsych* 9:2–10, 1976.

2. Scuvee-Moreau J and Dresse A. Effect of various antidepressants on the spontaneous firing rate of locus coeruleus and dorsal raphe neurons of the rat. *Europ. J. Pharmacol.* 57:219–25, 1979.

3. Dresse A and Scuvee-Moreau J. "Selective Action of the Tricyclic Antidepressants on the Spontaneous Firing of Noradrenergic or Serotonergic Cerebral Neurons." In *New Advances in the Diagnosis and Treatment of Depressive Illness*, series 531, pp. 112–116, edited by Mendlewicz J. Excerpta Medica, Intern. Congress, 1980.

4. Dahlstrom A and Fuxe K. Evidence for the existence of monoamine-containing neurons in the central nervous system. I. Demonstration of monoamines in the cell bodies of brain stem neurons. *Acta Physiol. Scand.* 62, suppl. 232:1–55, 1964.

5. Moore TY and Bloom FE. Central catecholamine neuron systems: anatomy and physiology of the norepinephrine and epinephrine systems. *Ann. Rev. Neurosci.* 2:113–68, 1979.

6. Maeda T and Dresse A. Possibilitiés d'étude trajet des fibres cérébrales monaminergiques chez le rat nouveau-né. *C.R. Soc. Biol.* 162:1626–29, 1968.

7. Graham RM and Aghajanian GK. Effects of amphetamine on single cell activity in a catecholamine nucleus, the locus coeruleus. *Nature* 234:100–2, 1971.

8. Aghajanian GK, Wang RY, and Baraban J. Serotonergic and non-serotonergic neurons of the dorsal raphe: reciprocal changes in firing induced by peripheral nerve stimulation. *Brain Res.* 163:169–75, 1978.

9. Moore RY and Bloom FE. Central catecholamine neuron system: Anatomy and physiology of the dopamine system. *Ann. Rev. Neurosci.* 1:129–69, 1978.

10. Bunney BS et al. Dopaminergic neurons: effect of antipsychotic drugs and amphetamine on single cell activity. *The J. Pharmacol. Exp. Ther.* 185:560–71, 1973.

11. Vanderhaeghen JJ et al. Immuno-histochemical localization of cholecysto-kinin and gastrine like peptide in the brain and hypophyse of the rat. *Proceedings of National Academy of Sciences,* U.S.A. 77:1190–94, 1980.

12. Quinaux N, Scuvee-Moreau J, and Dresse A. Inhibition of in vitro and in vivo uptake of noradrenaline and 5-hydroxytryptamine by five antidepressants; correlation with reduction of spontaneous firing rate of central monoaminergic neurones. *Naunyn-Schmiedeberg's Arch. of Pharmacol.* 319:66–70, 1982.

13. Ross SB and Renyi AL. Tricyclic antidepressant agents. I. Comparison of the inhibition of the uptake of ^{3}H-noradrenaline and ^{14}C-5-hydroxytryptamine in slices and crude synaptosome preparations of the midbrain-hypothalamus region of the rat brain. *Acta pharmacol. et toxicol.* 36:382–94, 1975.

14. Baumann PA and Maitre L. Blockade of presynaptic alpha 2 receptors and of amine uptake in the rat brain by the antidepressant mianserin. *Naunyn-Schmiedeberg's Arch. of Pharmacol.* 300:31–37, 1977.

15. Schacht U, Leven M, and Backer G. Studies on brain metabolism of biogenic amines. *Br. J. Clin. Pharmacol.* 4:77S–87S, 1977.

16. Ross SB and Renyi AL. Inhibition of neuronal uptake of 5-hydroxytryptamine and noradrenaline in rat brain by (Z)- and (E)-3-(4-bromophenyl)-N, N-dimethyl-3(3-pyridil)allylamines and their secondary analogues. *Neuropharmacol.* 16:57–63, 1977.

17. Starke K et al. Comparison of the effects of clonidine on pre- and post-synaptic adrenoreceptors in the rabbit pulmonary artery. *Naunyn-Schmiedeberg's Arch. of Pharmacol.* 285:133–50, 1974.

18. Cedarbaum JM and Aghajanian GK. Catecholamine receptors on locus coeruleus neurons: pharmacological characterization. *Europ J. Pharmacol.* 44:375–85, 1977.

19. Fabre LF and McLendon DMC. A double-blind study comparing the efficacy and safety of alprazolam with imipramine and placebo in primary depression. *Curr. Ther. Res.* 27(5)474–82, 1980.

20. Scuvee-Moreau J. Contribution expérimentale à l'étude du mode d'action des substances antidépressives. Thèse presentée pour l'obtention du grade de Docteur en Sciences Biomédicales Expérimentales, 1981.

21. Langer SZ. Presynaptic regulation of catecholamine release. *Biochem. Pharmacol.* 23:1793–1800, 1974.

22. Aghajanian GK and Cedarbaum JM. "Autoregulation of Central Noradrenergic Neurons." In *Catecholamine: basic and clinical frontiers.* 4th intern. catecholamine symposium. Asilomar, California, 1978.

22

Psychopharmacology and Suicidal Behavior

Stuart A. Montgomery, M.D. and Deirdre B. Montgomery

The number of hospital admissions following an incident of deliberate self-harm has risen steeply over the past 20 years and is still rising. Hospitals in England and Wales now provide care for some 2,000 cases of deliberate nonfatal self-poisoning every week. Proportionately, the increase has been highest in women; in younger women self-poisoning is the commonest cause of emergency admission to a medical ward.

The rate of "successfully" completed suicides probably has not changed very much. In the United Kingdom there was an apparent drop in the 70s that proved to be temporary. It is generally acknowledged that figures for suicide rates are hard to obtain and unreliable because they are open to reporting bias at several levels. Nevertheless, comparative suicide rates within the U.K. indicate that patients with a history of an attempt have a high rate of subsequent suicide. Estimates place the suicide rate in this group at 1–2% per annum, far in excess of the expected rate for the general population. Approximately 20% of patients will repeat their suicidal behaviour within a year.[1] Some patients are admitted several times in a year, and the size of the problem for medical care delivery systems is probably underestimated.

One means of preventing overdose often suggested is closer control of prescribing. There has been a substantial increase in the number of poisonings with psychotropic drugs since they became available, which has led to the belief that more discriminant prescribing could halt the rising number of self-poisonings. It is, however, unlikely to be a successful strategy since the fall in the misuse of one class of drugs—barbiturates—is balanced by a rise in poisonings by another, and probably only reflects a shift in prescribing habits. The proportion of poisonings by unprescribed drugs is reported to remain fairly constant at around 45%.

Despite the wealth of research, we still know very little about the causes of suicidal behaviour; it is difficult to envisage schemes for primary prevention. However, there is scope for primary prevention in the treatment of psychiatric illness associated with suicidal thoughts or acts. Retrospective analyses of presumed illness in successful suicides have estimated some 70% might have been suffering from depression at the time.[2] The methodology of such studies is not ideal because of the difficulty of avoiding bias inherent in all retrospective designs. Prospective surveys of hospital admissions following deliberate self-harm vary in their estimates of the degree of psychiatric illness presented. Gibbons et al. identified 25% of admissions as patients with psychiatric illness, operationally defined as in treatment or in need of treatment.[3] In Edinburgh, Kreitman found the largest category was personality disorders. Only 40% of admissions were diagnosed as suffering from a mental illness.[1]

It is well known that suicidal thoughts or acts are commonly found in depressive illness. A recent study of psychopathology in depressed patients in England and Sweden showed that suicidal *thoughts* were present in 91% of the English patients and 83% of the Swedish patients.[4] Suicidal *acts* were far less common and are not necessarily indicators of the severity of depression. The severity of the depression also does not appear to relate directly to the patient's readiness to put the thought into action and could not be used as a predictor of suicidal behavior. Several depression rating scales, including the Hamilton, give undue weight to a suicide act in according a severity rating to the depression.[5] The act is not necessarily an indicator of severity of depression, and in this respect, a depression rating scale such as the Montgomery and Asberg Depression Rating scale, which differentiates between thoughts and acts, is likely to give more valid ratings.[4]

While the exact relationship between suicide acts and depression is not clear, the treatment of suicidal thoughts is the treatment of the depression itself. Suicidal thoughts subside with the amelioration of the depression. In a recent study comparing two antidepressants,[6] the suicidal thoughts item of the Montgomery and Asberg Depression Rating Scale changed in the same direction as the response of the depressive illness, significantly correlating with overall change at $r = .87$.[6]

It is ironic that, in the treatment of depression, the clinician may give a group of patients known to be associated with suicidal risk the means to achieve this intent. The most common drugs associated with death in overdosage are the tricyclic antidepressants (TCAs), which are also the most commonly used in the treatment of depression. Common usage, however, only partly explains the phenomenon; it cannot obscure the relative lack of safety of the TCAs. Amitriptyline, for example, causes cardiotoxicity even in therapeutic doses and its cardiotoxicity in overdosage is well documented.

The risk attached to some of the antidepressant drugs has to be balanced against the risk attached to the depressive illness itself. The hazards associated with antidepressant treatment can be reduced by careful patient selection and careful drug selection. Clearly, where patients cannot be supervised and overdose is considered a risk, as for example in patients with a history of self-harm, a safer drug than the TCAs is preferred.

Levels of 5-hydroxyindoleacetic acid (5HIAA) have been shown to be lower in the brains of completed suicides, and studies in depressed patients have shown that there is an association between low levels of 5HIAA in the cerebrospinal fluid (CSF) and increased suicidal acts.[7,8] Clinical intervention studies in suicidal behavior are rather rare and it is of interest in this regard that zimelidine has been reported to have more effect in reducing suicidal thoughts than amitriptyline in the early stages of treatment.[6] Zimelidine is a 5HT uptake inhibitor which would be expected to raise the level of 5HIAA in the CSF.

Asberg et al. have proposed a bimodal distribution of 5HIAA suggesting the presence of a biological subgroup of serotonin depression.[9] The bimodality is questioned, but the association of lower levels of 5HIAA in the CSF and suicidal acts also has been reported by Asberg et al. and has been replicated by the same group.[10]

Our findings from a study of 49 depressed patients (carried out in an independent center) of a relationship between pretreatment levels of 5HIAA in CSF and a history of suicidal acts are in accord with the findings of Asberg et al., but at a lower level of significance (Fisher's exact test: $p = .053$). There was, however, a stronger relationship between pretreatment levels of homovanillic acid (HVA), the metabolite of dopamine, and suicidal acts (Fisher's exact test: $p < .01$).[11] A correlation between levels of 5HIAA and HVA has previously been noted, but the significance of the contribution of dopamine does not appear to have been taken sufficiently into account.[9,12] From the current findings it appears that the role of dopamine metabolism should be further investigated.

Treatment of suicidal thoughts in the absence of depression is an entirely different matter. Where systematic diagnoses have been applied to the group of patients with a history of self-harm, it becomes apparent that the largest category is that of personality disorders. Suicidal acts in this group of patients tend to be impulsive. They may sometimes but not invariably be associated with transient mood changes; this frequently brief lowering of spirits would not fulfill criteria for depressive illness. By and large this group of patients has not been regarded as suitable for antidepressant treatment.

Table 1 Intervention Studies in Suicidal Behaviour

Treatment		Design of Study	Study Period	Outcome
Psychiatric				
Greer & Bagley 1971	Retrospective	Follow-up comparing with Non-attenders (Inadequate control)	1–2 Years	Beneficial
Chowdhury, Hicks Krietman 1973	Prospective	Randomized standard or intensive follow-up	6 Months	No difference
Montgomery et al. 1979	Prospective	Placebo vs neuroleptic Double-blind	6 Months	Beneficial
Hawton 1980	Prospective	Domiciliary follow-up or standard O.P. department	1 Year	No difference
Montgomery et al. 1982	Prospective	Placebo vs anti-depressant Double-blind	6 Months	No difference
Psychotherapy				
Ettlinger 1979	Retrospective	Previous year (Inadequate Control)	1 Year	No difference
Liberman & Ekman 1981	Prospective	Behaviour therapy or insight orientated therapy	10 Days + 2 Year Follow-up	No difference
Social Work				
Oast & Zitrin 1975	Prospective	Social Worker Follow-up Non-attenders (Inadequate Control)	—	No difference
Gibbons et al. 1978	Prospective	Randomized standard care or intensive follow-up	1 Year	No difference

Health care workers find working with patients with personality disorders unrewarding; the patients tend to be hostile and uncooperative. They are difficult to follow up and their prognosis is generally poor; it is not surprising that there have been few controlled follow-up or intervention studies. Social work intervention, intensive outpatient supervision, and supportive psychotherapy have all been reported unsuccessful in reducing subsequent suicidal behavior.[12–18] Greer and Bagley reported that there was lower morbidity in the group who attended psychiatric follow up than those who did not;[15] but the finding is weakened by the influence of patient self-selection (Table 1).

Pharmacotherapy in patients with personality disorders is only now beginning to be investigated. Two placebo controlled long-term follow-up studies on the effects of drug therapy in reducing suicidal behavior have been reported.[19,20] In these studies, a more morbid group was selected than in earlier intervention trials; only patients with a history of multiple suicidal attempts prior to the index attempt were studied. Following the DSM III criteria the patients were diagnosed as having personality disorders, mainly borderline or histrionic, and not suffering from overt depression or schizophrenia. In the 58 patients treated with mianserin or placebo, there was no significant reduction in the number of suicidal acts during the 6-month treatment period with mianserin compared with placebo. However, in the flupenthixol–placebo study there was a significant reduction in the number of suicidal acts with flupenthixol at 4, 5, and 6 months (Table 2).

The apparent difference in effect of the two active compounds is interesting and there may be several explanations. Compliance is often a problem in personality disorders, and route of administration possibly gave flupenthixol an advantage over mianserin. The flupenthixol–placebo study protocol stipulated depot medication, whereas the mianserin study utilized oral dosing.

Nevertheless, it is interesting to speculate on the mechanism of action of flupenthixol in reducing suicidal acts. Although antidepressant properties have occasionally been claimed for flupenthixol, it is unlikely to be the reason for achieving its effect in this group of patients who were screened to exclude depressive or other psychiatric illness. This and the failure of the antidepressant in the parallel study suggest that something other than an antidepressant effect was operating. Similarly, any anxiolytic effect of flupenthixol is unlikely to be a sufficient explanation for the results.

The most important pharmacological action reported for flupenthixol is its effect on dopamine synthesis. Possibly, the effect on reducing suicidal behavior in personality disorders is mediated via the dopamine system. In this context it is perhaps apposite to note our finding of lower CSF HVA levels in depressed patients with a history of suicidal acts. Although care

Table 2 Outcome of 6 Months Prophylaxis with Flupenthixol Decanoate 20 mgs or Placebo Monthly Excluding 4 Dropouts on Active and 3 on Placebo Treatment

	Weeks in Study					
	4	*8*	*12*	*16*	*20*	*24*
Flupenthixol (n =14)						
Responders	13	12	11	11	11	11
Failures	1	2	3	3	3	3
Placebo (n =16)						
Responders	12	8	7	5	5	4
Failures	4	8	9	11	11	12
Fisher's exact probability	1.71	4,29	3.77	6.72[a]	6.72[a]	8.57[a]

[a] $p < .01$.

must be taken not to link the studies in personality disorders and the studies in depression, which have used quite different methodologies, the findings, taken together, strongly suggest that suicidal thoughts or acts may be mediated by the same system in personality disorders as well as in depression.

References

1. Kreitman N. In *Parasuicide* edited by Kreitman, p. 29. London: John Wiley & Sons, 1977.

2. Holding TA and Barraclough BM. Psychiatric morbidity in a sample of London coroner's open verdicts. *British Journal of Psychiatry* 127:133, 1975.

3. Gibbons JS et al. Evaluation of a social work service for self-poisoning patients. *British Journal of Psychiatry* 133:111, 1978.

4. Montgomery S and Asberg M. A new depression scale designed to be sensitive to change. *British Journal of Psychiatry* 134:382, 1979.

5. Hamilton M. Development of a rating scale for primary depressive illness. *British Journal of Social and Clinical Psychology* 6:278, 1967.

6. Montgomery SA et al. A double-blind comparison of zimelidine and amitriptyline in endogenous depression. *Acta Psychiatrica Scandinavica* Supplement 290, 63:314, 1981.

7. Shaw DDM, Camps FE, and Eccleston EG. 5 Hydroxytryptamine in the hindbrain of depressive suicide. *British Journal of Psychiatry* 113:1407, 1967.

8. Asberg M, Traskman L, and Thoren P. 5-HIAA in the cerebrospinal fluid—a biochemical suicide predictor? *Archives of General Psychiatry* 33:1193–97, 1976.

9. Asberg M et al. "Serotonin depression" a biochemical subgroup with the affective disorders. *Science* 191:478, 1976.

10. Traskman L et al. Monoamine metabolites in cerebrospinal fluid and suicidal behaviour. *Archives of General Psychiatry* 6:631, 1981.

11. Montgomery SA and Montgomery DB. Pharmacological prevention of suicidal behaviour. *Journal of Affective Disorders* 4:291–98, 1982.

12. Van Praag HM and Korf J. Retarded depression and the dopamine metabolism. *Psychopharmacologia* 19:199, 1971.

13. Oast S and Zitrin A. A public health approach to suicide prevention. *American Journal of Public Health* 65:144, 1975.

14. Gibbons JS et al. Evaluation of a social work service for self-poisoning patients. *British Journal of Psychiatry* 133:111–18, 1978.

15. Greer and Bagley C. Effect of psychiatric intervention in attempted suicide: A controlled study. *British Medical Journal* 1:310, 1971.

16. Hawton K. "Domiciliary and Out-patient Treatment Following Deliberate Self-poisoning." In *The Suicide Syndrome,* edited by Farmer R and Hirsch S. London: Croom Helm, 1979. pp. 244–58.

17. Ettlinger R. "A Follow-up Investigation of Patients after Attempted Suicide." In *The Suicide Syndrome*, edited by Farmer R and Hirsch S. London: Croom Helm, 1980. p. 167.

18. Liberman R and Eckman T. Behaviour therapy vs insight-oriented therapy for repeated suicide attempters. *Archives of General Psychiatry* 38:1126–30, 1981.

19. Montgomery SA et al. Maintenance therapy in repeat suicidal behaviour: A placebo controlled trial. Proceedings X International Congress for Suicide Prevention, Ottawa, pp. 227–29, 1979.

20. Montgomery D, Roy D, and Montgomery S. Mianserin in the prophylaxis of suicidal behaviour—a double blind placebo controlled trial. Proceedings XI International Congress of Suicide Prevention, Paris, 1981.

23

Some Clinical Evidence Supporting the Possible Involvement of Neurotransmitter Receptor Sensitivity Changes in the Action of Antidepressant Drugs During Longer-Term Treatment

Dennis L. Murphy, M.D. Larry J. Siever, M.D., Robert M. Cohen M.D., Benjamin F. Roy M.D., and David Pickar, M.D.

Among psychoactive agents, antidepressant drugs differ from stimulants such as amphetamine or sedatives such as barbiturates in the several-week delay in onset of their therapeutic actions. Only minimal clinical changes of any type, except slight sedation, occur during the first 5–10 days of full dose administration, and antidepressant effects may not become evident until 15–25 days after the initiation of treatment. This time lag is a characteristic of antidepressant drugs of widely divergent chemical structure and of apparently different cellular sites of initial biochemical effects, including the tricyclic and related compounds, the monoamine oxidase (MAO) inhibitors, and lithium.

Proposed explanations for this lag time between the initiation of drug treatment and clinical antidepressant response have been many. They range from the time-dependent requirements for the synthesis of new neurotransmitter-related enzymes or other proteins to psychological reequilibration or relearning processes. Recently, interpretations based upon adaptional changes in neurotransmitter receptor responsivity following longer term drug administration have been widely discussed.[1-5] Receptor-based alterations are an especially interesting possibility because prominent receptor changes during antidepressant drug administration have been found in the neurotransmitter systems most clearly implicated in the affective disorders—the noradrenergic and serotonergic systems—and a clear time dependency upon long term rather than acute antidepressant drug administration has been repeatedly demonstrated. In addition, time-dependent changes in brain noradrenergic receptor numbers have been found to accompany the administration to rodents of the whole spectrum of antidepressant treatments, including the uptake inhibiting and non-uptake inhibiting tricyclics, the MAO inhibitors, and even repeated electroshock administration.[1-5]

There has been little systematic exploration of time-dependent changes accompanying antidepressant drug treatment in man, other than, of course, the behavioral rating of therapeutic effects and side effects during clinical trials with these agents. In particular, only a handful of studies evaluating the possible involvement of alterations in neurotransmitter receptor function in antidepressant drug responses in man have been reported. In this chapter we will review some data from recent studies from our group investigating biological changes during the course of longer term treatment with several MAO-inhibiting antidepressant agents of the 2-propynlamine type. We will then attempt to interpret this generally indirect data in terms of recent studies of the time-dependent effects of these drugs and other antidepressant agents on neurotransmitter-related events, especially on amine receptors and other processes possibly relevant to the mode of action of these drugs.

Strategies and Results

Clinical Antidepressant Effects of Clorgyline and Other 2-Propynlamine MAO Inhibitors

Clorgyline is an MAO inhibitor that has been found to have antidepressant effects according to the results of three random assignment, double-blind studies in England and the United States.[6-8] Clorgyline is of special investigational interest because it is a highly selective inhibitor of MAO type A, which is principally responsible for the oxidative deamination of serotonin and norepinephrine, while it has lesser effects on dopamine, phenylethylamine, and other substrates deaminated to a greater extent in man by MAO type B.[9] Two structurally related compounds, deprenyl and pargyline, are partially selective inhibitors of the MAO-B enzyme.[9]

Most of the data summarized below was obtained from studies investigating the effects of clorgyline, 20–40 mg/day, given under double-blind conditions to patients with primary depression as defined by Research Diagnostic Criteria (RDC).[8,10] The patients received placebo capsules prior to and following the 4-week trials with clorgyline. Clorgyline was generally given initially in divided doses totaling 30 mg/day; dosage was changed upon the development of side effects, chiefly orthostatic hypotension. A smaller number of patients received pargyline in two studies using either 30 mg/day or 90 mg/day, or deprenyl in doses of 10 mg/day.

As previously stated, clorgyline administration in patients studied on our clinical research unit led to significant antidepressant effects as measured on both observer-rated and self-rated scales.[8,10] Pargyline administration, in contrast, was associated with significantly smaller antidepressant effects in fewer patients. Although clinical depression ratings had decreased to some extent in the second and third week of clorgyline administration, the changes did not become statistically significant or reach their maximum differences until the fourth week of treatment (Figure 1).

A nearly equal lag period was also observed for another behavioral effect of clorgyline and pargyline—the occasional precipitation of excess behavioral activation in the form of hypomanic or manic episodes.[11] All of the patients who developed this side effect in this study, as well as those in a previous study on the same research unit with another MAO inhibitor (phenelzine), did so after a minimum of 22 days of drug administration.[12] The only exception to this time lag occurred in a few patients who had received a different MAO inhibitor less than 3 weeks before beginning the second trial, during which the hypomanic or manic episode occurred. The possibility that pretreatment may have sensitized these individuals is discussed elsewhere.[11]

Cardiovascular Changes During Longer Term MAO Inhibitor Administration

A time lag in the onset of other clinical phenomena besides the mood changes was also observed with these MAO inhibitors. Clorgyline treatment in these patients led to reductions in systolic, diastolic, and mean arterial blood pressure (Table 1)[13,14] (Roy B et al., in preparation). Lesser changes occurred during pargyline and deprenyl administration. Greater changes were observed in blood pressures measured when standing than when sitting. This orthostatic hypotension, which was clinically symptomatic in approximately one-fourth of the patients, developed gradually during the 4-week period of clorgyline administration, with the greatest difference between sitting and standing pressures becoming evident in the final week of drug treatment and in the subsequent week following clorgyline discontinuation (Figure 2) (Roy B et al., in preparation).

The time course of blood pressure change tended to parallel the time course of onset of clinical antidepressant effects, as illustrated in the case example of a typical patient presented in Figure 3. Depression symptoms began to reappear and blood pressure returned toward pretreatment levels after a 7–10 day lag time following cessation of treatment. This patient had

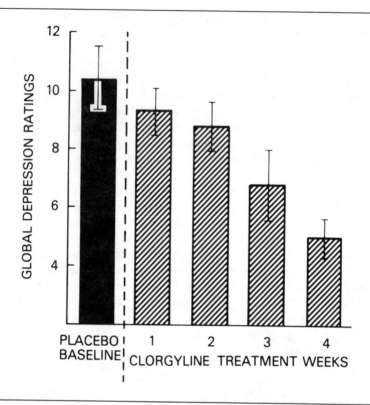

Figure 1 Time course of the development of clinical changes in patients responding to clorgyline, 20–40 mg/day

moderate hypertension prior to treatment and is illustrative of another finding noted in our initial report; namely, that patients with mild to moderate hypertension were among those patients with the most marked antidepressant responses to the MAO inhibitors.[8]

Some further evidence for an assocation between the blood pressure reductions and clinical antidepressant effects was found in the significant positive correlation ($r = + .58$, $p < .05$) between the reduction in Hamilton depression scale ratings and the reduction in standing blood pressure in the final week of clorgyline administration.[14] Correlation coefficients of similar magnitude between blood pressure changes and therapeutic effects have been found for several of the self-rated scales used in this study, including the Beck Depression Scale and the Profile of Mood States (POMS) depression factors.[14]

Sleep Changes During Longer Term MAO Inhibitor Administration

The most marked effect of most MAO inhibitors on EEG-monitored sleep patterns is a near total suppression of rapid eye movement (REM) sleep. This change has been noted previously with non-selective MAO inhibitors such as phenelzine,[15] but not with the MAO-B selective inhibitor, deprenyl, which produced only a 15% reduction in REM sleep.[16] In a recent study from our group, both clorgyline and high doses (90 mg/day) of pargyline produced essentially complete (97–100%) REM sleep suppression.[15] As indicated in Figure 4, this effect typically took from 7 to 10 days after the initiation of clorgyline administration to become complete. Similarly, there was a 7- to 10-day lag period after stopping clorgyline before REM sleep returned to pretreatment levels. Note that although the time course for this change in REM sleep is clearly delayed beyond the 4–24 hour period needed for MAO inhibition to become essentially (> 90%) complete,[13,16] the REM sleep alteration occurs earlier than both the mood and cardiovascular alterations. This raises the question of a sequence of changes involving possibly different mechanisms being required for these different drug effects.

Changes in the Pressor Response to Clonidine During Longer Term Antidepressant Drug Administration

A more direct examination of the question of possible processes involved in the different time-dependent effects of clorgyline has recently been conducted by L. Siever and coworkers using a pharmacologic challenge approach to assess the status of the noradrenergic neurotransmit-

Table 1 Mean Standing Arterial Pressure Changes Following Four Weeks' Treatment with MAO-Inhibitors

	Mean Arterial Blood Pressures (torr)
Clorgyline, 30 mg/day (N = 17)	− 14.0 ± 1.1[a]
Pargyline, 90 mg/day (N = 9)	− 14.6 ± 1.7[a]
Pargyline, 30 mg/day (N = 4)	− 6.3 ± 2.0
Deprenyl, 10 mg/day (N = 3)	+ 6.5 ± 1.3

[a] $p < .01$, paired t-test

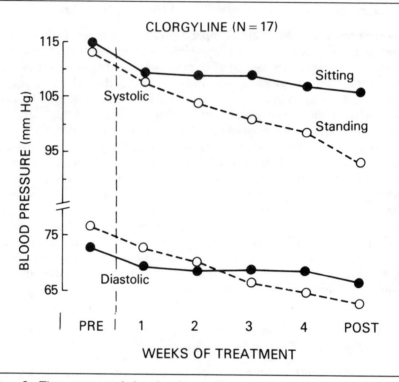

Figure 2 Time course of the development of blood pressure reductions in patients receiving clorgyline, 20–40 mg/day
Note: In particular, note the progressive increase in orthostatic hypotension as indicated by the gradual decreases in systolic pressure measured after standing.

ter system in man.[17-19] This particular study utilized clonidine, a centrally acting adrenergic agent which in low doses produces a hypotensive response. This blood pressure lowering effect appears to be due to clonidine's action as an α_2-adrenergic agonist because this hypotensive response can be induced in animals by local application of clonidine to the locus coeruleus, where α_2-adrenergic autoreceptors mediate an inhibitory feedback on noradrenergic activity.[20,21]

Depressed patients examined prior to clorgyline administration manifested a reduction in mean arterial pressure following a single clonidine dose. The maximum reduction was attained approximately 1 hour after administration. When clonidine administration was repeated after 4 weeks' treatment with clorgyline, nearly complete attenuation of the clonidine hypotensive response occurred:[17,18] However, after clorgyline administration for only 3 days, a hypotensive response equal to that found in the control, pre-clorgyline period was observed. A case example of this response is illustrated in Figure 5. As also noted in this figure, treatment with the tricyclic antidepressant, imipramine, for 4 weeks also led to a blockade of the clonidine-induced hypotensive response. Overall, a consistent, highly statistically significant attenuation of the clonidine response has been found during longer term, but not short-term, clorgyline administration to 9 patients with an intermediate level of blockade observed after 10 days of treatment.[18]

Two briefly reported investigations of patients treated with desmethylimipramine chronically also found diminished hypotensive responses to clonidine.[22,23] However, no evaluation was made of whether this change might also be observable after acute administration of desmethylimipramine. This presents a problem in assessment because the decreased hypotensive response to clonidine after tricyclic drug administration in animals has been interpreted as representing a direct blockade of α-adrenergic receptors.[24,25] The results from the clorgyline study in depressed patients, however, provide evidence that the antagonism of the clonidine

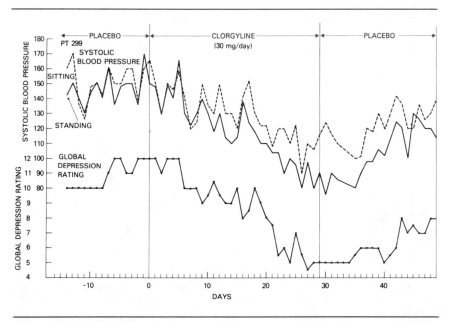

Figure 3 Correspondence between the time course of blood pressure reductions and clinical antidepressant changes in a 45-year-old woman treated with clorgyline in average doses of 30 mg/day

response may well represent a subsensitization of brain α_2-adrenergic receptors resulting from chronic but not acute MAO inhibition.[17,18]

Possible Delayed Onset of Changes in the Pressor Response to Tyramine and in Plasma Norepinephrine Reductions During Chronic MAO Inhibitor Administration

Preliminary data suggest that another effect of clorgyline administration, the potentiation of the pressor response to intravenously administered tyramine, may possess a time lag in reaching its maximum change. Clorgyline administration for 4 weeks leads to an average 30-fold increase in sensitivity to tyramine as reflected in the reduced dose of intravenously administered tyramine required to raise systolic blood pressure 30 mmHg after chronic clorgyline treatment.[26,27] In contrast, patients studied after acute (1-day) clorgyline administration showed only a 2-fold tyramine potentiation response.[26] Case examples (Table 2) from studies in progress indicate that after 1 week of clorgyline treatment, the tyramine pressor response attained approximately 50% of the maximum change observed subsequently in this patient after 4 weeks of clorgyline treatment at a daily dose of 30 mg/day.[28]

Similarly, clorgyline treatment for 1 week did not yield as great a reduction in plasma norepinephrine concentration (another effect of chronic clorgyline administration[26,27]), as that found after 4 weeks of

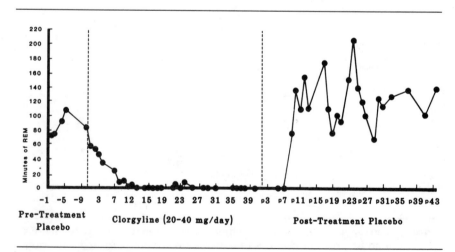

Figure 4 Time course of rapid eye movement (REM) sleep reductions during clorgyline administration

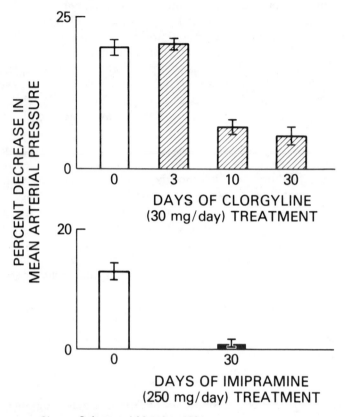

ALTERED BLOOD PRESSURE RESPONSE TO CLONIDINE FOLLOWING CHRONIC ANTIDEPRESSANT TREATMENT

Siever, Cohen and Murphy, 1981

Figure 5 Differential hypotensive responses to clonidine (4μm/kg) during short-term and longer term treatment with clorgyline, 30 mg/day, and during imipramine administration, 250 mg/day
Source: Siever, Cohen, and Murphy, 1981.

treatment, while clorgyline treatment for 1–4 days led to fairly rapid reductions in plasma and urinary MHPG concentrations.[27,28]

Discussion and Conclusions

Attempts to interpret the possible biochemical mechanisms involved in clinical effects of antidepressant drugs have grown exceedingly complex.

Traditional explanations have been based upon a potentiation of the effects of norepinephrine and/or serotonin by inhibition of neurotransmitter uptake in the case of the tricyclics, or by impairment in amine degradation in the case of the MAO inhibitors. Most recent theorizing, however, has focused on the effects of these agents that develop only after chronic administration and that, in many instances, appear to reflect adaptive changes in some aspects of noradrenergic function. These effects include apparent reductions in brain postsynaptic noradrenergic receptors measured both directly by receptor ligand binding approaches and functionally by assessment of their sensitivity to the stimulation by norepinephrine of cyclic AMP production. Reductions in adrenergic β-receptors or β-receptor-mediated cyclic AMP formation, for example, have been identified as a common alteration produced by essentially all clinically effective treatments, including some drugs which possess neither amine uptake-inhibiting nor MAO inhibiting potency as well as some which result from nonpharmacological manipulations, as in the case of electroshock (Table 3).[1,3,30,31] Data from other approaches also suggest that chronic antidepressant drug administration leads to alterations in noradrenergic function as assessed via measurements of the synthesis and turnover of norepinephrine and as reflected in a decreased rate of firing in neurons in norepinephrine-containing cell bodies in the locus coeruleus.[32-34]

In the case of the MAO inhibitors, and specifically clorgyline (the focus of our clinical studies), R. M. Cohen and coworkers have carried out a series of studies specifically examining changes in brain noradrenergic receptors during acute, semiacute, and chronic drug administration.[31,36]

Table 2 Changes in Blood Pressure Responses to Tyramine Following Short-Term and Longer Term Clorgyline Administration, and Following Clorgyline Discontinuation

Clorgyline Treatment Time Interval	Patient	Tyramine Pressor Sensitivity (Fold-Increases Over Baseline)
1 day	A	1.3
	B	2.8
1 week	C	19.2
4 weeks	A	34.7
	B	29.3
	C	38.0
	D	37.1
1 week postdrug	D	5.0
2 weeks postdrug	D	4.0

Table 3 Drug and Electroconvulsive Shock Effects on β-Adrenergic Receptors and/or Norepinephrine-Stimulated Cyclic AMP Accumulation in Rodent Brain Resulting from Chronic Treatment.[1,3,30,31]

Chronic Treatment	Dosage (mg/kg)	Duration (days)	Effect
Imipramine	20	5–20	Reduction
Amitriptyline	20	14	"
Desipramine	5–20	7–56	"
Clomipramine	20	7–14	"
Mianserin	30	14	"
Zimelidine	30	7–14	"
Iprindole	10	28–56	"
Nialamide	40	21	"
Pargyline	25	21	"
Clorgyline	1	21	"
Phenelzine	15	21	"
Electroconvulsive Shock	—	14	"

Significant reductions in numbers of β-adrenergic receptors assessed using ^{3}H-dihydroalprenolol as the binding ligand were found following 21 days of treatment with clorgyline and also with the non-selective MAO inhibitor phenelzine, but not with the MAO-B inhibitor pargyline (which, although structurally similar to clorgyline, acts only as a weak inhibitor of norepinephrine degradation and has only weak antidepressant effects). β-adrenergic receptor numbers were unaltered after 3 days of treatment with 1 mg/kg/day clorgyline, while after 10 days and 21 days, maximum reductions were observed. Decreased numbers of α_1-adrenergic receptors measured with ^{3}H-WB4101 were also observed following a minimum of 10 days' treatment. Reductions in α_2-adrenergic receptors estimated from ^{3}H-clonidine binding were 14% at 3 days, 35% at 10 days, and reached a maximum reduction of 62% at 21 days.[31]

Antidepressant drugs also affect other neurotransmitter receptors. In addition to the changes noted above in α1-, α2-, and β-adrenergic receptors, brain serotonin, dopamine, and histamine receptor numbers are also reduced during the administration of tricyclics as well as some other antidepressant drugs.[1-5] The available data are less complete regarding these other neurotransmitter receptor changes; but because growing evidence is indicative of interactions among these and other neurotransmitter systems, the attribution of a relationship between a change in one receptor group and a behavioral change in depressed patient groups has become extremely difficult to verify.

The sequence and primacy of these receptor changes has only begun to be evaluated both among the various neurotransmitter systems and for the presynaptic versus postsynaptic alterations within one system. It remains to be defined whether the reductions in adrenergic receptor numbers observed during antidepressant drug administration are associated with a reduction in noradrenergic function in compensation for the acute effects of the treatments. Such an interpretation would be in keeping with the revised hypotheses for depression invoking dysregulation of catecholamine functions and, in one version, postulating an overactive, inefficient state of catecholaminergic synaptic function in endogenously depressed patients.[2,3,5] Alternatively, the functional state of central noradrenergic system might be interpreted as simply being reequilibrated by the changes produced by antidepressant treatment, perhaps establishing a new steady state that somehow might be beneficial. A net increase in the functional state in one or another neurotransmitter systems might also be postulated, depending upon the balance created between presynaptic and postsynaptic receptor sensitivity changes and other aspects of neuronal function. Questions such as these are very difficult to approach because the location of receptors quantitated in the usual binding assays remains unknown. In the case of adrenergic receptor subtypes, for instance, most α_2-adrenergic receptors may not, in fact, be presynaptically located or function as autoreceptors (as they have sometime been termed), because evidence from chemical lesioning studies of presynaptic catecholamine neurons using 6-hydroxydopamine show a minimal loss of binding sites for α_2-adrenergic receptor ligands.[35]

These anatomical and functional complexities are not possible to approach conclusively by the indirect clinical studies described in this chapter. Indeed, many factors that might account for differences in acute *versus* chronic effects of antidepressant drugs in man have not yet been fully addressed. These factors range from simple pharmacokinetic bases for delays in drug effects, including time required to reach effective concentrations in brain caused by such factors as low or gradually increasing dosage patterns; drug metabolism effects; and drug transport capacities at tissue barriers; as well as more complicated cellular response characteristics. In the case of the material reviewed in this chapter, we have obtained information indicating that human mitochondrial MAO-B is $> 90\%$ inhibited in a peripheral tissue within 4 hours of oral administration of one of the 2-propinylamine MAO inhibitors, pargyline.[13] Animal data also indicate that clorgyline is a highly lipid soluble substance that readily penetrates into brain, with a rapid inactivation of MAO-A within a period of several hours.[9] This has not been verifiable in our patients because of the lack of a readily sampled tissue source of MAO-A in man.

The data summarized in Table 4 suggest a likely sequence of early, somewhat delayed, and late biological consequences of chronic antidepres-

Table 4 Physiological Changes Accompanying Acute Versus Chronic MAO Inhibitor Treatment in Man

	Acute	Chronic	Drug[a]
Antidepressant effect	0	+++	C; N-S
Switch into mania	0	+	C,P; N-S
Blood pressure reduction	+	+++	C,P; N-S
REM sleep reduction	+	+++	C,P; N-S
Platelet MAO-B inhibition	+++	+++	P,D; N-S
Plasma and urine MHPG reduction	++	+++	C,P; N-S
Clonidine-induced hypotension	++	0	C
Tyramine-induced hypertension	+	+++	C>P>D; N-S

[a] Drugs: C, clorgyline; P, pargyline; D, deprenyl; N-S, non-selective MAO inhibitors.

sant drug treatment. Some of the changes may simply represent the gradual development of the full primary effects of the drugs as effective concentrations become maximal. Others may well represent early secondary metabolic alterations to a primary effect; and yet others may represent secondary, adaptational events, including neuro-transmitter receptor changes. The most direct evidence suggestive of a receptor-based change in human brain resultant from chronic clorgyline administration is the alteration in the hypotensive response to clonidine found after chronic but not acute MAO inhibition.[17,18] This clinically observed change may well be the functional manifestation of the changes in adrenergic receptors observed during chronic, low-dose clorgyline administration in animals.[31,36] Although very preliminary, these data illustrate the potential for illuminating possible mechanisms of action of antidepressant drugs in man, and further suggest the crucial importance of examining and correlating the sequential development of biological and behavioral changes during the course of chronic drug treatment in patients.

References

1. Creese I and Sibley DR. Receptor adaptations to centrally acting drugs. *Ann Rev Pharmacol Toxicol* 21:357–91, 1981.

2. Cohen RM et al. Presynaptic noradrenergic regulation during depression and antidepressant drug treatment. *J Psychiatr Res* 3:93–105, 1980.

3. Charney DS, Menkes DB, and Heninger GR. Receptor sensitivity and the mechanism of action of antidepressant treatment. *Arch Gen Psychiatry* 38:1160–80, 1981.

4. Campbell IC et al. "Neurotransmitter-related Adaptation in the Central Nervous System Following Chronic Monoamine Oxidase Inhibition." In *Monoamine Oxidase: Structure, Function, and Altered Functions*, edited by Singer TP, Von Korff RW, and Murphy DL, pp. 517–30. New York: Academic Press, 1979.

5. Siever LJ et al. "Norepinephrine in the Affective Disorders and their Treatment. II. Receptor Assessment Strategy." In *Norepinephrine: Clinical Aspects*, edited by Lake CR, Ziegler MG. Baltimore: Williams & Wilkins, in press.

6. Herd JA. A new antidepressant—M and B 9302. A pilot study and a double-blind controlled trial. *Clin Trials* 6:219–25, 1969.

7. Wheatley D. Comparative trial of a new mono-amine oxidase inhibitor in depression. *Br J Psychiatry* 117:573–74, 1970.

8. Lipper S et al. Comparative behavioral effects of clorgyline and pargyline in man: A preliminary evaluation. *Psychopharmacology* 62(2):123–28, 1979.

9. Murphy DL. Substrate-selective monoamine oxidases: Inhibitor, tissue, species and functional differences. *Biochem Pharmacol* 27:1889–93, 1978.

10. Murphy DL et al. "Selective Inhibition of Monoamine Oxidase Type A: Clinical Antidepressant Effects and Metabolic Changes in Man." In *Monoamine Oxidase Inhibitors: The State of the Art*, edited by Youdim MBH and Paykel ES. New York: John Wiley & Sons, 1981. pp. 189–205.

11. Pickar D et al. Behavioral disturbances during the administration of selective and non-selective MAO inhibitors to depressed patients. *Arch Gen Psychiatry* 39:535–48, 1982.

12. Murphy DL et al. Platelet and plasma amine oxidase inhibition and urinary amine excretion changes during phenelzine treatment. *J Nerv Ment Dis* 164:129–34, 1977.

13. Murphy DL et al. Selectivity of clorgyline and pargyline as inhibitors of monoamine oxidases A and B *in vivo* in man. *Psychopharmacology* 62:129–32, 1979.

14. Murphy DL et al. "Cardiovascular Changes Accompanying Monoamine Oxidase Inhibition in Man." In *Function and Regulation of Monoamine Enzymes: Basic and Clinical Aspects*, edited by Usdin E, Weiner N, and Creveling C. Hampshire, England: MacMillan, 1981. pp. 549–60.

15. Cohen RM et al. REM sleep suppression induced by selective MAO inhibitors. *Psychopharmacology* 78:137–40, 1982.

16. Felner AE and Waldmeier PC. Cumulative effects of irreversible MAO inhibitors *in vivo*. *Biochem Pharmacol* 28:995–1002, 1979.

17. Siever LJ, Cohen RM, and Murphy DL. Antidepressants and α_2-adrenergic autoreceptor desensitization. *Am J Psychiatry* 138:681–82, 1981.

18. Siever LJ, Uhde TW, and Murphy DL. Possible subsensitization of α_2-adrenergic receptors by chronic monoamine oxidase inhibitor treatment in psychiatric patients. *Psychiatry Res* 6:293–302, 1982.

19. Siever LJ, Uhde TW, and Murphy DL. "Strategies for Assessment of Noradrenergic Receptor Function in Patients with Affective Disorders." In *Neurobiology of the Mood Disorders*, edited by Post RM, and Ballenger JC. Baltimore: Williams & Wilkins, in press.

20. Zandberg P, DeJong W, and deWeid D. Effect of catecholamine-receptor stimulating agents on blood pressure after local application in the nucleus tractus solitarii of the medulla oblongata. *Eur J Pharmacol* 55:43–56, 1979.

21. Crews FT and Smith CB. Presynaptic alpha receptor subsensitivity after long-term antidepressant treatment. *Science* 202:322–24, 1978.

22. Checkley SA et al. A pilot study of the mechanism of action of desipramine. *Br J Psychiatry* 138:248–51, 1981.

23. Charney DS et al. "Presynaptic Adrenoreceptor Sensitivity in Depression." *New Research Abstracts of the 134th Annual Meeting of the American Psychiatric Association*, May 1981, NR 12.

24. van Zwieten PA: The reversal of clonidine-induced hypotension by protriptyline and desipramine. *Pharmacology* 14:227–31, 1976.

25. Svensson TH, Bunney BS, and Aghajanian GK. Inhibition of both noradrenergic and serotonergic neurons in brain by the α-adrenergic agonist clonidine. *Brain Res* 92:291–306, 1975.

26. Pickar D et al. Tyramine infusions and selective MAO inhibitor treatment. I. Changes in pressor sensitivity. *Psychopharmacology* 74:4–7, 1981.

27. Pickar D et al. Tyramine infusions and selective MAO inhibitor treatment. II. Interrelationships among pressor sensitivity changes, platelet MAO inhibition and plasma MHPG reduction. *Psychopharmacology* 74:8–12, 1981.

28. Murphy DL et al. "Psychoactive Drug Effects on Plasma Norepinephrine and Plasma Dopamine β-Hydroxylase in Man." In *Catecholamines: Basic and Clinical Frontiers*, edited by Usdin E, Kopin I, and Barchas J. New York: Pergamon Press, 1979. pp. 918–20.

29. Pickar D et al. Alterations in noradrenergic function during clorgyline treatment. *Comm Psychopharmacol* 43:379–86, 1981.

30. Kellar KJ et al. Electroconvulsive shock and reserpine: Effects on β-adrenergic receptors in rat brain. *J Neurochem* 37:830–36, 1981.

31. Cohen RM et al. Changes in alpha- and beta-receptor densities in rat brain as a result of treatment with monoamine oxidase inhibiting antidepressants. *Neuropharmacology* 21:293–98, 1982.

32. Segal DS, Kuczenski R, and Mandell AJ. Theoretical implications of drug-induced adaptive regulation for a biogenic amine hypothesis of affective disorder. *Biol Psychiatry* 9:147–59, 1974.

33. Rosloff BN and Davis JD. Decrease in brain NE turnover after chronic DMI treatment: No effect with iprindole. *Psychopharmacology* 56:335–41, 1978.

34. Svensson TH and Usdin T. Feedback inhibition of brain noradrenaline neurons by tricyclic antidepressants: α-Receptor mediation. *Science* 202:1089–91, 1978.

35. U'Prichard DC, et al. Multiple apparent alphanoradrenergic receptor binding sites in rat brain: Effect of 6-hydroxydopamine. *Mol Pharmacol* 16:47–60, 1979.

36. Cohen RM et al. Chronic effects of a monoamine oxidase-inhibiting antidepressant: Decreases in functional alpha-adrenergic autoreceptors precede the decrease in norepinephrine stimulated cyclic AMP systems in rat brain. *J of Neuroscience* 2:1588–95, 1982.

Circadian Rhythm Disturbances in Affective Illness and Their Modification by Antidepressant Drugs

Thomas A. Wehr, M.D., Anna Wirz-Justice, Ph.D., and Frederick K. Goodwin, M.D.

Virtually all functions in living systems undergo cyclic changes; the time period of these cycles can range from microseconds to months or years. The most prominent cycles in physiological functions are circadian, that is, they approximate the natural 24-hour light-dark cycle of our environment. In this chapter, we will review evidence which emphasizes the importance of circadian rhythms in major depressive illness and in its pharmacological treatment. The results of circadian studies in depressed patients will be integrated with findings on the effect of chronic antidepressant treatment on the activity–rest cycle in hamsters and with data on the effect of chronic administration of these drugs on circadian rhythms in neurotransmitter receptors.

Circadian Rhythms in Depression

The human circadian system has been considered to consist of at least two endogenous, self-sustained oscillators: a strong one controlling body temperature, REM sleep propensity, and cortisol secretion; and, coupled to it, a weak one controlling the sleep–wake cycle and sleep-related neuroendocrine activity.[1,2] Studies conducted under "free-running" conditions (i.e., in the absence of external time cues) indicate that the inherent propensity of these putative oscillators is to run somewhat slower (longer) than 24 hours. Ordinarily, the longer than 24-hour rhythm of the coupled oscillator system is adjusted to precisely 24 hours by periodic environmental stimuli, such as dawn light, which acts on the oscillators through their connections to the eye. Light acting on circadian oscillators is also involved

333

in the regulation of seasonal and annual biological rhythms.[3,4] Phase-shift experiments and rapid transmeridian travel can temporarily disturb the normal phase-relationships between the two circadian oscillators and their overt rhythms. When humans are experimentally deprived of external time cues under free-running conditions, the two oscillators may spontaneously desynchronize and oscillate with unequal periods.[2] The intrinsic periods of the driving oscillators partly determine the timing of circadian rhythms relative to one another and the day–night cycle; for example, an oscillator with a fast intrinsic rhythm will entrain to the day–night cycle with a more advanced phase position than an oscillator with a slow intrinsic rhythm.

It is reasonable to assume that such a system of oscillators may become abnormal as a result of disease or may be altered by treatment interventions. Either the intrinsic periods of the oscillators could be altered, or changes could occur in the coupling between oscillators or in their entrainment to the external day–night cycle. These changes might affect the phase-position of circadian rhythms entrained to the day–night cycle or even their capacity to be entrained at all.

The hypothesis that circadian rhythm disturbances might be involved in affective illness originally evolved from consideration of four clinical features of depression: early morning awakening, diurnal variation in symptom severity, seasonality, and cyclicity of the illness. Early awakening may indicate that the timing or phase of a circadian rhythm is abnormally early. Diurnal variation, seasonality, and cyclicity are manifestations with different periodicities of the inherent rhythmicity of depression itself. The recurrent nature of the illness has been repeatedly confirmed by epidemiological studies. Characteristically, the illness remits spontaneously and recurs at some future time.[5,6] It has been hypothesized that such long-term cycles of relapse and remission could occur if affective episodes resulted from an abnormal internal phase relationship between two circadian rhythms, and if at least one of those rhythms escaped from entrainment to the day–night cycle and was free running in and out of phase with the other rhythm.[7,8]

Extensive studies of sleep patterns in affective illness shed light on these hypotheses. EEG sleep studies indicate that the timing of rapid eye movement (REM) sleep within a night's sleep is *phase-advanced* in depressives;[9] one possible cause of this abnormality is a corresponding phase-advance in the circadian rhythm of REM sleep propensity. In light of this finding we retrospectively analyzed published data describing a variety of physiological and biochemical circadian rhythms in depressives and were surprised to find a rather consistent phase-advance of patients' circadian rhythms compared with controls (Figure 1).[10] These results are compatible with the REM sleep finding, and with a circadian rhythm phase-advance hypothesis of depression.

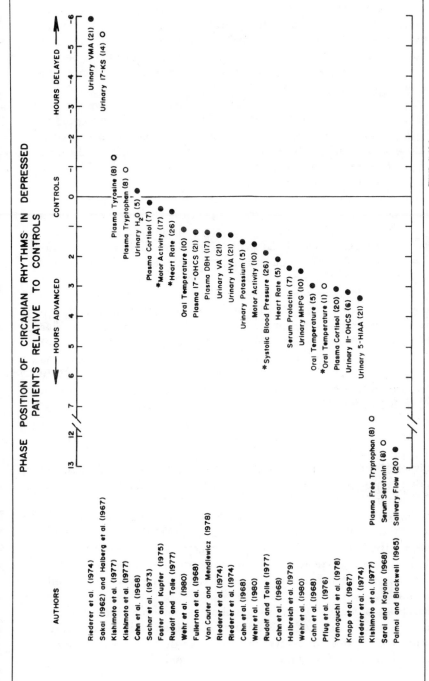

Figure 1 Early timing (phase-advance) of circadian rhythms in depressives compared with controls

Source: Wehr and Goodwin, 1981.

Note: Phase was defined as the time of the peak (acrophase) of a cosine function, $f(t)$ = mean + amplitude × cos (frequency $X t$ + phase), fitted to published data by the method of least squares. Open circles indicate studies where no data were obtained during sleep. Asterisks indicate studies where control group was not normal.

Because of the close association between circadian rhythms in REM sleep, body temperature, and cortisol secretion, a phase-advance in the latter two rhythms in depressives would tend to support the circadian phase-advance interpretation of the REM sleep abnormalities. Several studies of temperature and cortisol rhythms in depressives support the hypothesis.

With regard to temperature, our studies of manic-depressive patients during a depressive phase of their illness show a phase-position approximately 1 hour advanced compared with controls. Because of the advance, temperature was significantly lower early in the night and significantly higher later in the night in depressives compared with controls.[11] These results are in accord with those of Cahn et al. but not Lund et al., who found early temperature minima not only in depressives but also in some controls.[12,13] Longitudinal studies of the temperature rhythm are of interest because a patient can serve as his own control, and the process of change in circadian phase can be correlated with change in clinical state. Pflug studied a patient with recurrent depressions for over a year and found marked advances in the phase-position of the circadian temperature rhythm in association with depressive episodes.[14] Both the San Diego group (Kripke et al. and Atkinson et al.) and our group have studied longitudinal changes in temperature rhythms in rapidly cycling manic-depressive patients.[8,15] In our three patients, the point of maximal phase-advance of the circadian temperature rhythm coincided with the switch into the depressive phase of the mood cycle.[16] Temperature phases progressively advanced around the clock in two of Kripke's patients, as they cycled in and out of depression. In summary, some cross-sectional and longitudinal studies of the circadian temperature rhythm tend to support the idea that the early timing of REM sleep in depression is related to a phase-advance of a circadian oscillator.

Doig et al. noted that the onset of active cortisol secretion occurred earlier; that is, was phase-advanced in depressives.[17] Subsequent studies of fairly large numbers of patients by Fullerton et al., Conroy et al., and Yamaguchi et al. indicated that the 24-hour pattern of cortisol secretion is advanced.[18-20] (Sachar et al., however, found no shift in the timing of the rhythm.[21]) In the Fullerton et al. study, the degree of phase-advance of the cortisol rhythm was correlated with the severity of the depression. It is important to note that a change in waveform accompanies change in timing of the cortisol rhythm.

Alterations of neurotransmitter metabolism have been implicated in the pathophysiology of affective disorders. Circadian rhythms of neurotransmitter metabolites in depression are therefore of special interest. Riederer et al. studied urinary metabolites of serotonin (5HIAA), dopamine

(HVA), and norepinephrine (VMA, VA). [22] Our analysis of their results shows that 3 of the 4 rhythms are phase-advanced in depressives compared with controls. Our group studied urinary MHPG, a norepinephrine metabolite partially of central origin, and found the circadian rhythm to be approximately 3 hours phase-advanced in depressed manic-depressive patients compared with controls.[11] This finding has recently been replicated by Giedke et al.[23]

Although a circadian oscillator controlling REM sleep and other circadian rhythms appears to occupy an abnormally early phase-position relative to the sleep–wake cycle in depression, there is very little experimental evidence about the significance of this finding. Is the phase disturbance central to the pathophysiology of the illness, or is it merely an epiphenomenon? Advancing the time of sleep relative to the REM-temperature-circadian rhythm would "correct" the depressive phase disturbance; if the phase disturbance were part of the pathophysiology of the illness, such a procedure might be expected to induce a remission. Our group conducted such an experiment with a depressed manic-depressive woman with a history of prolonged stable depressions.[24] On two separate occasions, when her sleep period was advanced 6 hours earlier than its usual 11 P.M. to 7 A.M. time, so that she was sleeping from 5 P.M. to 1 AM (or 11 A.M. to 7 P.M. after the second shift), she experienced a rapid and complete remission for almost 2 weeks. She eventually relapsed each time apparently because the REM-temperature-circadian rhythm gradually adjusted to the shifted schedule and reestablished the preexisting phase-advance. Two additional patients showed complete responses, and two other patients showed less dramatic, partial responses to the procedure.

Possibly related to this procedure are reports of another type of intervention used with depressed patients—partial sleep deprivation in the second half of the night; in most cases, waking depressed patients several hours earlier than usual (e.g., 1:30 A.M.) has an antidepressant effect.[25] In these experiments, the time of waking is advanced without a corresponding shift in the time of going to sleep—a partial sleep deprivation. Waking patients during the first half of the night has little antidepressant effect.[26]

If being awake in the second half of the night relieves depression, then being asleep in the second half of the night may somehow sustain it. This interpretation implies that an early morning circadian phase that is sensitive to sleep may help to trigger depression. If the sleep-sensitive phase is associated with the REM-temperature-cortisol rhythm, depression may occur because a phase-advance in these rhythms causes the sensitive phase to advance from the first hours of waking into the last hours of sleep (Figure 2).

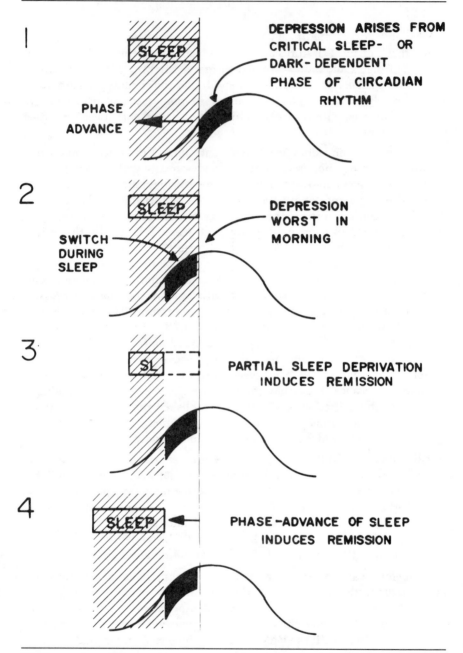

Figure 2 Hypothesis: Depression occurs in susceptible individuals when sleep interacts with a sleep-sensitive phase of circadian temperature rhythm that is normally associated with the first hours of waking but becomes advanced into the last hours of sleep. Partial sleep deprivation in the second, but not the first, half of the night induces transient depressive remission.

The Effects of Antidepressant Drugs on the Rest-Activity Cycle in Hamsters

If phase-advance of a circadian oscillator is involved in the pathophysiology of major depression, then it is reasonable to hypothesize that antidepressant drugs might alter or reverse the abnormally advanced oscillator. In other words, these drugs could work by delaying the phase-position of the REM-temperature-cortisol circadian rhythm relative to the sleep period. The controlling oscillator of this rhythm is by far the strongest oscillator and is, therefore, less easily phase-shifted than the controlling oscillator of the sleep–wake cycle. As in jet lag, correction of the phase-position of the REM-temperature-cortisol rhythm might require 1 or 2 weeks or longer.

We are unaware of any convincing findings about the effects of psychoactive drugs on the human circadian system. However, our group and others have conducted several types of animal experiments that indicate that antidepressants such as monoamine oxidase inhibitors, tricyclic antidepressants, and lithium delay the phase-position of various circadian rhythms, and may do so by lengthening the intrinsic period of their driving oscillator.[27] All of these experiments are preliminary, may not be specific for antidepressant drugs, and could be interpreted in other ways; nevertheless, nearly all of the animal results are consistent with such a prediction.

In our studies, locomotor activity in female hamsters was studied in a computer-based system designed for long-term collection and analysis of motor activity data.[28] The tricyclic antidepressant, imipramine, and the monoamine oxidase inhibitor, clorgyline, were administered chronically under free-running conditions. The main effect was to lengthen the period.[29,30]

Effects of Chronic Antidepressant Treatment on Circadian Rhythms in Neurotransmitter Receptors

Lengthening of the circadian period can be expected to delay the phase-position of circadian rhythms in the entrained condition.[4] In separate experiments we have shown that both clorgyline and imipramine delay the phase-position of the circadian rhythms of those neurotransmitter receptors that have been the focus of study in investigations of the mode of action of antidepressant drugs.[31,32]

First it was established that there are daily rhythms in α- and β-adrenergic, cholinergic, dopaminergic, opiate, and benzodiazepine receptor numbers (not in apparent affinity). The circadian rhythm for the α- and β-adrenergic receptor is illustrated in Figure 3.

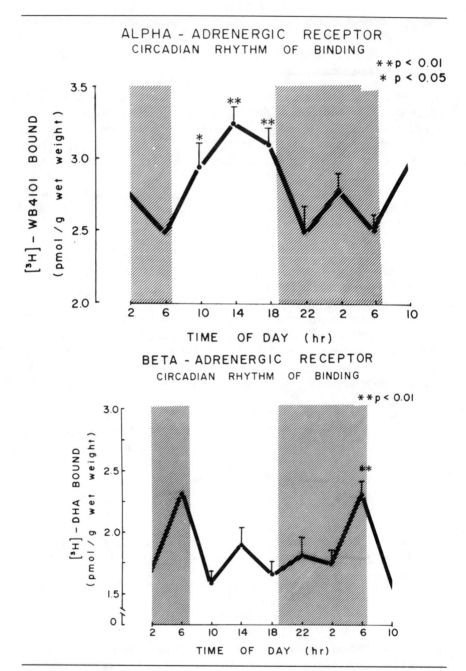

Figure 3 Specific binding to the α-(A)- and β-(B)-adrenergic receptor at 6 time points throughout the 24-hour day in April

Source: Kafka et al., 1981.

Note: Each point represents the mean ± S.E.M. of 6–7 animals; 3 points are repeated with S.E.M. to illustrate the rhythm more clearly without an arbitrary cut-off time. The shaded area represents the dark phase of the LD cycle. Statistical analysis with an ANOVA was followed by calculation of the least-squares difference to distinguish significant differences between time points ($P < .01^{**}$ and $P < .05^{*}$).

The extent of change throughout the day is of the same order of magnitude as that previously reported following chronic treatment with a variety of drugs. The rhythms persist in constant darkness with a change in waveform indicating that brain receptor circadian rhythms are endogenous but also may be subject to direct (masking) effects of light. In addition to the obvious methodological implications for receptor research, the physiological significance of these brain receptor rhythms and the functional

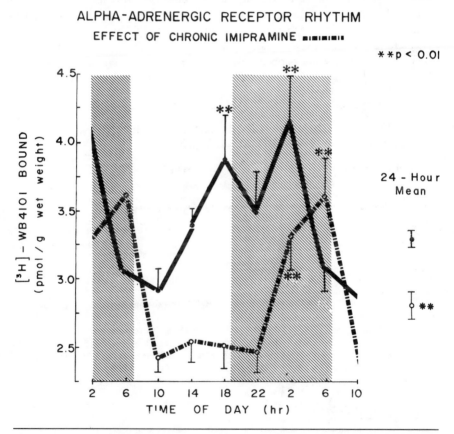

Figure 4 Circadian rhythm in binding of the α-adrenergic antagonist ^{3}H-WB4101 (.39 nM) in controls (-) and after chronic imipramine treatment (-.-) (10 mg/kg/day for 3 weeks) in June
Source: Wirz-Justice et al., 1980.
Note: The means ± S.E.M. of 7 animals at each of the 6 time points measured are shown. Three time points are repeated without S.E.M. to give a clearer picture of the temporal pattern without an arbitrary cut-off time. The shaded area is the time of lights off. Statistical analysis: ANOVA for each group indicated the existence of significant changes with time (controls, $p < .006$, imipramine-treated, $p < .001$). The 24-hour mean of imipramine-treated rats was also lower than that of controls (Student's t-test** $p < 0.001$).

importance of their phase relationships to one another and to the light–dark (LD) cycle remain to be elucidated.

Chronic treatment with clorgyline or imipramine changed all the temporal characteristics (waveform, amplitude, 24-hour mean, and phase) of these receptor rhythms in animals entrained to a 24-hour LD cycle. The changes were different in magnitude in that peak binding occurred later than in controls. For example, peak β-adrenergic receptor binding occurred 8–12 hours later, after chronic clorgyline or imipramine. The shift in peak binding phase position in other receptors was 4–8 hours later. The effect of chronic imipramine on the alpha receptor rhythm is illustrated in Figure 4;[29,45] similar data for the other receptor studies are summarized by estimating shifts in phase-position in Figures 5 and 6.[1,30–32,45]

The effects of antidepressant drugs on the rest–activity cycle and on receptor rhythms seem especially striking in light of a substantial body of

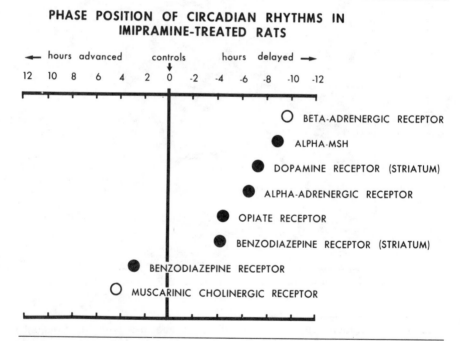

PHASE POSITION OF CIRCADIAN RHYTHMS IN IMIPRAMINE-TREATED RATS

Figure 5 Effects of imipramine/clorgyline on the phase positions of brain neurotransmitter receptor rhythms in rat brain

Note: Circles indicate the times of peaks (acrophases) of cosine function $[f(t) = + a \cos (wt + o)]$ fitted to group data at different times of day. Acrophases for treated animals are compared to controls for each receptor rhythm. Open circles indicate that the 24-hour rhythm changed from a unimodal to a bimodal pattern; in these cases estimation of phases may be unreliable. In general, the drugs delay the phase position of the brain neurotransmitter rhythms.

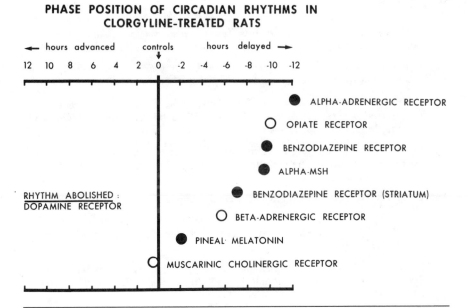

PHASE POSITION OF CIRCADIAN RHYTHMS IN CLORGYLINE-TREATED RATS

Figure 6 Effects of imipramine/clorgyline on the phase positions of brain neurotransmitter receptor rhythms in rat brain

Note: Circles indicate the times of peaks (acrophases) of cosine function [$f(t) = + a \cos (wt + o)$] fitted to group data at different times of day. Acrophases for treated animals are compared to controls for each receptor rhythm. Open circles indicate that the 24-hour rhythm changed from a unimodal to a bimodal pattern; in these cases estimation of phases may be unreliable. In general, the drugs delay the phase position of the brain neurotransmitter rhythms.

earlier data attesting to the remarkable temporal stability of circadian oscillators in the face of endogenous or exogenously induced changes in the chemical milieu of the brain.[33] Whether the changes reviewed here are specific to antidepressant agents or whether they might be produced by other psychoactive drugs is an important but as yet unanswered question.

A circadian theory of affective illness is attractive because it can integrate clinical phenomena (such as early awakening, diurnal variation in mood, and response to sleep deprivation) and epidemiological features (such as seasonality and cyclicity) with the effects of psychotropic drugs. Circadian studies suggest new animal models of depression and new models for development of drugs based on agents which directly manipulate the circadian system.

The concepts outlined in this chapter have been developed more fully in a recent book [TA Wehr and FK Goodwin (Eds.), *Circadian Rhythms in Psychiatry*. Boxwood Press, 1982], which integrates a wide range of recent developments in this relatively new field.

References

1. Weitzman ED and Czeisler CA. In *Biological Rhythms and Their Central Mechanism.* Edited by Suda M, Hayaishi O, and Nakagawa H. Amsterdam: Elsevier, 1979.

2. Wever RA. In *The Circadian System of Man: Results of Experiments Under Temporal Isolation.* New York: Springer-Verlag, 1979.

3. Gwinner F. "Animal Rhythms: Perspective and Circannual Systems." In *Handbook of Neurobiology: Biological Rhythms,* edited by Aschoff J. New York: Plenum Press, 1981. pp. 381–410.

4. Pittendrigh CS and Daan S. A functional analysis of circadian pacemakers in nocturnal rodents. I. The stability and lability of spontaneous frequency. *J Comp Physiol* 106:223–52, 1976.

5. Goodwin FK and Jamison KR. *Manic-Depressive Illness.* New York: Oxford University Press, 1982.

6. Zis AP and Goodwin FK. Major affective disorder as a recurrent illness. *Arch Gen Psychiatry* 36:835–39, 1979.

7. Halberg F. "Physiologic Considerations Underlying Rhythmometry, With Special Reference to Emotional Illness." In *Symposium Bel-Air III.* Geneva: Masson et Cie, 1968.

8. Kripke DF, et al. Circadian rhythm disorders in manic-depressives. *Biol Psychiatry* 13:335–50, 1978.

9. Vogel GW et al. Improvement of depression by REM sleep deprivation: New findings and a theory. *Arch Gen Psychiatry* 37:247–53, 1980.

10. Wehr TA and Goodwin FK. "Biological Rhythms and Psychiatry." In *American Handbook of Psychiatry,* edited by Arieti S and Brodie HKH. New York: Basic Books, 1981.

11. Wehr TA, Muscettola G, and Goodwin FK. Urinary 3-methoxy-4-hydroxy-phenylglycol circadian rhythm: Early timing (phase advance) in manic-depressives compared with normal subjects. *Arch Gen Psychiatry* 37:257–63, 1980.

12. Cahn HA, Polk GE, and Huston PE. Age comparison of human day-night physiological differences. *Aerospace Med* 39:608–10, 1968.

13. Lund R and Schulz H. The relationship of disturbed sleep in depression to an early minimum of the circadian temperature rhythm. Abstracts of the 12th CINP Congress, Goteborg, Sweden, p. 23, 1980.

14. Pflug B, Erikson R, and Johnsson A. Depression and daily temperature: A long-term study. *Acta Psychiat Scand* 54:254–66, 1976.

15. Atkinson M, Kripke DF, and Wolf SR. Autorhythmometry in manic-depressives. *Chronobiologia* 2:325–35, 1975.

16. Wehr TA, Gillin JC, and Goodwin FK. "Sleep and Circadian Rhythms in Depression." In *New Perspectives on Sleep Research,* edited by Chase M. New York: Spectrum Press, 1983.

344

17. Doig RJ et al. Plasma cortisol levels in depression. *Brit J Psychiat* 112:1263–67, 1966.

18. Fullerton DT et al. Circadian rhythm of adrenal cortical activity in depression. *Arch Gen Psychiatry* 19:674–88, 1968.

19. Conroy RTWL, Hughes BD, and Mills JN. Circadian rhythm of plasma 11-hydroxycorticosteroid in psychiatric disorders. *Brit Med J* 3:405–07, 1968.

20. Yamaguchi J, Maeda K, and Kuromaru S. The effects of sleep deprivation on the circadian rhythm of plasma cortisol levels in depressive patients. *Folia Psychiatrica et Neurologica Japonica* 32:479–87, 1978.

21. Sachar EJ et al. Disrupted 24-hour patterns of cortisol secretion in psychotic depression. *Arch Gen Psychiatry* 28:19–24, 1973.

22. Riederer T et al. The daily rhythm of HVA, VMA, (VA) and 5-HIAA in depression syndrome. *J Neural Trans* 35:23–45, 1974.

23. Giedke H, Gaertner HJ, and Mahal NA. Unpublished observation.

24. Wehr TA et al. Phase advance of the circadian sleep-wake cycle as an antidepressant. *Science* 206:710–13, 1979.

25. Schilgen B and Tolle R. Partial sleep deprivation as therapy for depression. *Arch Gen Psychiatry* 37:267–71, 1980.

26. Goetze U and Tolle R. Antidepressive wirkung des partiellen schlafentzuges warend der 1. Halfte der nacht. *Psychiatria Clin* 14:129–49, 1981.

27. Engelmann W. A slowing down of circadian rhythms by lithium ions. *Zeitschrift fur Naturforschung* 28:733–36, 1973.

28. Morgan N et al. A computer-based animal activity monitoring system. Unpublished manuscript.

29. Wirz-Justice A et al. Antidepressant drugs slow circadian rhythms in behavior and brain neurotransmitter receptors. *Psychopharmacol Bull* 16(4):45–47, 1980.

30. Wirz-Justice A, Wehr TA, and Groos G. In *Vertebrate Circadian Systems: Structure and Physiology.* Edited by Aschoff J, Daan S, and Groos G. Berlin: Springer-Verlag, 1981.

31. Wirz-Justice A et al. Clorgyline delays the phase position of circadian neurotransmitter receptor rhythms. *Brain Res*, in press.

32. Wirz-Justice A, Kafka MS, and Naber D. Circadian rhythms in rat brain, α- and β-adrenergic receptors are modified on chronic imipramine. *Life Sci* 27:341–47, 1980.

33. Pittendrigh CS and Calderola PC. Proceedings of the National Academy of Sciences, USA, 70:2697, 1973.

34. Sakai M. Diurnal rhythm of 17-ketosteroid and diurnal fluctuation of depressive affect. *Yokohama Med Bull* 11:352–67, 1962.

35. Halberg F, Vestergaard P, and Sakai M. Rhythmometry on urinary 17-ketosteroid excretion by healthy men and women and patients with chronic schizophrenia: Possible chronopathology in depressive illness. *Archives d'Anatomie, d'Histologie, d'Embryologie Normale et Experimentale* 51:301–11, 1967.

36. Kishimoto H. The biochemical studies of manic-depressive psychosis: I. The circadian rhythm of plasma tryptophan, tyrosine and cortisol, and its clinical significance. *Yokohama Med Bull* 28:23–28, 1977.

37. Foster FG and Kupfer D. Psychomotor activity as a correlate of depression and sleep in acutely disturbed psychiatric inpatients. *Am J Psychiatry* 132:928–31, 1975.

38. Rudolf GAE and Tolle R. Circadian rhythm of circulatory functions in depressives and on sleep deprivation. *Int Pharmacopsychiatry* 12:174–83, 1977.

39. VanCauter E and Mendlewicz J. 24-hour dopamine-beta-hydroxylase pattern: A possible biological index of manic-depression. *Life Sci* 22:147–56, 1978.

40. Halbriech U, Grunhaus L, and Ben-David M. Twenty-four-hour rhythms of prolactin in depressive patients. *Arch Gen Psychiatry* 36:1183–86, 1979.

41. Knapp MW, Keane PM, and Wright JG. Circadian rhythm of plasma 11-hydroxycorticosteroids in depressive illness, congestive heart failure and Cushing's syndrome. *Brit Med J* 2:27–30, 1967.

42. Sarai K and Kayano M. The level and diurnal rhythm of serum serotonin in manic-depressive patients. *Folia Psychiatrica et Neurologica Japonica* 22:271–81, 1968.

43. Palmai G and Blackwell B. The diurnal pattern of salivary flow in normal and depressed patients. *Brit J Psychiatry* 111:334–38, 1965.

44. Kafka MS, Wirz-Justice A, and Naber D. Circadian and seasonal rhythms in α- and β-adrenergic receptors in the rat brain. *Brain Res* 207:409–19, 1981.

45. Weitzman ED et al. Reversal of sleep-waking cycle: Effect on sleep stage pattern and certain neuroendocrine rhythms. Transactions of the American Neurological Association 93:153–57, 1968.

Withdrawal Effects Following Lithium Maintenance Treatment

Helmfried E. Klein, M.D., Waldemar Greil, M.D., and Pola Engel-Sittenfeld, Ph.D.

Introduction

The efficacy of lithium therapy for acute mania is well documented, as is its use as maintenance treatment to prevent recurrent affective episodes, mania, and depression.[1-15] The evidence so far is contradictory regarding lithium's effectiveness in treating acute depression.[16-18] Presently, lithium is being used in several other disorders, such as cyclothymia, alcoholism, and aggression.[19-22]

Most of the side effects of lithium—gastrointestinal irritation, fine hand tremor, and skin reactions—are reversible.[23-28] The renal effects, which include polyuria, polydipsia, and nephrogenic diabetes insipidus are usually benign;[29,30] however, kidney lesions, histological changes, and impaired urine concentrating ability have been reported.[31-34]

This chapter summarizes a controlled trial that the authors conducted to investigate various psychopharmacological, psychological, and biochemical variables during long-term lithium treatment and during a period when lithium medication was interrupted.

Methods

Twenty-one outpatients (13 female, 8 male) were admitted to the study. The mean age of the patients was 43 ± 15 years, ranging from 21 up to 63 years. Patients had been on lithium maintenance therapy for a minimum of 7 months and up to 10 years, with a mean period of 3.9 ± 2.3 years. The lithium serum concentration averaged $.68 \pm .24$ mmol/l, while the lowest level reached .3 and the highest .9 mmol/l. These patients were studied by means of several psycho-pathological alien and self-rating scales and by various psychological and biochemical tests. At the end of a 5-week placebo period an identical set of assessments was repeated as it was again following the reinstitution of a 5-week lithium application (Table 1).

Results

Psychopathological Findings

Within 5–15 days on placebo, 11 patients relapsed into severe psychotic states with hostile, manic, paranoid, retarded-depressive, and hypochondric-depressive syndromes. Two patients were regarded to need hospitalization; five had to be treated with neuroleptic and antidepressant medication on an outpatient basis; and in the remaining four cases, stabilization was regained by lithium alone. An important finding is that

Table 1 Psychiatric, Psychological, and Biological Scales and Tests Used for Patient Assessment

Lithium Maintenance Treatment	5 Weeks Placebo	5 Weeks Lithium
	Psychiatric Assessments	• HAMILTON—Depression Rating Scale • AMP—Scale • Global Assessment Scale
	Psychological Assessments	• HAWIE/ZUEWIE[a] • $d_2{}^\sim$ - Brickenkamp • Tapping • Creativity (VKT-Schoppe) • EWL—Mood Scale • MMPJ Saarbrucken • Holtzman-Inkblot—Technique (HJT) • Social Adjustment Scale (SAS)
	Biological Assessments	• Thyroid—Tests (T_4, T_3, TSH, basal and stimulated) • Prolactin • Vasopressin

Note: VKT = Verbal Creativity Test; EWL = Eigenschafts Wörterliste; AMP = Arbeitsgemeinschaft fuer Methodik und Dokumentation in der Psychiatric.
[a] HAWIE (Hamburg-Wechsler—Intelligenz Test fuer Erwachsene)/ZUEWIE (Zuerich-Wechsler—Intelligenz Test fuer Erwachsene). The German version of the WAIS (Wechsler Adult Intelligence Scale) and a parallel test form.

Table 2   Effects of Lithium and Placebo According to Three Assessment Systems

	Psychopathology Mean ± S.D. (n=21)			
	Lithium	*Placebo*	*Lithium*	
GAS	81.2	58.6	76.7	(Mean)
	±12	±27.9	±16.8	(S.D.)
	p<.0001		p<.0001	(t-Test)
AMP	3.9	17.3	5.8	(Mean)
	±4.7	±16.3	±6.7	(S.D.)
	p<.0005		p<.005	(t-Test)
HDRS	3.5	11.0	4.7	(Mean)
	±4.9	±10.9	±4.4	(S.D.)
	p<.002		p<.005	(t-Test)

Note: HDRS=Hamilton Depression Rating Scale; AMP=Rating Systems of the Arbeitsgemeinschaft fuer Methodik und Dokumentation in der Psychiatric; GAS= Global Assessment Scale.

various psychopathological syndromes erupting after lithium withdrawal corresponded to the previous feature of the disease of the individual patient.

The mean scores of the GAS, AMP, and HDRS show the highly significant clinical deterioration during placebo and also the prompt but insufficient improvement when lithium was reinstituted following the 5-week period (Table 2). The majority of those patients not relapsing into psychotic states (n =10) reported anxiety, nervousness, increased irritability and alertness, sleep disturbances, and occasionally elated mood. These minor symptoms began several days after lithium withdrawal and endured 1–2 weeks.

The high relapse rate was unexpected. Therefore, we retrospectively analyzed the case histories in an attempt to detect those patients prone to prompt relapse of psychosis after lithium withdrawal. It appeared that those patients who clinically were not fully stabilized during lithium maintenance therapy, might bear a higher risk to relapse. An operational criteria served to characterize a group of high-relapse patients for whom antidepressants or neuroleptics were indicated during maintenance therapy within the last 12 months before interruption of lithium treatment. The other group was characterized as not needing additional medication or just needing minor tranquilizers.

Of the 7 patients in need of additional antidepressive or neuroleptic medication during their maintenance treatment, 6 relapsed; while only 5 out of 14 of the comparison group experienced psychotic symptoms (Table 3). This difference reached statistical significance (Fisher's exact probability test: $p < .05$).

Table 3 Incidence of Relapse by Patients Using Additional Medication During Maintenance Therapy Compared to Patients Using No or Little Additional Medication

Additional Medication During Maintenance Lithium	Clinical Effects After Lithium Withdrawal	
	No Relapse	Relapse
No or Minor Tranquilizer	9	5
Neuroleptics or Antidepressants	1	6

Note: Fisher's exact probability test: p < .05.

Psychological Findings

Seventeen patients were able to complete the psychological test-battery during lithium and during placebo treatment. Patients were randomly assigned either first to be tested during lithium and then during placebo treatment, or in a reverse sequence. This sequence was to exclude the biasing factor of learning by test repetition.

Patients showed a significantly reduced IQ of performance when tested under lithium as compared to placebo (Table 4). This holds true independently whether the first testing was under placebo or under lithium. The differences in verbal intelligence are not consistent and group comparison does not reach statistical significance. Furthermore, significant performance reductions were observed by the Holtzman Inkblot Test taken during lithium treatment. Patients appeared to be less aware of the colored picture they were exposed to and needed significantly longer time for interpretation (Table 4). Although various psychological variables differed

Table 4 Results of Psychological Test-Battery During Lithium and Placebo Treatments

	Lithium	Placebo	p
WAIS[a]			
IQ:performance	97.7	103.8	<.0007
IQ:total	102.5	106.0	<.0004
HIT[b]			
Color	14.9	22.4	<.05
Reaction time	17.4	14.2	<.02

[a] Wechsler Adult Intelligence Scale.
[b] Holtzman Inkblot Test.

350

statistically to a significant extent, the actual differences were small and the clinical significance may be questioned.

Biological Findings

Mean group values of all biological parameters studied, except T_3, remained within the normal range during each of the three study periods.

The ratio of T_4/TBG (Thyroxine/thyroxine binding globuline) is regarded by endocrinologists as a very sensitive parameter in indicating changes of thyroid function. This quotient shows, like the other hormone-

Table 5 Biological Effects of Lithium and Placebo Treatments

	Lithium		*Placebo*		*Lithium*
T_4 $\mu g\%$	7 ± 1.8	n.s. (p<.1)	8 ± 3.1	p<.03	6.5 ± 2.3
T_3 ng%	174.7 ± 38.5	n.s.	183.7 ± 40.6	p<.005	149.9 ± 37.0
TBG ng%	2.1 ± 0.5	p<.05	1.9 ± 0.6	n.s.	2.0 ± 0.7
T_4/TBG	$3.4 \pm .7$	p<.005	4.2 ± 1.1	p<.0005	$3.2 \pm .6$
TSH $\mu U/ml$	$1.9 \pm .8$	p<.001	$.9 \pm .3$	p<.002	$1.4 \pm .4$
ΔTSH $\mu U/ml$	14.0 ± 8.7	p<.0005	4.5 ± 4.4	p<.001	9.9 ± 6.5

values listed in Table 5, the thyreostatic action of lithium. An interesting exception is formed by the T_3 values, which are clearly above the normal range. This may reflect the organism compensating for the down-regulated values of thyroid hormones by increasing T_3 excretion. Furthermore, it is striking that the thyreostatic effects of lithium are promptly reversed when lithium medication is discontinued.

Various biological variables studied in this trial show that reinstituted lithium treatment is more powerful to produce changes than long-term lithium therapy. This may simply reflect adaptive mechanisms of individuals exposed to chronic drug treatment.

Table 6 Effect of Lithium on Prolactin

	Li	*Pla*	*Li*
PRL	161	163	202
	n.s.	p<.05	
ΔPRL	1189	794	1170
to TRH	p<.05	p<.05	

Note: $n = 12$; PRL [μU/ml].

This adaptive mechanism is also shown by the prolactin values (Table 6). Lithium increases basal values of prolactin to a significant extent only if given acutely. However, if prolactin is stimulated by TRH, both during chronic and acute lithium treatment, prolactin values are significantly elevated compared to the placebo period. This action may reflect a neuroleptic-like antidopaminergic action of lithium.

Since most patients treated with lithium suffer increased thirst, it seemed particularly interesting to study vasopressin levels because this hormone is known to regulate the concentration abilities of the kidney. Again, changes became only statistically significant compared to placebo if lithium was applied acutely (Table 7). It has to be emphasized that these changes were not biased by changes of the osmolality of blood.

Conclusion

The immediate onset of psychotic symptoms suggest that rebound effects are due to lithium withdrawal rather than a spontaneous recurrence of the underlying disease while the protective effects of lithium were lacking. It also may demonstrate that lithium is exerting a constant psychoactive effect and that its action is not purely prophylactic, limited to preventing a hypothetical episode of an underlying affective disorder. These findings suggesting that lithium withdrawal may trigger psychotic states in a considerable number of patients is in accordance with a report by Small et al., who found 5 patients relapsing within 6 weeks after lithium withdrawal, although previously they were well stabilized on lithium.[35]

Table 7 Effect on Vasopressin Levels During Lithium and Placebo Treatments

Lithium	*Placebo*	*Lithium*
3.2 ± 1.2	3.4 ± 1.3	3.9 ± 1.2
n.s.	p<.05	

Note: $n = 16$; [pg/ml].

Alexander et al. tried lithium therapy in schizophrenic patients and reported that 4 out of 7 responders relapsed within 2 weeks after lithium withdrawal.[36] Lapierre reported a 20% relapse rate with mania in cyclothymic patients after experimental lithium withdrawal of only 5 days.[37]

It is generally assumed that if lithium maintenance is no longer indicated in an individual patient it may be stopped abruptly with no adverse effects. Schou reported neither abstinence phenomena nor any accumulation of relapses (rebound) during the period immediately after discontinuation of lithium.[1] Sporadic reports in the literature and our own findings, however, seriously question this widely accepted assumption.[35,37,38] It may be suggested that a stepwise withdrawal of lithium along with intensive supervision may be a more adequate approach to preventing relapse.

References

1. Schou M. *Lithium Treatment of Manic Depressive Illness. A Practical Guide,* p. 27. Basel: S. Karger, 1980.

2. Baldessarini RJ and Lipinski JF. Lithium salts: 1970–1975. *Ann Int Med* 83:527–33, 1975.

3. Davis JM. Overview: Maintenance therapy in psychiatry: II. Affective disorders. *Am J Psychiat* 133:1–12, 1976.

4. Gershon S and Shopsin B, eds. *Lithium: Its Role in Psychiatric Research and Treatment.* New York: Plenum, 1973.

5. Jefferson JW and Greist JH. *Primer of Lithium Therapy.* Baltimore: Williams & Wilkins, 1977.

6. Johnson FN, ed. *Lithium Research and Therapy.* London and New York: Academic Press, 1975.

7. Schou M et al. The treatment of manic psychoses by the administration of lithium salts. *J Neurol Neurosurg Psychiat* 17:250–60, 1954.

8. Goodwin F, Murphy DL, and Bunney WE. Lithium carbonate treatment in depression and mania. *Arch Gen Psychiat* 21:486–96, 1969.

9. Prien RF, Caffey EM Jr., and Klett CJ. Comparison of lithium carbonate and chlorpromazine in treatment of mania. *Arch Gen Psychiat* 26:146–53, 1962.

10. Shopsin B et al. Psychoactive drugs in mania. *Arch Gen Psychiat* 32:34–42, 1975.

11. Johnson G et al. Comparative effects of lithium and chlorpromazine in the treatment of acute mania. *Br J Psychiat* 119:267–76, 1971.

12. Angst J et al. Lithium prophylaxis in recurrent affective disorders. *Br J Psychiat* 116:604–14, 1970.

13. Baastrup PC et al. Prophylactic lithium: A double-blind discontinuation. *Lancet* 2:326–30, 1970.

14. Coppen A et al. Prophylactic lithium in affective disorders. *Lancet* 2:275–79, 1971.

15. Prien RF, Klett CJ, and Caffey EM, Jr. Lithium prophylaxis in recurrent affective illness. *Am J Psychiat* 131:198–203, 1974.

16. APA Task Force. Current status of lithium therapy. *Am J Psychiat* 132:997–1006, 1975.

17. Mendels J. Lithium in the treatment of depression. *Am J Psychiat* 133:373–78, 1976.

18. Bennie EH. "Lithium in the Management of Acute Depressive Illness." In *Lithium in Medical Practice,* edited by Johnson FN and Johnson S. Baltimore: Univ. Park Press, 1978. pp. 41–46.

19. Rifkin A et al. Lithium Carbonate in emotionally unstable character disorder. *Arch Gen Psychiat* 27:519, 1972.

20. Kline NS et al. Evaluation of lithium therapy in chronic and periodic alcoholism. *Am J M Sc* 268:15–19, 1974.

21. Merry J et al. Prophylactic treatment of alcoholism by lithium carbonate. *Lancet* 2:481–83, 1976.

22. Sheard MH et al. The effect of lithium on impulsive aggressive behavior in man. *Am J Psychiat* 133:1409–12, 1976.

23. Amdisen A and Schou M. Biochemistry of depression. *Lancet* 1:507, 1967.

24. Kirk L, Baastrup PC, and Schou M. Propranolol treatment of lithium-induced tremor. *Lancet* 2:1086–87, 1973.

25. Kallet JM et al. Beta blockade in lithium tremor. *J Neurol Neurosurg Psychiat* 38:719–21, 1975.

26. Lapierre YD. Control of lithium tremor with propanolol. *Canad Med J* 114:619, 1976.

27. Rifkin A et al. Lithium-induced folliculitis. *Am J Psychiat* 130:1018–19, 1973.

28. Yoder FW. Acneiform eruption due to lithium carbonate. *Arch Dermatol* 111:396–97, 1975.

29. Angrist BS et al. Lithium-induced diabetes insipidus-like syndrome. *Comp Psychiat* 11:141–46, 1970.

30. MacNeil S and Jenner FA. "Lithium and Polyuria." In *Lithium Research and Therapy,* edited by Johnson FN. London and New York: Academic Press, 1975.

31. Hestbech J et al. Chronic renal lesions following long-term treatment with lithium. *Kidney Internat* 12:205–13, 1977.

32. Burrows GD, Davies B, and Kincaid-Smith P. Unique tubular lesions after lithium. *Lancet* 1:1310, 1978.

33. Bucht G and Wahlin A. Impairment of renal concentrating capacity by lithium. *Lancet* 1:778, 1978.

34. Hansen HE et al. Renal function and renal pathology in patients with lithium-induced impairment of renal concentrating ability. *Proc Eur Dialysis Transpl Assn* 14:518–27, 1977.

35. Small JG, Small IF, and Moore DF. Experimental withdrawal of lithium in recovered manic-depressive patients: A report of five cases. *Am J Psych* 127:1555–58, 1971.

36. Alexander PE, Kammen DP, and Bunney WE. Antipsychotic effects of lithium in schizophrenia. *Am J Psych* 136:283–87, 1979.

37. Lapierre YD, Gagnon A, and Kokkinidis L. Rapid recurrence of mania following lithium withdrawal. *Biological Psychiatry* 15:859–64, 1980.

38. Wilkinson DG. Difficulty in stopping lithium prophylaxis. *Brit Med J* 1:235–36, 1971.

26

Response to Long-Term Lithium Treatment: Research Studies and Clinical Implications

Paul Grof, M.D., Ph.D.

Introduction

The question of response to stabilizing lithium treatment is increasingly important because it appears that lithium is used too indiscriminately in the current medical practice. This is certainly true for Canada; I could give a number of specific examples from Southern Ontario. During my visits to various teaching centers in the United States I have had an opportunity to see many patients in teaching sessions with psychiatric residents, and could not avoid the conclusion that indiscriminate lithium use is also a problem in the United States. This very likely reflects some of the misconceptions about which patients actually achieve stabilization on long-term lithium treatment.

Evidently, clinicians have developed a kind of reflex in their mind to think of lithium as soon as they see a patient with any recurrent mood disorder. This is rather unfortunate for our patients. Despite general belief, lithium actually has very little, if any, direct effect on moods, abnormal or normal. However, as systematic research over the past 20 years has shown, lithium can be very useful in clinical conditions that typically present with abnormal moods; that is why the connection between lithium and moods has been established in the clinician's mind.

Indiscriminate use of lithium reflects persistence of some of the clinical concepts (e.g., the concept of target symptoms), which were quite useful for treatment selection in the past but have since outlived their usefulness. The target symptom approach did provide a useful approximation for selecting certain psychoactive drugs to treat some acute psychiatric conditions. This approach, however, is not justified when it comes to treatment selection for long-term use where results are much more dependent on the nature and the course of the illness than on symptoms.

Predictors of Stabilization

Imagine a lady who has had 4 episodes of severe depression within the past 3 years. If she is placed on long-term lithium treatment in adequate dosage there are several possible outcomes. The resulting change can be best described in terms of the change in frequency of the episodes. The episodes (1) may disappear completely (complete response); (2) they can be reduced in frequency (partial response); or (3) they can show no reduction in frequency, with or without improved severity of illness (no response).

Over the years we have systematically investigated the question of which patients achieve stabilization on long-term lithium treatment and how to identify responders in advance. The first series focused on identifying the variables that discriminate between excellent responders and those who fail. The details of our strategy and findings are described elsewhere and they are not essential for understanding our main conclusions.[1-3] All patients selected for the studies were severely and frequently ill enough to require long-term treatment with medication. Patients included in these studies covered a wide range of recurrent affective disorders and were diagnosed in the first series by the diagnostic criteria of Feighner et al. and in the prospective study by Research Diagnostic Criteria (RDC) as described by Spitzer and coworkers.[4,5]

By several methodological maneuvers we optimized the detection of differences between those who benefit and those who don't. First, we defined the response stringently in terms of change in the frequency of episodes; second, we initially focused on clear-cut responders and nonresponders; and third, we put major effort into excluding false responders and nonresponders. False responders are patients who improve, usually temporarily, but the improvement is unrelated to lithium treatment. False nonresponders are common in lithium studies; they fail because of inadequate treatment with lithium and their failure confuses the study results.

Employing this strategy, we systematically compared excellent and poor responders on a large number of clinical, biological, and psychosocial variables. In particular, we investigated those characteristics which have been associated with lithium response in the literature, but found it impossible to extract from the literature a consistent description of the lithium responder, except that typical manic depressive patients tend to respond.[6–8] Of a large number of biological and psychosocial variables under study, we eventually came up with only six variables which consistently and replicably discriminated responders from nonresponders. When the data were analyzed in a multivariate way, most of the variables reported in the literature as associated with lithium response showed no connection with lithium stabilization.

The variables consistently associated with good response were as follows: First, the diagnostic subtype—there was a significant association between the response and the diagnosis of a primary affective disorder. The second important variable was the quality of the free interval (remission). This quality was determined before initiating long-term lithium treatment, by interviewing the patient at his best, when he or she was as free of abnormal moods as possible in the given case. A good quality of remission was significantly associated with a striking benefit from lithium. Such complete remission meant that the patient, at his best, was functioning well at work and in the family, and was not displaying any significant psychopathology at the interview. Nonresponders, on the other hand, frequently showed poor or questionable quality of remission. Third, we found reproducible association between lithium stabilization and the frequency of episodes during the 2 years preceding lithium. Excellent response was associated with low frequency of episodes, typical of most uncomplicated primary affective disorders, and dropped sharply where frequency of episodes exceeded four per year. A high frequency of episodes was much more common in the nonresponsive group. Fourth, as described already by others, genetic factors showed a significant link with achieved stabilization.[9] Family history positive for primary affective disorders was significantly associated with good response to lithium. Fifth, the presence of M antigen in the MNS's blood group system was more frequently noted among the responders. And finally, the MMPI profile determined at the patient's optimum functioning was of particular value. An abnormal optimum MMPI profile is a very strong indication that the patient will not achieve full stabilization on lithium treatment alone.[10] This finding is so clear-cut that an abnormal MMPI profile taken at the patient's optimum functioning can reliably serve in the clinical decision for individual patients. Although a normal MMPI profile with none of the scales exceeding the score of 70 is significantly more common among the lithium responders, this finding appears to have primarily statistical relevance: a normal profile does not give a strong assurance that an individual patient will stabilize.

Once we controlled for the major determinants of lithium response, it became clear that a number of other patient characteristics are unrelated to lithium response: variables such as sex, age, age at treatment, age at first episode, platelet MAO values, red cell lithium, and others.

A Common Denominator for Lithium Stabilization

When one finds several variables associated with lithium response, the question naturally arises whether some or all possess a common denominator. A series of multivariate analyses show that three variables account for most of the explainable variance in the material. The main contribution comes from quality of free interval, diagnosis, and recent frequency of episodes. In this respect the results confirm the clinical experience of many investigators that the core factors of lithium stabilization are the variables that can be seen as clinical characteristics of typical primary affective disorders (i.e., of a typical manic depressive): a good quality of free interval, a frequency of one or two episodes per year, and acute psychopathology that meets the criteria for primary affective disorders.

The additional three variables—MMPI profile at optimum, M antigen, and family history positive for primary affective disorders—maintain their significant association with lithium stabilization probably mainly through the above three major variables. For example, a normal MMPI profile at optimum is another expression of a good quality of free interval. Once the major three variables are entered into multivariate analyses, the three additional variables explain only a small amount of additional variance indicating that most of the predictive information is already contained in the clearly episodic course, the frequency of episodes, and the diagnosis. Furthermore, when all six variables are analyzed, it becomes clear that there are variables actually unrelated to the result of lithium stabilization: the platelet MAO values, red cell lithium concentration, and the number of previous episodes the patient experienced.[11,12] The hierarchical structure of these variables vis-à-vis the lithium stabilization perhaps explains the controversy in the literature about lithium response. Obviously, if the major critical variables are not taken into account, the investigator is likely to find differences between responders and nonresponders that are statistical artifacts and are not reproducible.

To sum up, our search for the root factors of lithium stabilization indicated that, of the variables we studied, it is the quality of free interval, typical frequency of episodes, and the diagnosis of primary affective disorder which are at the basis of the response.

Qualifications

Before we draw practical implications from these findings, it is important to stress several points. Without such qualifications, our findings could be misunderstood and so unwillingly contribute to the confusion already existing in the literature on lithium response. Any clinician who has experience with lithium therapy will recall several patients who have done well on lithium and yet do not fit the above criteria. This illustrates the complexity of the problem and the need for the following qualifications. First of all, we have been studying only one type of lithium effect in man, that of a stabilizing effect on recurrencies of abnormal moods. Other beneficial effects of lithium have been documented: the value of lithium in the treatment of acute mania, an anti-aggressive effect, symptomatic improvement in schizophrenics, reduced desire for alcohol abuse, and so on.

This variety of clinical effects of lithium should not come as a surprise in view of the large number of established biological effects of lithium. Some of these clinical effects are probably related to each other; for instance, the acute anti-manic and long-term stabilizing effects. Other benefits may possibly have different underlying mechanisms, and the clinical observations indeed suggest that some of the clinical effects of lithium are unrelated to each other. Thus, it is important to keep in mind the fact that clinical improvement on lithium treatment does not mean that we are dealing with the same phenomenon as the stabilizing treatment for abnormal moods.

Second, we have investigated the benefits from pharmacological effects of lithium on recurrencies and we took great pains to exclude false responders and false nonresponders. The obvious, but often forgotten fact is that the patient's well-being on lithium does not necessarily stem from a pharmacological benefit of lithium. Let us take an example of a patient with four recent episodes of affective illness. When the patient is placed on lithium and stays free of depression for a year, the natural assumption is that he is benefiting from lithium. A closer follow-up may show that the patient actually is a chronic neurotic with superimposed depressive decompensations under environmental stress. The assumption that he should have had another recurrence is based on our knowledge of the statistics for primary affective disorders, and the recurrence risks for depression secondary to a neurosis have not been well mapped yet. If the therapist has the courage to take the patient off lithium, he may find the patient does well for several years. In this case, the seeming benefit of lithium was based on an overestimation of the anticipated affective morbidity. If such false responders are included in the data they blur the picture.

Other examples of seeming benefit from lithium take place when inappropriate doses of antidepressants are discontinued at the time when lithium treatment is initiated, or in patients who temporarily respond to the nonspecific, psychological effect of a rigid monitoring schedule of lithium treatment.

Similarly, if patients get worse or psychotic after they have been taken off lithium, it does not necessarily mean that they had been stabilized on lithium. This is reflected in Klein's chapter in this book. High rates of prompt relapses off lithium (about 50%) have also been reported by other investigators and are usually explainable, if one keeps in mind the variety of lithium effects.[12] In some schizoaffective patients lithium does not produce stabilization of mood but has a symptom-ameliorating effect resembling an antipsychotic action. When these patients are taken off lithium, they can promptly go into a full-blown psychotic excitement. However, as mentioned in Chapter 1, the pattern of relapses is much lower if one discontinues lithium in well-stabilized primary affective disorders. Such patients will gradually experience recurrencies in a pattern that follows a predictable statistical curve. These observations again illustrate the complexity of the phenomena which, to date, have been included under the oversimplified concept of "lithium responses."

Third, in our study we have paid attention only to the change in the frequency of recurrencies. Our approach is feasible and reproducible, but it misses more subtle improvements in the severity of illness that may take place even with an unchanged relapse rate. Such improvements may be seen as clinically significant by both patient and therapist.

Finally, in the interest of interpretable research, all patients in our studies were treated with lithium only; not in combination with antidepressants and antipsychotics, which is frequently the case in clinical practice. Medications other than lithium were given only while the patients were experiencing an acute episode. To clarify the relationship between lithium treatment and the outcome, no other medications except hypnotics were given when patients were not acutely disturbed. In many other studies, the vast majority of patients on lithium receive other medications, which poses a problem for interpreting the observed changes. Our findings pertain to stabilization achieved by the long-term administration of lithium alone.

A Prospective Study

The results of our series of studies raised several concerns. For one thing, when one returns to the literature on lithium response, one is struck by the lack of agreement on the characteristics of a lithium responder. In addition, it is well accepted that findings from multivariate analyses can be considered valid only if the identified variables can perform well on an independent set of data. Thus, we had to conclude that the only way to separate real findings from possible statistical artifacts was to test the findings in a prospective study.

For this purpose, each new referral who was scheduled for long-term lithium treatment on clinical grounds, was carefully assessed in our clinic. Such assessment provided data regarding the patient's research diagnosis, quality of free interval, episode frequency during the 2 preceding years, family history, MMPI profile at optimum, and the blood groups. In other words, the patient was assessed specifically with regard to all the variables we found to discriminate between responders and nonresponders. The values of each patient were then keyed into a computer program that compared the specific characteristics of each new patient with those of the original group of patients with well-established response. In essence, the computer program performed a discriminant function analysis and included a new referral (i.e., not yet classified member). Such analysis resulted in a value expressing the likelihood that the new patient belongs to a lithium response group. The obtained discriminant score was used as the expression of the probability of the new patient's response. By comparing each new patient with the bank of earlier response data, the computer in fact predicted lithium response.

Finally, once the new patient had been treated with lithium for an adequate period, the treatment outcome was determined by a psychiatrist who was not aware of the computer predictions. To date, 35 new patients have completed stabilizing lithium treatment that was adequate in dosage and in length, so that the computer-predicted and the clinically observed responses can be compared. Of the 35 predictions, 29 proved correct and 6 wrong, with both groups being approximately equal in responders and nonresponders. This result can be expressed as a "hit rate" of 83%.

In launching this study in 1978, we were unexpectedly helped by the major concerns which developed around the side-effects of long-term lithium treatment at that time. This provided us with a number of referrals from clinicians who had already made up their minds about placing the patient on long-term lithium, but wanted help with detailed psychiatric and medical assessment of the patient. We could answer such specific requests without revealing our assessment of the patient's lithium responsiveness.

The preliminary results of the prospective studies suggest that the response to stabilizing long-term lithium treatment is a predictable event for most recurrent affective disorders, and that our earlier findings on the predictive variables can be considered validated.

Practical Implications

It is now clear that by placing a patient on long-term lithium, the clinician is making a serious decision. The benefits of lithium treatment can be dramatic, yet in recent years we have been learning more about various side-effects of long-term lithium treatment. Surprisingly, responders and nonresponders differ not only in the benefit from lithium but also in the way they tolerate it. Recent data has supported the earlier clinical impression that lithium nonresponders actually have a higher frequency of side-effects such as a significantly increased urine volume during lithium treatment.[13]

Many clinicians maintain that there is no need to carefully search for lithium-responsive patients. One can simply place patients on lithium treatment and observe what happens, in a trial-and-error manner. The difficulty with this approach is that the decision to place a patient on long-term lithium is not a neutral one: To treat or not to treat with lithium is not a decision without consequences. Treating what clearly is a lithium nonresponsive condition with long-term lithium is a problematic practice; such patients are not only deprived of more effective alternatives, but are also more vulnerable to some side-effects and, in addition, they may be psychologically harmed by false hopes.

Thus, it makes good sense to assess the patient carefully and comprehensively, on the basis of all information available about the patient, when considering a patient for long-term lithium treatment. If one cannot be sure about the lithium responsiveness and a diagnosis other than primary affective disorder is likely, one should explore whether other suitable treatments have already been fully utilized. On the other hand, if one may comfortably conclude that other suitable treatment alternatives have been adequately tried and have failed, it makes good sense to place the patient on a therapeutic trial of lithium. However, the clinician should be clear in his mind that he is starting a therapeutic trial with all that such a trial involves: the goal should be defined, a trial should be time-limited, and the clinician should keep reassessing the outcome. If the patient's condition does not have lithium-responsive characteristics, one should keep reassessing whether the patient is indeed better on lithium or better off it. To clarify this issue a trial for several months off lithium may be eventually needed. Finally, if an apparently suitable patient is not responding to long-term lithium treatment, the adequacy of the treatment (dosage and length) and the diagnosis should be reviewed.

On paper these suggestions seem all too obvious. Unfortunately, under the strain of everyday practice they are frequently forgotten. Otherwise, how could one explain that there are so many patients around who have had a "therapeutic trial of lithium" for 3 or 5 or even 10 years?

Lithium vs. Carbamazepine Responders

Carbamazepine was first reported as a successful stabilizing treatment for recurrent affective disorders in Japan.[14] More recently, that work has been confirmed and expanded by Robert Post and coworkers.[15]

Naturally, any therapeutic program that works systematically with recurrent affective disorders gradually accumulates a sizable group of lithium nonresponsive patients. Therefore, since 1978 we have been exploring the value of carbamazepine in our clinic. Our experience so far included fewer than 20 long-term treated patients. However, all of our carbamazepine patients have been already studied on other treatments for several years and therefore each of them can provide valuable information.

In addition, our experience with assessing and predicting lithium response allows us to use a similar clinical model for investigating carbamazepine treatment. Most of our patients went on carbamazepine because they failed on lithium treatment. Other patients responded well to lithium but decided to try carbamazepine because they wanted to avoid some troublesome lithium side-effects. Our early findings suggest that lithium and carbamazepine responders come from two different populations. Patients who previously achieved stabilization on lithium did not benefit from carbamazepine, despite adequate treatment and adequate blood levels. Conversely, our carbamazepine responders had failed on long-term lithium treatment. Some psychiatrists suggest that there is possibly a third group of patients who do not benefit from lithium or carbamazepine alone but achieve stabilization on a combination of both. We have not seen such a case yet.

Very recently Drs. MacCrimmon, Livingstone, and I and some coworkers have embarked on a project testing the hypothesis that patients who will respond to long-term treatment with carbamazepine can be identified electroencephalographically. Pilot findings support such a hypothesis; however, we are still at the initial stage.

Summary

Preliminary results of a prospective study of the response to stabilizing lithium treatment suggest that the response is predictable for most patients. The epitome of an excellent lithium responder is a patient with a good quality of remissions, a moderate frequency of recurrences, and diagnosis of primary affective disorder. If the MMPI profile taken at the patient's optimum is abnormal, the chances of stabilization of lithium alone are greatly reduced. In addition, the responders more frequently have family history of primary affective disorder and a positive M antigen. The characteristics of the responding patients are not widely appreciated and lithium is probably overprescribed in Canada and the United States. Our very early experience with carbamazepine suggests that the responders to lithium and carbamazepine probably come from two different populations of affective disorders.

References

1. Grof P et al. Predicting the responses to long-term lithium treatment. *L'Encephale,* in press.

2. Grof P et al. "Clinical and Laboratory Correlates of the Response to Long-term Lithium Treatment." In *Origin, Prevention and Treatment of Affective Disorders,* edited by E. Stromgren and M Schou. London: Academic Press, 1979. pp. 28–40.

3. Grof P et al. "Responders and Nonresponders to Long-term Lithium." In *Vth. World Congress of Psychiatry, Abstracts,* p. 327. Mexico City, 1971.

4. Feighner JP. Diagnostic criteria for the use in psychiatric research. *Arch. Gen. Psychiat.* 26:57–63, 1972.

5. Spitzer PL, Endicott J, and Robbins F. Research diagnostic criteria. *Arch. Gen. Psychiat.* 35:837–44, 1978.

6. Carroll B. "Prediction of Treatment Outcome with Lithium." In *Lithium: Controversies and Unresolved Issues.* Excerpta Medica, World Congress Lecture Series, 1979. pp. 171–97.

7. Ananth J and Pecknold JC. Prediction of lithium response in affective disorders. *J. Clin. Psychiat.* 39:95–199, 1978.

8. Petursson H. Prediction of lithium response. *Compr. Psychiat.* 20:226–41, 1979.

9. Mendlewicz J, Fieve RR, and Stallone F. Relationship between effectiveness of lithium therapy and family history. *Amer. J. Psychiat.* 130:1011–13, 1973.

10. Lane J et al. The MMPI in the prediction of response to lithium stabilization. *L'Encephale,* in press.

11. Grof P et al. "Platelet Monoamine Oxidase in Affective Disorders." *Abstract, Proceedings of the 1st. CCNP Annual Meeting,* edited by DJ McClure. Pfizer, Montreal, 1979.

12. Lapiere YD, Gagnon A, and Kokkinidis L. Rapid recurrence of mania following lithium withdrawal. *Biol. Psychiat.* 15:859–64, 1980.

13. Grof P, Hux M, and Dressler B. "Kidney Function and Response to Lithium Treatment." *Progress in Neuro-Psychopharmacology and Biological Research* 5:491–94, 1982.

14. Takezaki N and Hanaoka N. The use of carbamazepine (tegretol) in the control of manic depressive psychosis and other manic depressive states. *Clin. Psychiat.* 13:173–83, 1971.

15. Post RM, Ballanger JC, and Reus VI. "Effects of Carbamazepine in Mania and Depression." *The Scientific Proceedings, 131st. Annual Meeting, APA, New Research, Abstracts 7,* 1978.

27

Clinical Pharmacokinetics of Alprazolam, a Triazolo Benzodiazepine

David J. Greenblatt, M.D., Marcia Divoll, R.N., Darrell R. Abernethy, M.D., Ph.D., and Richard I. Shader, M.D.

Alprazolam (Figure 1) is a triazolo benzodiazepine derivative released for clinical use in the United States in late 1981. Its clinical efficacy has been evaluated in the treatment of both anxiety and depression.[1-3] This chapter describes some aspects of the pharmacokinetic properties of alprazolam in humans.

Analytic Techniques

Alprazolam, like its structural analogue triazolam, is a halogen-substituted benzodiazepine derivative. As such, its electronegative properties make it appropriate for quantitation by gas chromatography coupled with the sensitivity and specificity of the electron-capture detector.[4] Plasma samples are analyzed after addition of a triazolo benzodiazepine internal standard (Figure 1). Samples are extracted with an organic solvent at physiologic pH, and the organic phase is separated and evaporated to dryness. After reconstitution in a small amount of solvent, the redissolved residue is subjected to chromatography using a relatively nonpolar silicone liquid phase (1% OV–17), at high column temperatures (approximately 290°C). Both triazolam and alprazolam can be analyzed by this method (Figure 2). The linear relation between plasma alprazolam concentration and peak

Supported in part by Grant MH-34223 and Grant AM-MH 32050 from the United States Public Health Service. We are grateful for the assistance and collaboration of Ann Locniskar, Lawrence J. Moschitto, Jerold S. Harmatz, James Coleman, and Dr. Randall B. Smith.

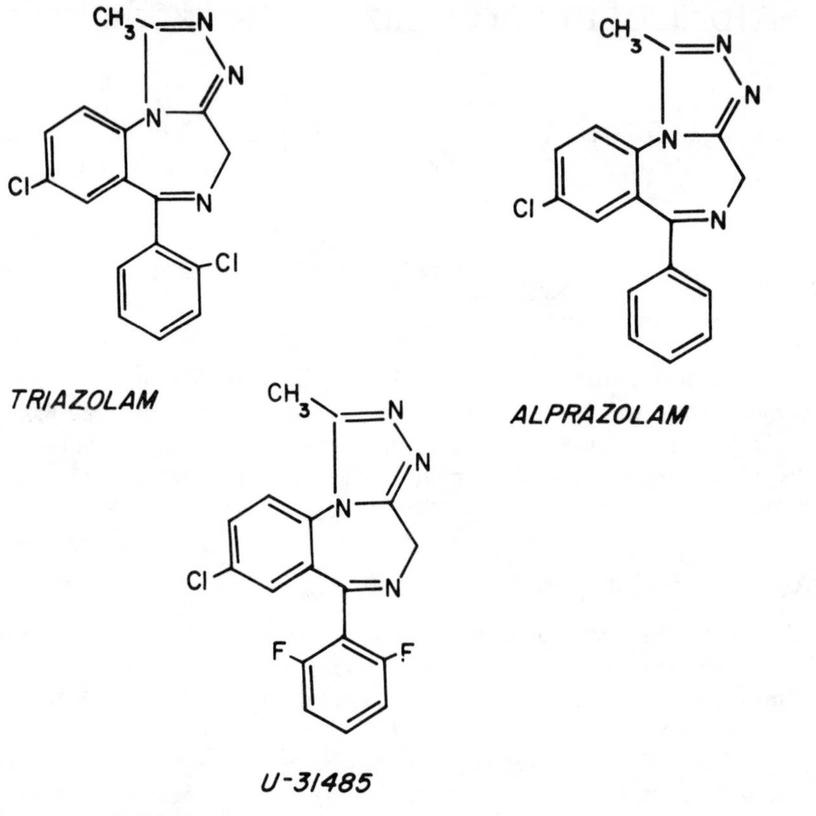

TRIAZOLAM

ALPRAZOLAM

U-31485

Figure 1 Structural formula of the triazolo benzodiazepine derivatives triazolam and alprazolam

Note: Also shown is the structure of U-31485, the triazolo benzodiazepine used as an internal standard for gas chromatographic assay.

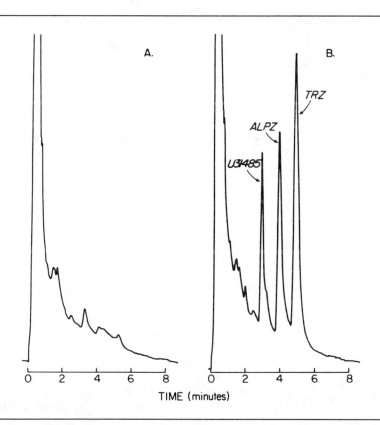

Figure 2 Left, chromatogram of a drug-free control plasma sample; right, extract of the same sample to which was added 10 ng/ml each of U-31485, alprazolam, and triazolam

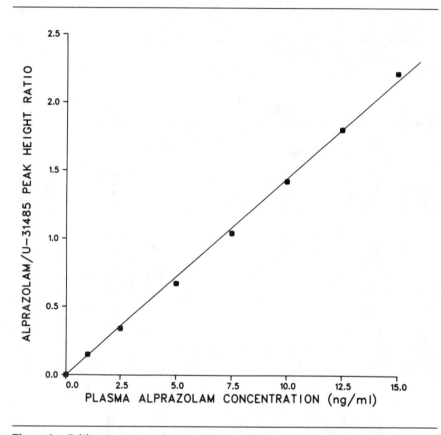

Figure 3 Calibration curve showing linear relation of plasma alprazolam concentration to the peak height ratio of alprazolam versus internal standard

height ratio of alprazolam to internal standard makes it possible to quantitate sub-nanogram quantities of alprazolam in human plasma samples (Figure 3).

Single Dose Pharmacokinetics

The metabolic biotransformation of alprazolam in humans appears to proceed mainly by hepatic oxidation.[5] The major hydroxylated metabolite may have pharmacologic activity. However, since the metabolite is cleared as fast as it is formed, accumulation of significant amounts in plasma apparently does not occur. Thus, the parent drug probably accounts for essentially all of the pharmacologic activity attributable to administration of alprazolam to humans.

The pharmacokinetic properties of single 1-mg oral doses of alprazolam have been evaluated in a series of healthy male and female volunteers from 20 to 80 years old.[6] After oral administration, absorption of alprazolam is reasonably rapid, with peak plasma levels usually attained within 2 hours of the dose (Figure 4). Alprazolam elimination then proceeds with a half-life ranging from 6 to 26 hours, depending on the age and sex of the subject. Half-life increases significantly with age in men, but is unrelated to age in women (Figure 5). The prolongation of half-life associated with old age in males is due to a reduction in total metabolic clearance, inasmuch as volume of distribution is not importantly altered by age (Figure 6). This is consistent with many previous studies of benzodiazepines biotransformed by oxidative mechanisms, including diazepam, desmethyldiazepam, desalkylflurazepam, and clobazam.[7-11] Half-life prolongation and reduced metabolic clearance occurs with old age in elderly males, whereas clearance is far less altered by age in women. Further, a given individual's ability to biotransform alprazolam via oxidation is consistent with that person's ability to biotransform other oxidized benzodiazepines.[12] (See Figure 7.)

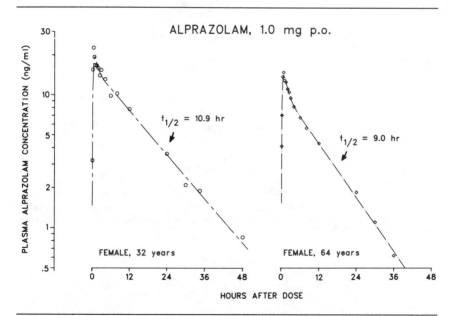

Figure 4 Plasma alprazolam concentrations and pharmacokinetic functions following administration of a single 1-mg oral dose of alprazolam to representative young and elderly female volunteers

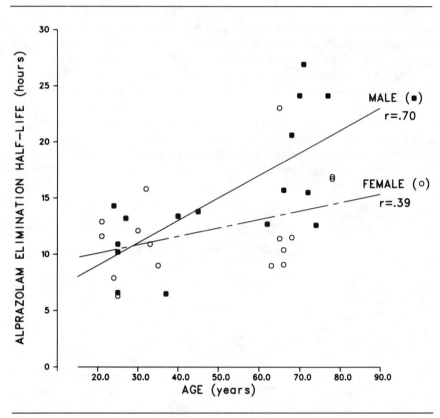

Figure 5 Relation of age to alprazolam elimination half-life in males and females
Note: A highly significant increase in half-life with age was noted in males, but age was not significantly related to half-life in females

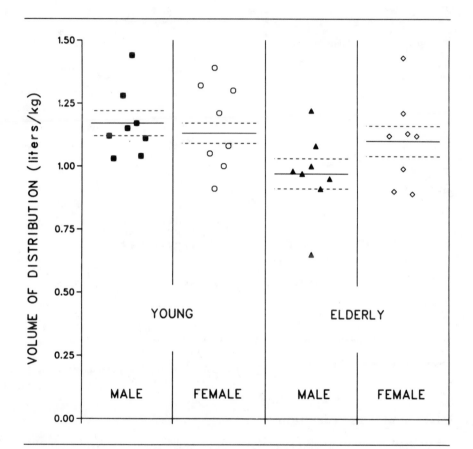

Figure 6 Relation of alprazolam volume of distribution to age and sex
Note: Individual and mean (±SE) values are shown for each group.

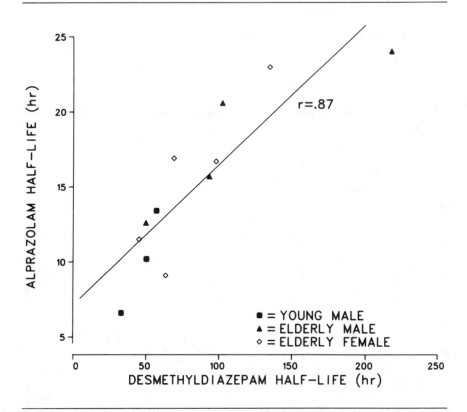

Figure 7 Relation of alprazolam elimination half-life to that of desmethyldiazepam among a series of volunteers who received single oral doses of both drugs
Note: Desmethyldiazepam was administered as either of its two precursor substances, clorazepate or prazepam. Solid line was determined by least-squares regression analysis.

Interaction with Cimetidine

As in the case of other benzodiazepines transformed by oxidation,[13–15] coadministration of cimetidine impairs the total metabolic clearance of alprazolam, inasmuch as cimetidine is a nonspecific inhibitor of hepatic microsomal oxidation. Therefore, coadministration of alprazolam with cimetidine can be expected to prolong elimination half-life because of reduction of total metabolic clearance (Figure 8), thereby leading to elevation of steady-state plasma concentrations during multiple-dose therapy. It should be emphasized, however, that the clinical implications of this interaction are not yet established for alprazolam or for any other benzodiazepine.

Multiple Dose Kinetics

Because the elimination half-life of alprazolam falls in the intermediate range relative to other benzodiazepines, multiple-dose therapy will lead to an intermediate degree of drug accumulation (Figure 9). Steady-state plasma concentrations in any given individual are approximately proportional to dose. A "therapeutic window" for alprazolam in the treatment of anxiety or depression is not yet established, but studies evaluating this question are now underway.

Clinical Implications

Studies to date characterize alprazolam as a benzodiazepine derivative biotransformed by oxidation, having an elimination half-life in the

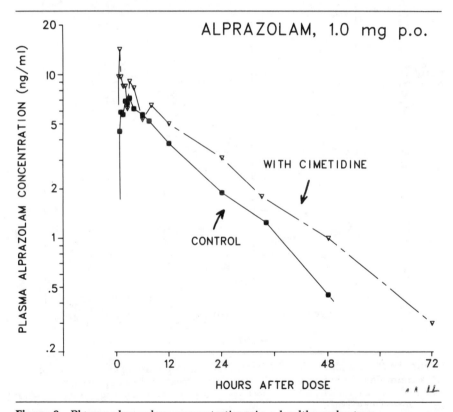

Figure 8 Plasma alprazolam concentrations in a healthy volunteer

Note: Volunteer was administered a single 1-mg oral dose on two occasions, once in the control state without coadministration of other drugs, and once during concurrent therapy with cimetidine, 300 mg every 6 hours. Coadministration of cimetidine prolonged the elimination half-life of alprazolam and reduced its metabolic clearance.

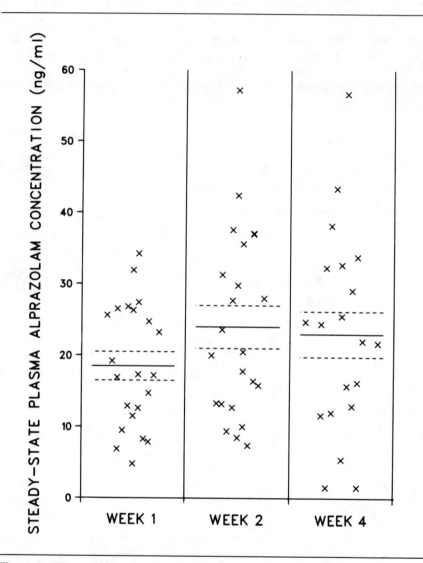

Figure 9 Plasma alprazolam concentrations during chronic alprazolam therapy in a controlled clinical trial of this drug in the treatment of depression

Source: We are grateful to Dr. Joe Mendels for his permission to illustrate data from this study of which he is principal investigator.

Note: Doses ranged from 2 to 5 mg per day. Individual and mean (±SE) values are shown at weeks 1, 2, and 4 of the study.

intermediate range. Based on these properties, it can be expected that twice or three times daily dosage will be appropriate in clinical practice. As is the case with other benzodiazepines transformed by oxidation, reduced clearance of alprazolam can be anticipated in patients with severe liver disease, in those taking cimetidine or other microsomal inhibitors, and in elderly individuals of the male gender. It is possible that reduced dosage of alprazolam will be appropriate in these clinical situations, although this has not been clearly established in clinical investigations.

References

1. Greiss KC and Fogari R. Double-blind clinical assessment of alprazolam, a new benzodiazepine derivative, in the treatment of moderate to severe anxiety. *J Clin Pharmacol.* 20:693–99, 1980.

2. Cohn JB. Multicenter double-blind efficacy and safety study comparing alprazolam, diazepam and placebo in clinically anxious patients. *J Clin Psychiatry* 42:347–51, 1981.

3. Fabre LF and McLendon DM. A double-blind study comparing the efficacy and safety of alprazolam with imipramine and placebo in primary depression. *Curr Ther Res.* 27:474–82, 1980.

4. Greenblatt DJ et al. Electron-capture gas chromatographic analysis of the triazolobenzodiazepines alprazolam and triazolam. *J Chromatogr.* 225:202–7, 1981.

5. Eberts FS et al. Disposition of [14] C-alprazolam, a new anxiolytic-antidepressant, in man. *Pharmacologist* (Abstract) 22:279, 1980.

6. Greenblatt DJ et al. Alprazolam kinetics in the elderly: Relation to antipyrine disposition. *Arch Gen Psychiatry,* in press.

7. Greenblatt DJ et al. Diazepam disposition determinants. *Clin Pharmacol Ther.* 27:301–12, 1980.

8. Allen MD et al. Desmethyldiazepam kinetics in the elderly after oral prazepam. *Clin Pharmacol Ther.* 28:196–202, 1980.

9. Shader RI et al. Effect of age and sex on disposition of desmethyldiazepam formed from its precursor clorazepate. *Psychopharmacol.* 75:193–97, 1981.

10. Greenblatt DJ et al. Kinetics and clinical effects of flurazepam in young and elderly noninsomniacs. *Clin Pharmacol Ther.* 30:475–86, 1981.

11. Greenblatt DJ et al. Clobazam kinetics in the elderly. *Brit J Clin Pharmacol.* 12:631–36, 1981.

12. Greenblatt DJ et al. Antipyrine kinetics in the elderly: Prediction of age-related changes in benzodiazepine oxidizing capacity. *J Pharmacol Exp Ther.* 220:120–6, 1962.

13. Klotz U and Reimann I. Delayed clearance of diazepam due to cimetidine. *N Engl J Med.* 302:1012–14, 1980.

14. Desmond PV et al. Cimetidine impairs elimination of chlordiazepoxide (Librium) in man. *Ann Int Med.* 93:266–68, 1980.

15. Klotz U and Reimann I. Influence of cimetidine on the pharmacokinetics of desmethyldiazepam and oxazepam. *Eur J Clin Pharmacol.* 18:517–20, 1980.

28

Clinical Predictors of Treatment Response: An Update

Robert O. Friedel, M.D.

This chapter will review the major advances in recognizing predictors of response to tricyclic antidepressants (TCAs) since the review by Bielski and Friedel in 1976.[1] At that time we reviewed all prospective, double-blind controlled studies that evaluated predictors of response of depression to either imipramine or amitriptyline. Most of the selected studies evaluated the association of the specific symptom with a patient's global or "depressed mood" response to a tricyclic, whereas some studies measured change in the symptom itself, independent of global improvement. In that review it was held that the first approach more accurately measures improvement of the patient's depressive syndrome. Most studies utilized a placebo group, permitting identification of specific drug effects through significant drug placebo differences. The lack of a placebo group was considered to confound the specific drug effect with other factors, such as spontaneous remission and placebo response, and was noted when appropriate. The predictive variables examined in the review were demographic, personality, past history, family history, course of illness, symptom, diagnosis, and biochemical. Because the studies reviewed utilized widely divergent methodologies to investigate different patient types for different purposes, it was difficult to correlate the resulting data. Usually, only findings significant at the $p < .05$ level were presented and results tabulated in an effort to extract clinically useful conclusions.

A summary of the consistent findings from those studies of predictors of TCA response is given in Table 1. The variables found to predict for imipramine response were insidious onset, weight loss, middle and late onset insomnia, psychomotor retardation, upper socioeconomic class, and

Table 1 Comparison of Clinical Predictors of Antidepressant Response

	Response	*Non-Response*
Bielski-Friedel (1976)		
Imipramine	Insidious onset Weight loss Middle, late insomnia Psychomotor retardation	Neurotic, hypochondriacal, hysterical traits Multiple prior episodes Delusions
Amitriptyline	Anorexia Middle, late insomnia Psychomotor retardation Psychomotor agitation	
Nelson-Charney (1981)	Psychomotor retardation Loss of interest Emotional withdrawal	Delusions Psychomotor agitation
Kupfer-Spiker (1981)		Anxiety Delusions Agitation Bipolar depressive illness

low urinary MHPG levels. The presence of neurotic, hypochondriacal, and hysterical traits, multiple prior episodes, and delusions predicted for a response to imipramine that was no better than to placebo. Response to amitriptyline therapy differed only in that insidious onset, weight loss and *low* urinary MHPG were absent from the list and replaced by anorexia and *high* urinary MHPG levels. Lack of response to amitriptyline was predicted by the same factors as were found for imipramine.

Two advances in the field since the time of that review have resulted in an increased understanding of the clinical variables predictive of antidepressant response. The most important factor has been the marked increase in emphasis on the use of operational diagnostic criteria, especially the Feighner Criteria, the Research Diagnostic Criteria (RDC), and DSM III Criteria for major depressive disorders.[2-4] All three have been closely scrutinized for validity from various perspectives, including that of treatment response. In comparing the classic predictors of response of affective disorder to somatic interventions such as drug therapy and electroconvulsive therapy (ECT), it became apparent that the new classification systems resulted in heterogenous populations. For example, a patient could meet Feighner Criteria for primary affective disorder or DMS III Criteria for major depressive disorder without demonstrating symptoms which had emerged from the drug treatment literature as predictive of good therapeutic response. DSM III and the RDC do include "melancholia" and "endogenous" subtypes of major depressive disorder which contain many of the classic symptoms usually associated with response to antidepressant therapy. However, patients meeting these criteria still appear to constitute a heterogenous population and show varying responsiveness to tricyclic therapy.[5] The second development in this field has been the increased number of reports supporting psychomotor retardation as a predictor of positive response to TCAs and confirming previous findings that delusions are a strong predictor of nonresponse to tricyclics when used alone.

In the area of psychomotor retardation, Nelson and Charney recently published an extensive review of the literature dealing with the symptoms of major depressive illness to determine those symptoms which best characterize the syndrome of endogenous depression.[6] The authors grouped the descriptive literature on this entity into factor analytic studies, cluster analytic studies, discriminant function studies, symptom frequency studies, instrumental measures, and treatment response studies. Based on treatment response data and neurochemical evidence, they concluded that endogenous or "autonomous" depression may exist in at least two states— a retarded anhedonic type and an agitated delusional type. The authors state that the symptom most strongly associated with autonomous depression is psychomotor change, with retardation a strong predictor of TCA response, and agitation a moderate predictor of response to antipsychotic agents used in combination with antidepressants. The authors also concluded that there is moderate evidence that loss of interest and emotional withdrawal also predict for response to TCAs. Symptoms of weight loss and middle and late onset insomnia were judged to have only slight predictive value for response to tricyclics.

At the time of our review in 1976, there was still some question regarding the power of the presence of delusions to predict nonresponse to TCAs used alone. As noted at the time, early investigators had observed that depressed patients with delusions responded less well to TCAs than otherwise similar patients who did not manifest this symptom.[7,8] However, these observations were largely ignored until Glassman et al. reported that delusional unipolar depressives were less responsive than nondelusional unipolar depressives when treated with imipramine.[9] Since then, a number of additional studies have supported these findings. Avery and Lubrano have recently reviewed the 1964 report by De Carolis et al., which compared high-dose imipramine with ECT treatment of depression in 437 patients.[10,11] Whereas 83% of depressed patients with delusions responded to ECT, only 40% responded to imipramine. Also 70% of nondelusional patients responded to imipramine, a significantly larger proportion than found in the delusional group. Simpson et al. evaluated the response of depressed patients to 150 mg or 300 mg per day of imipramine.[12] Of 15 patients with delusions, 10 received 150 mg (5 were response failures) and 5 received 300 mg (2 were response failures). This response rate was significantly poorer than that of the nondelusional patients studied. Charney and Nelson retrospectively analyzed the course, symptoms, treatment response, and personality of 54 delusional and 66 nondelusional unipolar depressed patients, and found that only 2 of 9 delusional patients responded to treatment with tricyclic antidepressants, while 25 of 37 had good treatment outcome with a tricyclic-antipsychotic combination, and 9 of 11 responded favorably to ECT.[13] A similar study compared the treatment response of patients who met RDC criteria for unipolar endogenous major depressive disorder.[14] Only 3 of 18 patients with delusions and/or hallucinations responded to TCAs alone *versus* 17 of 23 nonpsychotic patients. Psychotic patients who failed to respond to TCAs later had a favorable response to ECT or an antipsychotic-antidepressant combination. In a recent study, Kupfer and Spiker examined the factors which predict nonresponse to amitriptyline in a well-defined group of 76 inpatients with a diagnosis of major depressive syndrome based on clinical data.[15] Cognitive disorganization, anxiety, and depression, as rated by the patients, appeared to be significant predictors of nonresponse. Anxiety has been reported previously as a predictor of nonresponse to tricyclics and of response to monoamine oxidase inhibitors.[16-18] Agitation, as defined by RDC, also was a strong predictor of nonresponse, a factor which appeared to be independent of the patient's delusional status. Of the 17 patients who demonstrated delusions, 5 were complete responders, 5 were partial responders, and 7 were judged to be nonresponders. It was concluded that the presence of delusions, based on clinical diagnosis and supported by self-ratings of cognitive disorganization, contributed to nonresponse, although the presence of delusions alone did not statistically predict nonresponse. Finally, patients defined by RDC as having a Bipolar II depressive subtype did not respond to TCAs as well as unipolar patients. This finding is consistent with reports that patients with bipolar illness had a significantly poorer long-term response to imipramine than to lithium and no better than to placebo.[19,20]

The only report that contradicts these findings is flawed methodologically in that the criteria for "psychotic depressions" were broadly defined and most likely included patients who were not delusional or psychotic.[21] Therefore, the data emerging in this area strongly support the conclusion that patients with major depressive disorder with melancholia and with delusions are less likely to respond well to treatment with tricyclic antidepressants alone than to an antipsychotic-antidepressant combination or to ECT.

To summarize, it appears that the Feighner Criteria, Research Diagnostic Criteria, and *DSM-III* Criteria for major depressive disorder define a heterogenous population of patients and are all of little value in defining a population of patients responsive to antidepressant treatment. The use of the endogenous subtype of the RDC or the melancholic subtype of *DSM-III* criteria does result in populations of patients who are more likely to demonstrate symptoms predictive of antidepressant response, but not with as much precision as is currently possible using specific symptoms emerging from the treatment outcome literature. Based on these data, the strongest clinical predictor of tricyclic response in depressed patients appears to be psychomotor retardation, and to a lesser extent loss of interest, emotional withdrawl, middle and late onset insomnia, and weight loss (Table 1). Delusions appear to be a strong predictor of nonresponse to tricyclics, but predict response to an antipsychotic-tricyclic combination or to ECT.

Finally, it seems important to recognize these symptom predictors in order to interpret the results of current treatment outcome studies that evaluate such variables as drug plasma levels, cognitive therapy and pharmacotherapy-psychotherapy interactions.[22–26]

References

1. Bielski RJ and Friedel RO. Prediction of tricyclic antidepressant response: A critical review. *Arch. Gen. Psychiatry* 33:1479–89, 1976.

2. Feighner JP et al. Diagnostic criteria for use in psychiatric research. *Arch. Gen. Psychiatry* 26:57–63, 1972.

3. Spitzer DS, Endicott J, and Robins E. Research diagnostic criteria. *Arch. Gen. Psychiatry* 35:773–82, 1978.

4. American Psychiatric Association. *Diagnostic and Statistical Manual of Mental Disorder*, 3rd ed. Washington, DC: APA, 1980.

5. Nelson JC, Charney DS, and Quinlan DM. Evaluation of the DSM-III criteria for melancholia. *Arch. Gen. Psychiatry* 38:555–59, 1981.

6. Nelson JC and Charney DS, The symptoms of major depressive illness. *Am. J. Psychiatry* 138:1–12, 1981.

7. Friedman C, DeMowbray MS, and Hamilton V. Imipramine (Tofranil) in depressive states. *J. Ment. Sci.* 107:948–53, 1961.

8. Hordern A et al. Amitriptyline in depressive states: Phenomenology and prognostic considerations. *Brit. J. Psychiat.* 109:815–25, 1963.

9. Glassman AB, Kantor SJ, and Shostak M. Depression, delusions, and drug response. *Am. J. Psychiatry* 132:716–19, 1975.

10. Avery D and Lubrano A. Depression treated with imipramine and ECT: The De Carolis study reconsidered. *Am J. Psychiatry* 136:559–62, 1981.

11. De Carolis V et al. Imipamina ed elettroshock nella terapie delle depression: Analisis clinico-statistica dei risultati in 437 case. *Sistema Nervoso* 1:29–52, 1964.

12. Simpson GM et al. Two dosages of imipramine in hospitalized endogenous and neurotic depressives. *Arch. Gen. Psychiatry* 33:1093–1102, 1976.

13. Charney DS and Nelson JC. Delusional and non-delusional unipolar depression: Further evidence for distinct subtypes. *Am J. Psychiatry* 138:328–33, 1981.

14. Frances A et al. Psychotic depression: A separate entity? *Am. J. Psychiatry* 138:831–33, 1981.

15. Kupfer DJ and Spiker DG. Refractory depression: Prediction of non-response by clinical indicators. *J. Clin. Psychiatry* 42:307–12, 1981.

16. West ED and Dally PJ. Effects of iproniazid in depressive syndromes. *Brit. Med. J.* 1:1491–94, 1959.

17. Robinson DS et al. Clinical pharmacology of phenelzine. *Arch. Gen. Psychiatry* 35:629–35, 1978.

18. Quitkin F, Rifkin A, and Klein DR. Monoamine oxidase inhibitors. *Arch. Gen. Psychiatry* 36:749–64, 1979.

19. Prien RF, Klett CJ, and Caffey EM, Jr. Lithium carbonate and imipramine in prevention of affective episodes. *Arch. Gen. Psychiatry* 29:420–25, 1973.

20. Prien RF, Klett CJ, and Caffey EM, Jr. Lithium prophylaxis in recurrent affective illness. *Am. J. Psychiatry* 131:198–203, 1974.

21. Quitkin F, Rifkin A, and Klein DR. Imipramine response in deluded depressive patients. *Am. J. Psychiatry,* 135:806–11, 1978.

22. Risch SC, Huey LY, and Janowsky DS. Plasma levels of tricyclic antidepressants and clinical efficacy: Review of the literature - Part I. *J. Clin. Psychiatry* 40:6–16, 1979a.

23. Risch SC, Huey LY, and Janowsky DS. Plasma levels of tricyclic antidepressants and clinical efficacy: Review of the literature - Part II. *J. Clin. Psychiatry* 40:58–69, 1979b.

24. Kovacs M et al. Depressed outpatients treated with cognitive therapy of pharmacotherapy: A one-year followup. *Arch. Gen. Psychiatry* 38:33–39, 1981.

25. Weissman MM. The psychological treatment of depression: Evidence for the efficacy of psychotherapy alone in comparison with, and in combination with pharmacotherapy. *Arch. Gen. Psychiatry* 36:1216–69, 1979.

26. Weissman MM et al. Depressed outpatients. *Arch. Gen. Psychiatry* 38:51–55, 1981.

Antidepressant Drug Therapy in the Elderly

Jonathan O. Cole, M.D.

The topic for this chapter is the result of my involvement in a series of studies of drug therapy in the depressed elderly carried out on "symptomatic volunteers." Patients with significant depressive symptoms responded to newspaper advertisements and were treated as outpatients at the Geriatric Psychopharmacology Laboratory run by Roland Branconnier and his associates. I have also consulted on the drug therapy of older depressed patients at McLean Hospital for the past 8 years. From this experiential base I have essayed a literature review and have come painfully face to face with the gross inadequacies of the literature in this field. It is remarkable how little firm knowledge exists about the special problems of antidepressant drug therapy in the elderly. One is left with a series of presumptions which may well be correct but are not adequately proven. Compared to non-elderly adult depressed patients:

1. Elderly depressions are a bit less likely to respond to (or tolerate) standard antidepressant drugs.
2. The elderly require lower dosages because:
   a. they metabolize drugs more slowly and develop adequate plasma levels on low dosages; or
   b. they have lower plasma protein levels and therefore more unbound drug; or
   c. they develop limiting side-effects at lower plasma levels; or
   d. they (the elderly) have more concomitant medical illnesses which make them more vulnerable to side-effects (or drug-drug interactions).

3. Given our current tricyclic antidepressant drugs, the elderly are more vulnerable to the following:

   a. orthostatic hypotension;

   b. cardiac rhythm disturbances including heart block and tachycardia;

   c. peripheral anticholinergic effects like dysuria, constipation, or dry mouth; and

   d. central anticholinergic affects like memory disturbances and deliria. In this case, there is a second presumption that preexisting organic brain deficit will make patients more vulnerable to central anticholinergic side-effects.

4. Electroconvulsive therapy (ECT) is used more often in the elderly either because drugs do not work or because ECT is judged safer.

5. Agitated depression in the elderly requires the use of antipsychotic drugs with or without added antidepressants.

6. Monoamine oxidase inhibitors are risky in the elderly.

7. Lithium carbonate causes more toxicity in the elderly.

8. Amphetamine-type stimulants may be helpful in elderly depressions.

One legitimate inference from some of the above presumptions is that the new heterocyclic antidepressants—without cardiac, blood pressure, or anticholinergic effects—should be clearly superior to older tricyclics for depressions in the elderly.

The real problem in assessing all these presumptions is that very few studies exist which, in fact, specifically study a preselected group of elderly depressions in controlled comparisons of standard and new antidepressants and placebo. I know of no parallel studies that compare results of studies in the elderly with studies in depressed younger adults.

In fact, I was only able to locate three placebo-controlled studies of antidepressant drug therapy in elderly patients. One by Gerner et al. at UCLA compares trazodone with imipramine and placebo in 60 outpatients over the age of 60, who met the Research Diagnostic Criteria (RDC) for unipolar depression.[1] The average dose of imipramine was 145 mg a day and the dose for trazodone was 305 mg a day by the fourth week. Both drugs were significantly more effective than placebo on the Hamilton Depression Rating Scale (HDRS) but not on global improvement ratings, or on the Beck Depression Scale, a self-report. Imipramine caused significantly more total side-effects and more anticholinergic side-effects than either trazodone or placebo, and more cardiovascular side-effects than placebo. Imipramine patients dropped out twice as frequently as patients on trazodone or placebo. Another study by Branconnier et al. compared amitriptyline, mianserin, and placebo with amitriptyline dosages going up to 150 mg and mianserin to 60 mg a day.[2] Patients were over 60 years of age, scoring 15 or more on the HDRS and at least 50 on the Zung Self-rating Depression Scale, and showed mild cognitive impairment on at least three of six neuropsychological tests. Seventy-five outpatients were studied. Overall, both active drugs were found to be superior to placebo on the HDRS, but no differences were found on the Zung or the Profile of Mood States (POMS). Global improvement ratings showed a weak trend (p < .18) favoring both drugs over placebo. A neuropsychological "impairment index," summing scores on nine neuropsychological tests, showed impairment on amitriptyline as compared with both mianserin and placebo at 3 and 5 weeks. Amitriptyline also significantly impaired performance on one of the nine tests, the quantitated Bender Gestalt Test. On electrocardiographic measures only a significant increase in pulse rate on amitriptyline was found: no prolongations of EKG intervals were detected. Mianserin caused significantly more drowsiness than placebo, while amitriptyline caused significantly more anticholinergic side-effects than mianserin or placebo. In an earlier study, Zung et al. compared imipramine with Gerovital (a parenteral procaine preparation) and placebo in a total of 30 depressed outpatients over 60.[3] The mean dose of imipramine over the 4-week treatment period was about 75 mg a day. Imipramine-placebo differences were not significant, but covariance analysis was not used; the dose was low and the sample size small.

One other study partially qualifies.[4] It compared methylphenidate with placebo in elderly patients selected for symptoms of fatigue plus two of four other qualifying criteria which included depression (POMS), confusion (POMS), reaction time slowing or lower digit symbol substitution test scores. Significant drug-placebo differences in favor of methylphenidate were found on the depression and confusion factors of the POMS, with higher baseline POMS depression predicting greater improvement on the active drug. The two neuropsychological measures did not show drug-placebo differences.

These studies chiefly show that placebo-controlled double-blind studies of antidepressant drugs in elderly depressed outpatients can be done and can show some drug-placebo differences. The clinician's rating of patient illness on the HDRS appear more sensitive than self-report measures in these older depressions. Salzman et al. suggest that the elderly's tendency to use denial as a defense may make self-report scales insensitive.[5]

None of the studies even approach the larger problem of possible differences, if any, in drug efficacy or side-effects in elderly *versus* younger depressions. The only study relevant to this issue is by Hordern et al., in which imipramine and amitriptyline are compared in a very large series of depressed female patients of all ages. In this study, amitriptyline was more effective than imipramine in patients 60–70 years of age.

The review articles on antidepressant efficacy are not helpful with respect to the influence of age on response to antidepressants. Bielski and

Friedel's 1976 review notes only six studies that seriously considered age as a predictor.[7] Two studies had better response to imipramine in patients over 40; one had poorer response to imipramine in postmenopausal women. Three studies found no predictive effects of age. Even if these results were clearer, they are not really relevant to the drug therapy of depressed patients over 60 or 65. Nelson and Charney's more recent review specifically excludes age as a determinant of diagnosis or drug response.[8] Avery and Winokur, in an extensive review of 609 charts of depressed psychiatric inpatients found better response to electroconvulsive therapy than to drugs in depressions over 60.

There is a little evidence that tricyclic plasma level adequacy ranges established in younger depressed patients also predict improvement on tricyclics in the elderly for nortriptyline and for doxepin.[10,11] Patients over 65 appear to metabolize imipramine (IMI), desipramine (DMI), and amitriptyline (AMI) less rapidly than do younger patients. In fixed dosage studies of amitriptyline and imipramine, plasma levels of AMI, IMI, and DMI were twice as high at steady-state in older patients. Nortriptyline (NT) levels were equivalent in the two age groups. These results for DMI and NT are confounded because their plasma levels are being influenced by their formation from IMI or AMI as well as by their metabolism. A more detailed pharmacokinetic study of nortriptyline in normal elderly volunteers confirmed that half-life and plasma clearance and volume of distribution β values were similar to those obtained in studies of young adults.[13]

Side-effects

Given that cardiac illness is more common in the elderly, how do antidepressants affect cardiac function in health or disease? Tricyclics are, in general, known to affect heart rate and intracardiac conduction and to produce orthostatic hypotension. Reviews by Glassman and Bigger and by Smith et al. agree that changes in heart rate are not large (increases of 3 to 16 beats per minute), occur more commonly perhaps with AMI and NT than with IMI and DMI, and could be of clinical significance only if coronary artery disease were present, in which case tachycardia might further reduce coronary blood flow and lead to or worsen angina.[14,15] Cardiac conduction is slowed, but this effect is only occasionally statistically detectable in averaged data from controlled studies. With NT, prolongation of the P-R interval on QRS complex occurs mainly at plasma levels above the therapeutic window. At ordinary nontoxic plasma levels of tricyclics, these conduction changes are clinically relevant mainly in patients with preexisting bundle-branch block. Orthostatic hypotension is not more severe or more common on tricyclics in elderly patients but can have more serious consequences because of the risk of fractures of perhaps coronary infarction. Nortriptyline seems less likely to cause orthostatic hypotension at "effective" plasma levels than does IMI.[14,15] Other tricyclics are less well studied. Sudden death may be associated with tricyclic use in patients with acute cardiac disease, but this is not adequately proven and is so infrequent as to be undetectable in ordinary controlled clinical trials of antidepressants in the elderly.

A record review suggests that confusional episodes are somewhat more likely to occur under drug therapy (antidepressants alone or in combination with antipsychotic and antiparkinsonian drugs) in elderly than in younger depressed patients.[16] A study of the effects of single dosages of amitriptyline (50 mg), trazodone (100 mg), and placebo in normal elderly volunteers found that AMI slowed reaction time and impaired ability to retrieve learned verbal material from secondary memory while leaving recognition of learned material intact.[17] Trazodone did not impair any neuropsychological test performances but did significantly increase self-report ratings on the fatigue scale of the POMS.

Discussion

The available studies generally support clinical experience. Depressed patients over 60 do, in fact, often respond to antidepressant drugs. The studies also suggest that newer heterocyclic drugs may have advantages in older depression because of their fewer and/or different side-effects.

The issue of possible differences in drug response or drug side-effects between older and younger depressions is not answerable at this point and may well be of only minor importance. Elderly depressions do benefit from drug therapy and do have side-effects. Clinicians do worry more about drug use in elderly patients; therefore, controlled studies of antidepressant drugs in the elderly are certainly worth doing. Phenelzine is a good example of the effect of the absence of such studies. Despite increasing and powerful clinical evidence that phenelzine is a potent antidepressant and its expanding use over the last 10 years, I know of no published modern studies of its efficacy and safety in the elderly. I have been able to persuade clinicians to use it occasionally in elderly depressed inpatients at McLean, but because of the possibility that phenelzine might somehow be unsafe, it has only been used in very treatment resistant, often demented, patients and positive clinical response has been rare. Georgeotas and collaborators have done two currently unpublished studies of monoamine oxidase inhibitors in depressed elderly patients, and Robinson has the impression that phenelzine is well tolerated in elderly patients with cardiac disease. Better studies available in the literature on the use of phenelzine or other monoamine oxidase inhibitors in the elderly could have settled this issue long ago, and, if these drugs are safe and effective in patients failing to respond to tricyclics, might have enabled a good many depressed elderly patients to have been adequately and usefully treated.

For the future, the main issues and design features necessary for studies of antidepressants in the elderly are identical to those used for ordinary adult depressions. Necessary special features include more attention to side-effects, particularly anticholinergic symptoms, orthostatic hypotension and confusion, measurement of plasma levels because of the possibility of delayed metabolism of drugs in the elderly, less aggressive dosage regimens, and more frequent electrocardiographic assessment.

The greater likelihood of concomitant or even depression-causing physical disease in the elderly makes a particularly thorough prestudy medical assessment of depressed patients necessary. Because most elderly patients are on various medications for physical problems, such patients need to be included, not excluded, from Phase III studies to see whether unsuspected drug-drug interactions do or do not occur.

A major problem in older depressions is the role of degrees of dementia in affecting response to antidepressants, as well as the possibility that some antidepressants might elevate mood but impair memory in elderly patients. The criteria are not available that might separate depressive pseudodementia, benign senile forgetfulness, brain dysfunction secondary to physical disease, early Alzheimer's Disease, or even occult early multi-infarct dementia.

References

1. Gerner R et al. "A placebo-controlled Double-blind Study of Imipramine and Trazodone in Geriatric Depression." In *Psychopathology in the Aged,* edited by Cole J and Barrett J New York: Raven Press, 1980. pp. 167–82.

2. Branconnier R, Cole J, and Ghazvinian S. The therapeutic profile of mianserin on mild elderly depressives. *Psychopharmacology Bulletin* 17:129–31, 1981.

3. Zung W et al. Pharmacology of depression in the aged: Evaluation of Gerovital, H.3 as an antidepressant drug. *Psychosomatics* 15:127–34, 1974.

4. Branconnier R and Cole J. "The Therapeutic Role of Methylphenidate in Senile Organic Brain Syndrome." In *Psychopathology in the Aged,* edited by Cole J and Barrett J New York: Raven Press, 1980. pp. 183–94.

5. Salzman C, Shader R, and Harmatz J. "Response of the Elderly to Psychotropic Drugs: Predictable or Idiosyncratic?" In *Aging. Volume 2.* edited by Gershon S and Raskin A New York: Raven Press, 1975. pp. 259–72.

6. Hordern A, Burt C, and Holt N. *Depressive States: A Pharmacotherapeutic Study.* Springfield, Ill: C.C. Thomas, 1965.

7. Bielski R and Friedel R. Prediction of tricyclic antidepressant response: A critical review. *Archives of General Psychiatry* 33:1479–89, 1976.

8. Nelson J and Charney D. The symptoms of major depressive illness. *American Journal of Psychiatry* 138:1–19, 1981.

9. Avery D and Winokur G. The efficacy of electroconvulsive therapy and antidepressants in depression. *Biological Psychiatry* 12:507–23, 1977.

10. Smith R, Reed K, and Leelavathi D: Pharmacokinetics and the effects of nortriptyline in geriatric depressed patients. *Psychopharmacology Bulletin* 16:54–56, 1980.

11. Friedel R. "The Pharmacotherapy of Depression in the Elderly: Pharmacokinetic Considerations." In *Psychopathology in the Aged,* edited by Cole J and Barrett J. New York: Raven Press, 1980. pp. 157–63.

12. Nies A et al. Relationship between age and tricyclic antidepressant plasma levels. *American Journal of Psychiatry* 134:790–93, 1977.

13. Dawling S et al. Nortriptyline therapy in elderly patients: Dosage prediction after single dose pharmacokinetic study. *European Journal of Clinical Pharmacology* 18:147–50, 1980.

14. Glassman A and Bigger J. Cardiovascular effects of therapeutic doses of tricyclic antidepressants. *Archives of General Psychiatry* 38:815–20, 1981.

15. Smith R et al. Cardiovascular effects of therapeutic doses of tricyclic antidepressants: Importance of blood level monitoring. *Journal of Clinical Psychiatry* 41:12, Sec. 2, 57–63, 1980.

16. Davies R et al. Confusional episodes and antidepressant medication. *American Journal of Psychiatry* 128:127–31, 1971.

17. Branconnier R and Cole J. Effects of acute administration of antidepressants on cognition, cardiovascular functions and salivation in the normal geriatric: A comparison of trazodone and amitriptyline. *Journal of Clinical Psychopharmacology* 1:825–85, 1981.

30

Treating Depressed Patients With Medical Problems

Leo E. Hollister, M.D.

Depression is ubiquitous, and the prevailing mood appears in a variety of disorders. Whether serious depressions represent a continuum from the sadness that all of us endure occasionally or represent a completely separate entity, which some prefer to call melancholia, is still uncertain, although recent evidence suggests the latter. Symptoms of depression may be determined culturally, but depressive illness exists throughout the world.

The initial complaint of depressed patients is quite often likely to be some common physical complaint rather than one of sadness, hopelessness, or a feeling of failure.[1] Some of the manifestations, such as fatigue, headache, insomnia, and gastrointestinal disturbances are similar to those produced by anxiety; others are more distinctive, such as anorexia and weight loss, bad taste in the mouth, chronic pain, loss of interest, inactivity, reduced sexual desire, and a general feeling of despondency. It can be appreciated readily that anxiety-depression can mimic many diseases or disorders. To make matters more complicated, these symptoms may be secondary to some other disease or disorder as often as they are primary symptoms.

When depression accompanies a physical illness or disorder, it is sometimes difficult to determine the precise etiologic relationship. Several possibilities exist:

1. The physical symptoms may be manifestations of depression itself, especially the common "masked depression," in which the presenting complaints are more often physical than they are psychological.

2. Depression may be secondary to some debilitating or life-threatening physical illness. Often depression is a perfectly appropriate response.
3. Depression may be primary in a vulnerable individual who just happens to have a coincidental physical problem. The latter may or may not have acted as a trigger for the primary depression.
4. The physical symptoms may mimic depression. Such a "pseudo-depression" may not require any specific treatment.

Given the frequency of depression and the frequency of acute or chronic illness in the population, it is evident that many instances of concurrent depression and physical illness are coincidental. Nonetheless, a number of different physical disorders and drugs have been rather consistently associated with depression. This association may confound the diagnosis of depression, if that is the presenting symptom, or confound the course of the physical illness. Thus, diagnostic distinctions must be made and appropriate treatment offered. We shall now consider some of those chronic illnesses and drugs that have been most often linked with mental depression. The most extensive recent review of the subject has been published elsewhere.[2]

Depression Associated with Drugs

Many drugs are now recognized as being "depressogenic." Given the widespread use of drugs and the estimated frequency of depression in the general population, it is not always easy to be certain that an association between drug treatment and depression is not fortuitous. However, patterns emerge that strongly suggest such an association.

Mental depression was one of the first side-effects of reserpine to be noted, being relatively common in normal persons. As the drug became popular for treating hypertensives, true endogenous depression was frequently encountered. Often no prior history of mental or emotional instability was obtained, yet the reaction could be prolonged and severe enough to lead to suicide.[3] As reserpine and similar drugs deplete the central nervous system aminergic neurones of norepinephrine, serotonin, and dopamine, the changed capacity for storage of these amines in the central nervous system could account for the depressive reaction. The reserpine-induced depression is the basis for the amine hypothesis of depression. Other drugs with similar effects on brain amines, such as methyldopa, have also been implicated in depressive reactions.[4] On the other hand, some antihypertensive drugs whose actions may be only peripheral (such as guanethidine or hydralazine) or uncertain as to their effects on brain amines (such as propranolol) have also been implicated. In the case of propranolol, 11 of 13 patients who had previously become depressed with reserpine were also depressed when on this drug.[5]

The most logical treatment, as it would be with any drug suspected of causing depression, would be to withdraw the drug. In the case of various sympatholytic antihypertensives, such a variety of other types of drugs are available that many times these drugs may be bypassed in treatment altogether. On the other hand, some sympatholytics may be less likely than others to make specific patients depressed. Finally, one might simply try lowering the dose. Preliminary experience suggests that even very small doses of a drug like reserpine may retain some antihypertensive effect without its depressogenic action.

Other drugs that affect central nervous system biogenic amines may also elicit depressive reactions. Phenothiazines have been implicated as precipitants of depression since their initial use in treating schizophrenic patients. At one point, phenothiazines were considered to be contraindicated in depressed patients. Reports of aggravation of depression by long-acting forms of fluphenazine decanoate or enanthate are difficult to ascribe uniquely to this particular phenothiazine or its dosage form.[6]

Unlike phenothiazines, which block access of dopamine to its receptors, levodopa increases dopamine while decreasing serotonin in brain. The latter action might precipitate depression. Report of two depressions among 125 patients treated with levodopa for Parkinson's syndrome, as well as the precipitation of psychoses, suggest that most mental effects of levodopa are bad.[7]

Depressions have been ascribed to use of benzodiazepines, most notably diazepam. Nothing in the pharmacology of these drugs suggests that they are truly depressogenic. As anxiety and depression are inextricable, it is more likely that depressed patients may be misdiagnosed as being anxious and treated with these drugs. As anxiety resolves, depression becomes more obvious.

Whether or not oral contraceptives cause depression is still unresolved. The estimated prevalence of depression in 2–5% of patients on these agents may not be higher than in an untreated similar population. Much higher prevalence rates have been found in some series of patients, or with some types of preparations. Depression and loss of libido occurred in 28% of patients treated with strongly progestational preparations; fatigue, lethargy, and other somatic symptoms were also common with oral contraceptives.[8] A previous history of a depressive reaction, a long course of treatment, or the use of preparations with high progestin content seem to predispose toward depressive reactions.[9,10] As the amounts of both progestins and estrogens in newer formulations of oral contraceptive combinations are decreasing, depression might be expected to occur less frequently in the future if a true causal relationship exists. Recent experience supports this possibility. The incidence of depression was found to be no higher in users of oral contraceptives than among matched controls. Increasing age, a higher level of neuroticism, and employment as a housewife predisposed toward depression in women.[11]

Nevertheless, it might be well to make inquiry about past depressions in the woman or in her family members whenever an oral contraceptive is prescribed. Those with positive histories might merit closer surveillance. One might even consider the use of 50 mg/day of pyridoxine as a prophylactic treatment.[12]

Drugs of abuse, such as alcohol, opiates, stimulants, and hallucinogens are frequently associated with depression. Some have averred that depression promotes abuse of the drug, that is, drugs are taken as a form of self-treatment. In the case of alcoholics, most of whom are observed in the immediate post-detoxification stage, cause and effect are difficult to distinguish. Secondary depression has been reported in 28–50% of alcoholics. Among 61 alcoholics seen for outpatient treatment in a mental health center, 59% were clinically depressed.[13] Among 70 patients with alcoholism, 39 were depressed. The onset of depression followed onset of alcoholism in 36 instances; thus, the majority of depressions in alcoholics are secondary.[14] No systematic studies have been done to determine the efficacy of tricyclics or lithium in treating these patients. When lithium is used in alcoholic patients with depression, decreased drinking may be observed.[15]

Depression associated with opiate abuse may be more apparent than real, for drug-induced lethargy and diminished affect could mimic depression. Depression has not been a prominent part of opiate withdrawal. Depression observed in methadone-maintained opiate-dependent individuals is less likely to be spurious. Among 35 such patients with depression, some favorable response was observed following treatment with a tricyclic antidepressant.[16] On the other hand, withdrawal from stimulants is often accompanied by definite depression, possibly either as a rebound from the preceding euphoric state or as a result of depletion of catecholamines. One has the distinct clinical impression that hallucinogens, especially LSD-25, evoke depressions frequently. Whether such depression results from a direct action of the drug or from an interaction between the drug and a particular personality (the "psychedelic" aspect of these drugs) is uncertain.

Other drugs that have been associated with depression include various barbiturates, corticosteroids, methysergide, indomethacin, amantadine, fenfluramine, and anticholinesterase insecticides. Drugs such as the sedatives may simply unmask an unrecognized depression and are not truly depressogenic. Corticosteroids may interact with a depressive personality. The other drugs, however, have various mechanisms of action that might be considered to be depressogenic.[17]

Depression Associated with Neurological Diseases or Disorders

Early in the course of the disease, multiple sclerosis may produce symptoms suggesting a neurosis or hysteria. Depression tends to occur later and is characterized by anxiety and irritability. Some of the episodic symptoms of the disease may suggest those of depression: fatigue, weakness, and bizarre complaints. The absence of a precipitating cause for depression and the uniformly poor response to treatment may suggest the real nature of the problem.[18]

Although it is often said that patients with Parkinson's disease are depressed, one cannot be sure whether the depression is real or mimicked by the manifestations of the illness. Lack of facial movement, lack of spontaneous speech or movements, and social withdrawal are some of the signs that may mimic depression. This is not to say that such patients, faced with a progressive and fatal illness, should not be depressed. They often are, and the severity is related to the degree of physical incapacity. In fact, the disease may obscure the recognition of depression. Levodopa treatment of Parkinson's disease may actually aggravate the depression.[19] If depression is treated with tricyclics, one may wish to decrease the amount of antiparkinson drug to avoid an excessive amount of central anticholinergic action.

Brain tumors, especially those affecting the temporal lobe, also may mimic depression. Headaches, vague paresthesias, and lapses of memory following inapparent seizures may suggest a diagnosis of depression before the real diagnosis is apparent. Patients with normal pressure hydrocephalus may present with an agitated depression. The classical symptoms of disorientation, gait disturbances, and urinary incontinence should alert one to the remediable problem.[20] Patients with senile brain disease or small strokes may show changes in personality that suggest depression. Some patients retain enough insight so that they are aware of their decline and become depressed on this account. Thus, even if a diagnosis of Alzheimer's disease is tenable, if the patient is also clearly depressed, that disorder should be treated. One can offer little treatment for the chronic brain syndrome. On the other hand, many depressed elderly show a pseudo-dementia picture that mimics Alzheimer's disease. The differential diagnosis between degenerative brain disease and depression in the elderly is extremely important. Doses of tricyclic antidepressants should be low in depressed elderly, who are extremely sensitive to the anticholinergic action as well as having a decreased ability to metabolize these drugs. Although monoamine oxidase (MAO) inhibitors might be thought of as reasonable drugs for treating elderly depressed patients, because of increased activity of the enzyme in the aging brain, these drugs are not often used.

Depressed patients with essential or familial tremor may have it aggravated when treated with tricyclic antidepressants. Tremor is a common side-effect of those drugs, probably secondary to their sympatho-mimetic actions. Propranolol may be tried, but one must be careful to make sure that it does not aggravate the depression.

Depression Associated with Metabolic-Endocrine Disorders

Menopause is probably the most common hormonal aberration, occurring in at least 50% of the population (or more if you subscribe to the notion of a male menopause). As it occurs at a time in life when depression is common, some think that depression may be the result of the estrogen (or androgen) deficiency and that this type of depression might be alleviated by hormonal replacement therapy. Research findings are contradictory. On the one hand, estrogens given to menopausal or postmenopausal women improved well-being and mental performance as compared with placebo-treated patients.[21] On the other hand, while estrogen treatment reduced wakefulness in perimenopausal women with insomnia, it had no specific effect on anxiety or depression, which were highly responsive to pla-cebo.[22] Still, many clinicians and patients feel that a trial of estrogen might be warranted in depressed menopausal women with other signs (hot flashes, vaginal atrophy, osteoporosis) of estrogen deficiency. The situation is even more complicated in men. Serial measurement of serum testoster-one levels does not indicate that androgen deficiency occurs in men during aging. As this is an epoch of life in which spontaneously occurring endogenous depression is frequent, one should not hesitate to employ tricyclic antidepressants or MAO inhibitors in such patients, using full doses to obtain the optimal antidepressant effect.

Depression in the postpartum period usually occurs within 2–4 weeks of delivery. Some patients may become depressed while still pregnant, while others may not become depressed until 2 or 3 months postdelivery. Postpartum depression is also of variable duration, ranging from 3 months to over a year. The sharp decline in hormone levels that occurs at delivery has been suggested as the cause of such depression, yet the variable onset is not entirely consistent with such a concept. Pyridoxine deficiency, which would decrease the conversion of tryptophan to serotonin by reducing decarboxylase activity, has been a postulated mechanism. Recent work suggests that pyridoxine deficiency does not occur in such patients.[23] If that is the case, then treatment with conventional antidepressants is indicated.

Depression during pregnancy should be managed, to the extent possible, without drugs. The general rule, that drugs should be used during pregnancy only for the well-being or to preserve th life of the mother holds. Depression can be a life-threatening disorder, however, so that if a choice has to be made, drug therapy should be tried. The evidence over a good number of years indicates little risk of increased dysmorphogenesis from antidepressants.[24]

Hypothyroid patients appear depressed; they are expressionless, apathetic, and slow in movements and speech. Yet the appearance of depression may not necessarily be associated with depressed affect. Many cases of suspected depression in this disorder may be spurious. Hyperthyroid patients look anxious, neurotic, confused, schizophrenic, or manic. The occasional patient with so-called apathetic hyperthyroidism may look depressed, but again it is questionable whether these instances represent true depressions. In either case, treatment for hypo- or hyperthyroidism is usually adequate to ameliorate the mental symptoms.[25]

As many as 60% of patients with adrenal insufficiency are said to be depressed. Once again, manifestations of the disorder, such as fatigue, weight loss, and diminished activity may mimic depression. Patients with hyperadrenocortical activity have a variety of mental disorders, the estimate being that 85% have some disorder. Depression is less common than a schizophreniform psychosis or mania. Possibly these aberrations represent idiosyncratic responses to the changed hormone levels. Treatment of the underlying disorder of the adrenal cortex usually remedies most of the associated emotional disorders.

Hyperparathyroidism presents with two kinds of psychiatric syndromes: (1) an organic psychosis with obtunded consciousness; and (2) a depressive syndrome with lethargy, fatigue, and lack of spontaneity. The diagnosis is readily made on the usual biochemical battery of tests now routinely ordered. Usually both types of disorder respond to surgical treatment with removal of the adenoma.[26]

Hypercalcemia may be a paraneoplastic syndrome caused by production of parathormone by the neoplasm. A variety of tumors have been associated with hypercalcemia. Seven of 12 patients with hypercalcemia secondary to malignant tumors had mental symptoms, 3 of whom were depressed. Efforts to reduce the hypercalcemia by intravenous saline, furosemide, prednisone, or mithramycin cause the mental state to return to normal.[27]

Depression Associated with Heart Disease

Almost all patients who suffer a myocardial infarct become depressed. If they were not, they would be crazy. This catastrophe threatens both one's life and one's lifestyle. For the first few days the patient is anxious, mainly about survival. Soon after, he becomes depressed, mainly concerned about his future abilities to work, to play, to make love, and to live his normal life expectancy. Such depression is realistically based and is best handled by empathetic counseling by a knowledgeable physician.[28] Fortunately, most patients who survive a week will merit a rather optimistic prognosis. I would personally prefer to err in the direction of being a Pollyanna than in the direction of being a Gloomy Gus.

Failure of a patient to resume the progression from severe invalidism to a near normal life may indicate depression. The patient who is reluctant to move lest he get anginal pain, who fears returning to work, and who has no interest in sexual activity may very well be depressed unrealistically. Such patients may represent instances in which the myocardial infarct was simply the precipitating cause for depression in someone vulnerable to the latter disorder. In that case, treatment with antidepressant drugs would be indicated. Normally, one would prefer to use these drugs, with their many autonomic nervous system actions and some degree of cardiotoxicity, only in patients whose infarcts have completely healed. As mentioned above, early depression is much more likely situational, so that drug treatment need not be a first resort.

Patients who have had cardiac surgery with valve replacement, or even with a heart transplant, occasionally become depressed. Whether such depression is more common than that which might occur spontaneously in a corresponding age group is uncertain. In any case, treatment is no different from what might be used under ordinary circumstances. One might wish to avoid the use of tricyclics in patients with delayed cardiac conduction times. An MAO inhibitor might be a more suitable antidepressant.

The extent to which tricyclic antidepressants are cardiotoxic is controversial. At therapeutic doses, patients frequently experience tachycardia, caused both by the anticholinergic and sympathomimetic effects of the drugs. Changes in cardiac conduction times and T-wave abnormalities may be seen on the electrocardiogram with slightly more than usual therapeutic doses. It is when deliberate or accidental overdoses are taken that cardiotoxicity becomes clearly evident, with the development of life-threatening ventricular arrhythmias. Sudden death, which occurs rarely with therapeutic doses, is probably related to the quinidine-like action of some antidepressants. In patients with existing heart disease, especially with prolonged cardiac conduction times, some of the "second-generation" antidepressants, such as amoxapine or maprotilene, may be safer.

Drugs, such as the tricyclic antidepressants, that block the amine pump may reverse the antihypertensive effects of guanethidine, clonidine, and methyldopa with resulting "rebound overshoot." Doxepin, and possibly some of the "second generation" antidepressants with less effect on the amine pump, may be less likely to produce this clinically important interaction.

Depression Associated with Surgery

Whether a true posthysterectomy syndrome exists is controversial. When 56 posthysterectomy patients were compared with 56 women who had other operations, depression was much more common in the former group. Fatigue, headaches, hot flashes, dizziness, disturbed sleep, dyspareunia, and urinary symptoms were also significantly more common in the posthysterectomy group. Forty-one of the patients were clinically depressed. Many of these symptoms, including depression, might be responsive to estrogen replacement treatment.[29] On the other hand, it may be that depression is more common preoperatively in such patients.[30] It would seem to be prudent to ascertain this before operation and to treat such patients with estrogen replacement or tricyclic antidepressants after surgery. Tricyclics might be considered first in patients with a preoperative history of depression.

A depressed patient being treated with tricyclic antidepressants or MAO inhibitors may be at greater risk from anesthetic complications owing to the anticholinergic and hypotensive effects of these drugs. Usually it is sufficient if the anesthetist is aware that these drugs are being taken. They should be discontinued for a few days before elective surgery.

Depression Associated with Infectious Diseases

While an occasional patient with a bacterial, fungal, or protozoal infection may become depressed, the association is likely to be only coincidental. In the case of viral infections, however, much clinical folklore suggests an association, but precious little hard evidence is at hand. Influenza, infectious mononucleosis, cytomegalic virus infections, viral hepatitis of various types, and herpes simplex infections have been reputed to be associated with depression, either during or following the illness.[31] The evidence is strongest in the case of infectious mononucleosis, where depression has been observed that is both temporary as well as long lasting.[32] Women are said to be more affected by infectious mononucleosis than are men.[33] Sympathomimetic stimulants such as dextroamphetamine, or monoamine oxidase inhibitors, such as tranylcypromine, may be effective treatments. Tricyclic antidepressants may be required for chronic depressions triggered by these viral illnesses.

Depression Associated with Kidney Disease

Depressions in victims of end-stage renal failure is common and usually based upon a psychological factor. However, in one study, 8 of 20 renal transplant patients had secondary depression. Corticosteroid therapy for immunosuppression and methyldopa treatment to control hypertension were suspected etiological factors.[34] Many cases of depression following renal transplantation are also explainable by psychological factors. Although psychotherapy may be more to the point, if the depression is resistant, or if it is severe, drug treatment is indicated. Alternate-day steroid dosage or choice of other antihypertensive drugs must be considered when the depression is suspected of being secondary to drugs.

If tricyclic antidepressants are used in patients with renal failure, the usual doses and dosage schedules are permissible, so long as doses are conservative. Very little of these drugs is excreted unchanged through the kidney.

Depression Associated with Nutritional or Electrolyte Disorders

Deficiencies of several water-soluble vitamins produce vague symptoms that can mimic depression. At various times, thiamine, pyridoxine, folic acid, ascorbic acid, and vitamin B-12 deficiencies have led to a diagnosis of depression. As such disturbances usually occur in the context of alcoholism, profound personal neglect, or severe illness, the clinical manifestations resembling depression are confounded by many extraneous influences. When the patient becomes anemic, either because of iron deficiency or the anemia accompanying folate or vitamin B-12 deficiency, the symptoms of fatigue, breathlessness, and slowed thinking can easily be confounded with depression.

A high prevalence of emotional disorders, primarily anxiety and depression, are seen among outpatients treated for obesity. Predisposing factors include an early onset of obesity, severe caloric restriction but not total fasting, and outpatient rather than inpatient treatment.[35] One might argue that sympathomimetic stimulants might be useful in such patients for their mood-elevating effects rather than for their anoretic actions.

Decreases in serum sodium or potassium levels, or increases in serum calcium levels, may simulate depression. Usually, these abnormalities are easily detected by the biochemical screening batteries frequently used these days. More often than not, they occur in the presence of evident physical illness, often being the result of the treatment of such illness.

Depression Associated with Malignancies

Some types of malignancies, especially those of the pancreas and gut, are associated with depression even before they become clinically evident. Such patients may be mistakenly treated for depression, usually without much success, until the signs of malignancy become clear. Unfortunately, by then it is often too late for any effective treatment. Thus, a middle-aged patient with no reasonable cause for depression, no prior history of depression, and a continuing poor response to drug treatment should be suspected of having cancer.

Depression Associated with Respiratory Disease

Patients with bronchial asthma, or chronic obstructive pulmonary disease associated with chronic bronchitis and emphysema, are more often anxious than depressed. Any drug that tends to obtund consciousness may decrease respiratory drive and precipitate acute respiratory failure in patients with advanced lung disease. Most tricyclic antidepressants have varying degrees of sedative properties, with the exception of protriptyline, which might be the drug of choice in such patients who are also depressed.

Depression Associated with Liver Disease

Although faced with a fatal illness, most patients with alcoholic hepatitis or cirrhosis seem to maintain remarkably good spirits. Drugs that obtund consciousness may precipitate hepatic encephalopathy, so such drugs, which include most tricyclic antidepressants, must be used with exceeding care. The matter is further complicated by the fact that hypoalbuminemia may lead to exaggerated effects of these highly protein-bound drugs and the liver disease decreases metabolism of such drugs. This situation probably applies equally to the MAO inhibitors as well as to the "second generation" antidepressants.

Depression as a Reaction to Physical Disorders

Although depression is an appropriate response to physical illnesses that threatens to end or drastically alter the patient's life, it should not be ignored. Depression may render a patient unwilling or unable to comply with his treatment regimen or even complicate the primary illness.

Patients with fatal or potentially fatal malignancies have every right to become depressed. The best management of such secondary depression is sympathetic counseling and support. If the depression does not respond to psychological measures, one would try antidepressant drugs. The latter may also be of some benefit in managing the chronic pain often associated with advanced cancer, either used alone or in conjunction with narcotic analgesics.

Stroke is still a common catastrophe of the middle and later years of life. A paralyzed or noncommunicative patient may very easily become depressed. The presence of a cerebrovascular disorder does not contribute to depression but the attendant disability does; severity of depression was as great in patients disabled with extracerebral disorders. The degree of depression was substantial in each group.[36] Such depressions are clearly secondary to the traumatic experience. Intensive efforts at rehabilitation may bolster the patient's spirits, especially if any progress is made. When depression persists, a trial of tricyclic antidepressants is in order. Doses must be small; consistently favorable responses are the exception.

Baldessarini and colleagues have recently evaluated nearly 40 age-matched hospitalized patients at a Boston rehabilitation center and the Massachusetts General Hospital for mood changes following stroke. Of these, 25 were recovering from stroke in the territory of the left ($n = 13$) or right ($n = 12$) middle cerebral artery; comparisons were made with surgical and medical patients ($n = 14$). All were evaluated for mood and for changes in appetite, sleep, and other vegetative functions by three independent experienced clinical investigators and rated for elements derived from the Hamilton Depression Rating Scale (HDRS) and Research Diagnostic Criteria for depression on a four-point severity scale. In addition, dexamethasone suppression tests, (DST) (1 mg of the steroid at 11:30 P.M. followed by assay of plasma cortisol at 4:00 and 11:00 P.M. the next day, with 5 ng/ml as the upper limit of a normal response) were carried out. The prevalence of moderate to severe mood, appetite and sleep disturbances were 48%, 32%, and 40% among stroke patients versus 0%, 0%, and 7%, respectively, among medical-surgical controls. Among stroke patients, the prevalence of more severe disturbances of mood and vegetative functions tended to be more prevalent among those with left hemispheric lesions (all of which were assessed quantitatively by computed tomography). The prevalence of abnormal ("positive") DST results was much higher in stroke patients than controls (52% versus 14%, $p < .05$). Abnormal DST results were associated strongly with moderate-to-severe disturbances of mood, appetite, and sleep ($p < .02$). The high output of cortisol and failure to suppress with dexamethasone appear to be state-dependent as the DST became normal with the disappearance of depressionlike symptoms in a small number of patients followed for several weeks, some of whom appeared to benefit from treatment with antidepressant drugs. These results suggest that depressionlike mood and vegetative changes are much more common after stroke than is generally appreciated and that these may be reversible and treatable, and may be evaluated usefully with the DST. (Remarks by Ross J. Baldessarini, M.D. in response to the author's presentation.)

Spinal cord injuries are another catastrophe, often affecting young persons. One might think that depressions associated with these injuries would be exceedingly difficult to treat. However, a more rapid than expected response to amitriptyline was observed in 9 severely depressed patients with spinal cord injury, 6 quadriplegic and 3 paraplegic.[37]

Treatment of end-stage renal failure has been revolutionized by dialysis and renal transplantation. Patients live longer but not necessarily better. Psychiatric disturbances are common among such patients, who have a high suicide rate. Depression is prominent and is often based on some psychological factor, such as one's dependence on a piece of machinery to keep one alive.

Disfiguring surgery that alters the patient's body image may produce depression. Mastectomy, hysterectomy, prostatectomy, limb amputations, and colostomies are such operations. Depression following mastectomy has been most thoroughly studied. Serious anxiety, depression, or sexual problems were noted in 29 of 75 (39%) of postmastectomy patients as compared with only 6 of 50 (12%) control patients. Only 6 of the mastectomy patients had a radical procedure, which is the most disfiguring. The possibility that radiotherapy might have contributed to depression was based on the observations of some patients that it made them feel exhausted and lowered their spirits.[38]

The reason for mastectomy may be of consequence. Among 69 patients in whom mastectomy was done for cancerous breast disease, 22% were judged to be moderately to severely depressed on the HDRS 2 years postoperatively. Among 91 patients in whom mastectomy was done for benign breast disease, such depression was present in only 8%. Evident signs of depression at the time of surgery was the best predictor of the long-term outcome.[39]

Nonetheless, some doubt the postmastectomy depression. Depression was found in 20% of 40 patients with breast cancer treated with mastectomy, but in 18% of 50 patients with other sorts of cancers. Thus, it was felt that mastectomy itself did not generally produce the depression.[40]

No matter. It still seems eminently sensible to counsel patients exposed to such an operation well in advance to avoid possible psychological complications. When such procedures have been done, the patients generally cope better with their altered state. Although drugs may be used to treat such postoperative depressions, one cannot be sure that their effects are specific.

Antidepressant Use at the Extremes of Life

An unfortunate sudden death in a child treated vigorously with imipramine for school phobia led to the restriction of 2.5 mg/kg as the maximum permissible dose of tricyclics in children. The main reason is that protein-binding of drugs in children is less than in adults, with more free drug available for pharmacologic action. Probably a similar restriction in dose should be applied to most "second generation" antidepressants.

The elderly, in whom depression is likely to be much more frequent, also require smaller doses. They, too, have decreased protein-binding as well as possibly decreased metabolism of these drugs. Conservative doses avoid peripheral anticholinergic side-effects, mental confusion, orthostatic hypotension, or possible cardiotoxicity, all potentially severe side-effects in the elderly. Some of the "second generation" drugs with less anticholinergic action or less cardiotoxicity may be the preferred agents in the elderly.

Summary

Depression may occur in a variety of medical situations. The signs of depression may be mimicked by physical illness, in which case proper diagnosis and treatment of the physical illness usually leads to resolution of the apparent depression. On the other hand, depression may complicate the physical illness and its appropriate treatment makes management of the medical problems easier. A variety of treatments are used, including the traditional ones of counseling and psychotherapy, as well as use of various drugs. All medical patients with depression should have an extensive drug history, as drugs are a common source of depressive reactions in such patients. When in doubt, all psychoactive drugs should be temporarily discontinued. The recognition of depression in medical patients is not difficult and leads to more successful treatment.

Some of the problems associated with the use of drugs for treating depression in patients with medical disorders may be mitigated by the "second generation" drugs that have less anticholinergic action or less cardiotoxicity. Yet, even with these advantages, these newer drugs have side-effects that may be hazardous. A drug may never be developed that has only the specific therapeutic action desired, but it would be nice to have a drug for treating depressed patients that was as well tolerated as are the benzodiazepines for treating anxiety. Whether some of the newer agents in this class will meet the test remains to be seen.

References

1. Davies B. Diagnosis and treatment of anxiety and depression in general practice. *Drugs* 6:389–99, 1973.

2. Altschule MD. Depression as seen by the internist. *D.M.* 24:1–47, 1977.

3. Hollister LE. Current concepts in therapy. Complications from psychotherapeutic drugs. II. *N. Engl. J. Med.* 264:345, 1961.

4. McKiney WT, Jr. and Kane FJ, Jr. Depression with the use of alpha-methyldopa. *Amer. J. Psychiatry* 124:80, 1967.

5. Waal HJ. Propranolol-induced depression. *Brit. Med. J.* 2:50, 1967.

6. DeAlarcon R and Craney MWP. Severe mood changes following slow-release intra-muscular fluphenazine injection. *Brit. Med. J.* 3:564, 1969.

7. Wagshul AA and Daroff RB. Depression during 1-dopa treatment. *Lancet* 2:592, 1969.

8. Grant ECG and Pryse-Davies J. Effect of oral contraceptives on depressive mood changes and on endometrial monoamine oxidase and phosphatases. *Brit. Med. J.* 3:777, 1968.

9. Changing oral contraceptives: Today's drugs. *Brit. Med. J.* 4:789–91, 1969.

10. Editorial. Advising the profession. *Brit. Med. J.* 4:755–56, 1969.

11. Fleming D and Seager CP. Incidence of depressive symptoms in users of oral contraceptives. *Brit J. Psychiatry* 132:431–40, 1978.

12. Malek-Ahmadi P and Behrmann PJ. Depressive syndrome induced by oral contraceptives. *Dis. Nerv. Syst.* 37:406–8, 1976.

13. Pottenger M et al. The frequency and persistence of depressive symptoms in the alcohol abuser. *J. Nerv. Ment. Dis.* 166:562–70, 1978.

14. Woodruff RA et al. Alcoholism and depression. *Arch. Gen. Psychiatry* 28:97–100, 1973.

15. Merry J et al. Prophylactic treatment of alcoholism by lithium carbonate: A controlled study. *Lancet* 1:481–82, 1976.

16. Woody GE, O'Brien CP, and Rickels K. Depression and anxiety in heroin addicts: A placebo-controlled study of doxepin in combination with methadone. *Am. J. Psychiatry* 132:447–50, 1975.

17. Whitlock FA and Evans LEJ. Drugs and depression. *Drugs* 15:53–71, 1978.

18. Goodstein RK and Ferrell RB. Multiple sclerosis - Presenting a depressive illness. *Dis. Nerv. Syst.* 38:127–31, 1977.

19. Mindham RHS, Mardsen CD, and Parkes JO. Psychiatric symptoms during 1-dopa therapy for Parkinson's disease and their relationship to physical disability. *Psychol. Med.* 6:23–33, 1976.

20. Rosen H and Swigar ME. Depression and normal pressure hydrocephalus: A dilemma in neuropsychiatric diagnosis. *J. Nerv. Ment. Dis.* 163:35–40, 1976.

21. Fedor-Freybergh P. Influence of estrogens on well-being and mental performance in climacteric and postmenopausal women. *Acta. Obstet. Gynec. Scand.* (Sppl 64), 1977.

22. Thomson J and Oswald I. Effects to estrogens on the sleep, mood and anxiety of menopausal women. *Brit. Med. J.* 2:1317–19, 1977.

23. Livingston JE, McLeod PM, and Applegarth DA. Vitamin B-6 status in women with post-partum depression. *Am J. Clin. Nutri.* 31:886–91, 1978.

24. VanBlerk GA, Majerus TC, and Myers RA. Teratogenic potential of some psychopharmacologic drugs: A brief review. *Int. J. Gynaecol Obstet* 17:339–402, 1980.

25. Taylor JW. Depression in thyrotoxicoses. *Am. J. Psychiatry* 132:552–53, 1975.

26. Noble P. Depressive illness and hyperparathyroidism. *Proc. Roy. Acad. Med.* 67:1066–67, 1974.

27. Weizman A et al. Hypercalcemia-induced psychopathology in malignant diseases. *Brit. J. Psychiat.* 135:363–66, 1979.

28. Kavanagh T, Shephard RJ, and Tuck JA. Depression after myocardial infarction. *Can. Med. Assoc. J.* 113:23–27, 1975.

29. Richards DH. A post-hysterectomy syndrome. *Lancet* 2:983–85, 1974.

30. Hunter DJS. Effects of hysterectomy. *Lancet* 2:1265–66, 1974.

31. Editorial. Low spirits after viral infections. *Brit. Med. J.* 2:440, 1976.

32. Hendler N and Leaky W. Psychiatric and neurologic sequelae of infectious mononucleosis. *Am. J. Psychiatry* 135:842–44, 1978.

33. Cadic M, Nye FJ, and Storey P. Anxiety and depression after infectious mononucleosis. *Brit. J. Psychiatry* 128:559–61, 1976.

34. McCabe, M and Corry RJ. Psychiatric illness and human renal transplantation. *J. Clin. Psychiatry* 39:393–400, 1978.

35. Stunkard AJ and Rush J. Dieting and depression re-examined. A critical review of ontoward responses during weight reduction for obesity. *Ann. Intern. Med.* 81:526–33, 1974.

36. Robins AS. Are stroke patients more depressed than other disabled subjects. *J. Chron. Dis.* 29:479–82, 1976.

37. Kine SP, Davis SW, and Sell GH. Amitriptyline in several depressed spinal cord-injured patients: Rapidity of response. *Arch. Phys. Med. Rehab.* 58:157–61, 1977.

38. Maguire GP et al. Psychiatric problems in the first year after mastectomy. *Brit. Med. J.* 1:963–65, 1978.

39. Morris T, Greer HS, and Pettingale KW. Psychiatric problems after mastectomy. *Brit. Med. J.* 1:1211–12, 1978.

40. Worden JW and Weisman AP. The fallacy of post-mastectomy depression. *Am. J. Med. Sci.* 273:169–75, 1977.

Psychotherapy in Comparison and in Combination with Pharmacotherapy for the Depressed Outpatient

Myrna M. Weissman, Ph.D.

Psychotherapy in the marketplace has been an ostentatious success. The practitioners, the consumers, and the psychotherapies have multiplied. At least 250 psychotherapies have been identified, administered by psychiatrists, psychologists, psychiatric social workers, nurses, clergy, and counselors for a variety of conditions including schizophrenia, snake phobias, alcoholism, distress, despair, and disinterest.

In the midst of this stunning success there has been only one flaw—that of credibility. For depression, where some type of psychotherapy combined with some type of pharmacotherapy is a common treatment, psychotherapy has begun to gain credibility from controlled clinical trials.

The scientific evidence for psychotherapy and drugs in the treatment of depression has received mixed reviews. Clinicians treating depressed patients are impatient with the researcher's reluctance to draw conclusions and inclination to call for more research. They are weary of the researcher's claim that properly designed trials have not been conducted; that the samples are too small or too poorly selected; that only a few treatments have been tested and not even those were sufficiently standardized.

Clinicians, having experience with depressed patients who have improved, feel justified in the use of these treatments. Moreover, they have to care for distressed persons and can't afford to delay acting until all the evidence is in. The clinician must act in the face of uncertainty and use whatever he or she believes will best relieve the patient's suffering. Even clinicians who keep abreast of the latest research evidence may have

This research was supported in part by Alcohol, Drug Abuse, and Mental Health Administration grant MH 26466 from the Clinical Research Branch, National Institute of Mental Health, Rockville, Maryland.

difficulty translating it into practice with patients who don't quite fit the inclusion and exclusion criteria of controlled trials.

The biologically oriented researcher is particularly sympathetic to this research, thanks to at least two ideologic biases about psychotherapy. First, there is a theoretical bias. They are skeptical about the relevance of psychosocial interventions in a disorder which their own research and that of others increasingly has demonstrated genetic and biochemical components.

Second, there is an empirical bias. Whereas they are aware of the overwhelming evidence for the efficacy of pharmacotherapy for depression, particularly the tricyclics, they are skeptical or unaware of the growing (albeit small) body of evidence for the value of psychotherapy in depression.

I would like to work at improving the dialogue with both clinicians and the biologists. The first issue—the interplay between psychosocial and biological genetic factors in a complex disorder such as depression —won't be dealt with here. This discussion could focus on the parallels between depression and other chronic, noninfectious medical disorders such as hypertension, heart disease, or arthritis. A useful epidemiologic concept that would highlight the parallels between these disorders would be that of relative risk; that is, the relative contribution of various risk factors (biological and psychosocial) which increase the probability of the onset or the exacerbation of the disorder.

Instead, this chapter will focus on the empirical evidence for psychosocial interventions—the growing body of scientific evidence for the efficacy of psychotherapy in comparison and in combination with pharmacotherapy in the treatment of ambulatory depression. For the clinician I will try to translate the available evidence into practice.

Recent Developments in Testing of the Psychotherapies

The acceleration in the development and scientific testing of the psychotherapies over the last decade account for this chapter. These developments, which are being used in the testing of psychotherapy, include the following:

1. Clinical trials with random assignment of patients to treatment;
2. Well-defined protocols with inclusion and exclusion criteria; specification of the amount, timing, and type of treatment; criteria for withdrawal of patients from treatment;
3. Incorporation of the new advances in psychopathology, including more reliable diagnostic measures;
4. Testing in diagnostically homogeneous patients in order to determine whether a particular psychotherapy is useful for a particular disorder;

5. Use of various control groups to compare against psychotherapy;
6. Evaluation of outcome by persons who are independent of and blind to the treatment condition;
7. Use of videotapes of psychotherapy sessions to independently assess the quality of the treatment and the outcome;
8. Use of standardized, quantified measures which cover a variety of outcome, including symptoms and social functioning;
9. Evaluation of the possible negative side-effects of psychotherapy;
10. Specification of the psychotherapies in procedural manuals which record the therapeutic techniques and their sequence to ensure that a uniform treatment and the one under study is being used consistently in the research, both within and between therapist;
11. Development of training programs for psychotherapists involved in clinical trials to ensure that the procedures specified in the manual are being transmitted.

As a result of these efforts, evidence for the efficacy and safety of psychotherapy and pharmacotherapy in comparison and in combination has been gradually accumulating. Increasingly sophisticated questions are now being answered about what psychotherapy, in combination with what tricyclic, in what sequence, produces what effect for which subtype of depressed patient.

Most of the clinical trials of psychotherapy have been conducted with ambulatory depressed patients who are not psychotic and do not experience manic episodes; that is, the nonbipolar depressed patient. This emphasis derives from the high prevalence and associated morbidity of ambulatory depression, and the economics of reimbursement. Against this background, the psychotherapies which have been designed and tested with the ambulatory depressed patient are described.

Description of the Psychotherapies

Although many types of psychotherapies are widely and appropriately used in depression, as of this writing, five therapies (cognitive, interpersonal, behavioral, marital, and group) have undergone scientific testing in clinical trials. To ensure homogeneity, depressed patients who meet the criteria of major depression as defined by the Research Diagnostic Criteria (RDC) * and the *Third Diagnostic and Statistical Manual* (DSM III) participated in the studies.

---

* The Research Diagnostic Criteria for the syndrome of major depression includes dysphoric mood, at least five other symptoms, persistence of at least two weeks, producing impairment of functioning or necessity of treatment, and occurring in the absence of schizophrenia or other disorders which may better explain the symptoms.[1]

Cognitive Therapy

Cognitive therapy, developed by Beck, is based on the assumption that the affective response in depression is determined by the way an individual perceives experience.[2] As a result of an emergence of maladaptive cognitive themes, the depressed patient tends to regard himself and his future negatively. Correction of negative concepts is expected to alleviate the depressive symptoms. For example, an extremely low self-concept can be treated by presenting a hierarchy of cognitive tasks, and through these tasks, demonstrating the invalidity of the patient's self-reproaches.

Interpersonal Psychotherapy

Interpersonal psychotherapy (IPT) assumes that the development of depression occurs in a social and interpersonal context and is determined by the interpersonal relations between the depressed patient and significant other.[3] Depression is seen as having three component processes: symptom formation, social adjustment, and personality. Interpersonal psychotherapy attempts to intervene in the first two, and does not claim to have an impact on enduring aspects of personality. The goals are to improve the quality of the patient's social and interpersonal functioning by enhancing ability to cope with internally and externally induced stresses, by restoring morale, and by helping the patient to deal with the personal and social consequences of the disorder. Thus far, techniques have been developed for the management of depressed patients with grief and loss, interpersonal deficits, interpersonal role disputes (usually marital disputes), and role transitions.

Behavioral Approaches

Behavior therapy explains the occurrence of depression as stimulus and response. Negative reinforcing events in the environment and lack of available positive reinforcements as well as the individual's own behavior elicit certain aspects of the depressive syndrome.[4] Several techniques based on behavioral concepts have been developed for depressed patients: social skills therapy, which emphasizes increasing assertiveness, verbal skills, and social adjustment; pleasant events therapy, which focuses on increasing pleasant and rewarding experiences; and self-control therapy, which emphasizes self-monitoring, self-evaluation, and self-reinforcement. This last technique serves to correct the depressed patient's problem in self-control in monitoring negative events and in making internal attributions of responsibility and excessive self-punishment.

Marital Therapy

Marital therapy attempts to alter the interaction between or among the marital partners. It is based on the assumption that the marital relation affects thoughts, feelings, and behavior, and that symptom removal can be achieved by changing the transactional marital system. Marital therapy can be individual, collaborative, concurrent, conjoint, combined or group. The theoretical base and a typology of marital types have been well summarized by Gurman and Kniskern.[5]

Group Therapy

In group therapy a trained psychotherapist and a group of patients attempt to effect changes in the emotional states, attitudes, and behavior of the patient. Currently, explicit definitions of techniques and descriptions of what occurs within the group format are lacking, although there are efforts to develop cognitive therapy in a group context.

Status of Development of the Five Psychotherapies

Cognitive therapy has been tested in seven trials; interpersonal psychotherapy in three trials; behavioral approaches in nine trials; marital and group therapy in one trial each.[6-8] Of the five therapies, only cognitive, interpersonal, and some of the behavioral techniques have been specifically designed for depressed patients. Procedural manuals are available only for the cognitive and interpersonal therapies; however, this is a rapidly moving field. Undoubtedly, other clinical trials, new therapies, and more procedural manuals are under development or being completed as of this writing.

Psychotherapy in Comparison to Drugs

There are seven completed studies from which information on psychotherapy in comparison with a tricyclic antidepressant can be drawn; all five of the psychotherapies are represented. Two studies found psychotherapy superior to drugs (cognitive therapy compared to imipramine in one study and behavior therapy compared to amitriptyline in the other) in attrition and symptom reduction for acute treatment of depressed patients.[6,8] One study found drugs (amitriptyline) and psychotherapy (IPT) about equal for acute symptom reduction. Three studies found drugs superior to psychotherapy (interpersonal, group, or marital) in the prevention of relapse or symptom reduction, but psychotherapy slightly superior to drugs in the enhancement of social functioning. The psychotherapy effect in one study

413

occurred only in patients who remained in treatment for 8 months without relapsing.

A recently published study conducted by the Medical Research Council, Brain Metabolism Unit, Edinburgh, Scotland, found cognitive therapy better than doctor's pharmacotherapy choice (usually amitriptyline or clomipramine) in general practice patients.[7]

The results on the comparisons of psychotherapy with drugs are equivocal for acute treatment. The treatments appear to be equal overall but to have different targets of action.

Psychotherapy in Combination with Drugs

Five completed studies tested the efficacy of psychotherapy (cognitive, interpersonal, marital, group) combined with a tricyclic antidepressant. All five studies show the superiority of combined treatment over a control group or over either treatment alone. In none of the studies were there negative interactions in combining drugs with psychotherapy. The effects of the two treatments together were additive.

In general, studies have found that the combination of psychotherapy and a tricyclic is better than either treatment alone or than no regular treatment. The combination provides a broader spectrum of action as each treatment may affect different domains.[9] Psychotherapy seems to have its effect on social and interpersonal areas and has a slower onset of action. Drugs have their effect on the vegetative symptoms of depression such as sleep and appetite, and have a more rapid onset of action.

Implications for the Management of Depression

The overall evidence thus far is in favor of combined treatment (drugs and psychotherapy) over either treatment alone for the ambulatory nonbipolar depressive. However, there is considerable variability in patients' acceptance and preference for the various treatments, and there are different types of depression. Some patients want only one of the treatments. They may be reluctant to take medication or may not wish to talk about personal matters. Other patients may be able to tolerate only one of the treatments regardless of preference. They may be intolerant of the medication's side-effects or have cognitive deficits or economic problems that make psychotherapy impractical. What research evidence can guide the management of the ambulatory depressive with drugs and psychotherapy?

Which Psychotherapy?

We cannot yet state how the psychotherapies compare to one another, nor can we offer guides on the basis of research data about the selection of a particular psychotherapy for the depressed patient. Such data will be forthcoming in the next 3–5 years.

Pharmacotherapy vs. Psychotherapy

The evidence comparing pharmacotherapy to psychotherapy is suggestive. Cognitive or behavioral therapy may be more efficacious than pharmacotherapy for the general practice patient. However, the patient who will not accept one treatment should not be denied the other, since the evidence shows that either treatment is better than no treatment. Moreover, several recent findings on the symptoms, social functioning, and diagnostic subtypes of patients from our own data and that of others can begin to guide the clinician's selection of an effective treatment.

The research evidence shows that pharmacotherapy is most efficacious on sleep disturbance and appetite loss, and that the effects on these symptoms are relatively early (1–4 weeks). Therefore, the patient whose depression is mostly manifest in these symptoms should not be denied an antidepressant.[9]

Alternatively, psychotherapy is most efficacious on suicidal feelings, guilt, loss of interest, and social and interpersonal problems, and is indicated for patients whose depression is mostly manifest in these areas. Psychotherapy has a later onset of action and the differential effects on social and interpersonal functioning may not be apparent for from 6 months to 1 year.

Recent findings by our group from the New Haven-Boston Collaborative study suggest that the RDC subtypes of endogenous and situational depression may be useful guides to treatment selection.[10]

Endogenous and situational depressions are defined by the RDC as follows:

1. **Endogenous major depressive disorder—** from groups A and B a total of at least four symptoms for probable, six for definite, with at least one symptom from group A.

   Group A. (1) Distinct quality to depressed mood, i.e., depressed mood is perceived as distinctly different from the kind of feeling the patient would have or has had following the death of a loved one; (2) lack of reactivity to environmental changes (once depressed the patient does not feel better, even temporarily, when something good happens); (3) mood is regularly worse in the morning; (4) pervasive loss of interest and/or pleasure.

   Group B. (1) Feelings of self-doubt or reproach or excessive or inappropriate guilt; (2) early morning awakening or middle of night insomnia; (3) psychomotor retardation or agitation (more than a mere subjective feeling of being slowed down or restless); (4) poor appetite;

(5) weight loss (two pounds a week over several weeks or 20 pounds in a year when not dieting); (6) loss of interest or pleasure (may not be pervasive) in usual activities or decreased sexual drive.

2. **Situational major depressive disorder**— illness has developed after an event or in a situation that seems likely to have contributed to the appearance of the episode at that time. In making the judgment the amount of stress inherent in the event or situation is considered, along with the cumulative effect of such stresses, and the closeness of the events to the onset or exacerbation of the depressive episode.[1]

In the New Haven-Boston clinical trial, 81 depressed patients were randomized into one of four treatments: combined amitriptyline and interpersonal psychotherapy, either treatment alone, or a nonscheduled treatment control group.[9] Of the 81 patients, 31 (40%) were diagnosed by the psychiatrist at the intake interview as situational only, and 20 (27%) as endogenous only.

The depressed patients diagnosed as situational only responded equally well to drugs, psychotherapy, or the combination and responded poorly to nonscheduled treatment. However, the combination of drugs and psychotherapy did not seem to offer more than psychotherapy alone.

The endogenous patients on the other hand, responded poorly to psychotherapy alone, which was no better than no scheduled treatment. The response in this group was best to the combination of drugs and psychotherapy. The relative lack of response to drugs alone may have been due to poor compliance; this study was begun in 1972 before plasma level monitoring of tricyclics was feasible. Future studies will incorporate plasma level tests.

These results are based on small samples and require replication. They suggest that the situational depressions respond well to either pharmacotherapy or psychotherapy but do not respond well to no treatment. The endogenous depressions, on the other hand, do not do well on psychotherapy alone and do best on the combination of drugs and psychotherapy.

Future Directions

Despite the progress, there are gaps in the data. There are many psychotherapies which, on the basis of clinical experience, we would expect to be quite efficacious in the treatment of depression but which haven't as yet been tested in clinical trials. We also do not know the value of the treatments described for the bipolar patient or for the psychotically depressed or hospitalized patient. One retrospective study, however, did suggest the value of couples therapy in conjunction with lithium in the management of married bipolar patients.[11] The couples in group therapy had a more benign posthospitalization course than those given minimum support.

There is, however, sufficient evidence from small, individually conducted clinical trials to launch a multicenter collaborative trial. Such a study has been designed by the staff at the Clinical Research Branch of the National Institute of Mental Health, in consultation with many experts, and is currently underway. This collaborative study involves three clinical sites and incorporates all of the recent scientific advances described for the conduct of clinical trials. In addition, a number of single-center clinical trials are currently underway. In the next 3 years data will become available from at least five studies in the United States. The next decade will bring clearer answers about which types of psychotherapies to use with which drugs, and for which depressed patients.

References

1. Spitzer RL, Endicott J, and Robins E. Research diagnostic criteria: Rationale and reliability. *Arch Gen Psychiatry* 35:773–82, 1978.

2. Beck A. *Cognitive Therapy and the Emotional Disorders.* New York: International Universities Press, Inc., 1976.

3. Klerman GL et al. "Manual for Short-Term Interpersonal Psychotherapy (IPT) of Depression." Fourth Revision, June 1979 (unpublished).

4. Lewinsohn P, Biglan A, and Zeiss A. "Behavioral Treatment of Depression." In *The Behavioral Management of Anxiety, Depression and Pain*, edited by Davidson P. New York: Brunner/Mazel, 1976. pp. 91–146.

5. Gurman AS and Kniskern DP. "Research on Marital and Family Therapy: Progress, Perspective and Prospect." In *Handbook of Psychotherapy and Behavioral Change: An Empirical Analysis*, edited by Garfield SL and Bergin AE, 2nd Edition. New York: John Wiley & Sons, 1979.

6. Weissman MM. Psychological treatment of depression: Evidence for the efficacy of psychotherapy alone, in comparison with and in combination with pharmacotherapy. *Arch Gen Psychiatry* 36:1262–69, 1979.

7. Blackburn IM et al. The efficacy of cognitive therapy in depression: A treatment trial using cognitive therapy and pharmacotherapy, each alone and in combination. *Brit J Psychiatry* 139:181–89, 1981.

8. McLean PD and Hakstian AR. Clinical depression: Comparative efficacy of outpatient treatment. *J Consult Clin Psychology* 47:818–36, 1979.

9. DiMascio A et al. Differential symptom reduction by drugs and psychotherapy in acute depression. *Arch Gen Psychiatry* 36:1450–56, 1979.

10. Prusoff BA et al. Research diagnostic criteria: Their role as predictors of differential response to psychotherapy and drug treatment. *Arch Gen Psychiatry* 37:796–801, 1980.

11. Davenport YB et al. Couples group therapy as an adjunct to lithium maintenance of the manic patient. *Amer J Orthopsychiatry* 47:495–502, 1977.

Index